Medical Aspects of Early Intervention

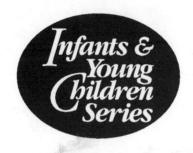

Edited by

James A. Blackman, MD, MPH

Professor of Pediatrics
Director of Research
Kluge Children's Rehabilitation Center and Research Institute
Department of Pediatrics
University of Virginia
Charlottesville, Virginia

AN ASPEN PUBLICATION®
Aspen Publishers, Inc.
Gaithersburg, Maryland
1995

Library of Congress Cataloging-in-Publication Data
Medical aspects of early intervention/
edited by James A. Blackman.
p.   cm.
Articles reprinted from Infants and young children.
Includes bibliographical references and index.
ISBN 0-8342-0648-X
1. Handicapped children—Rehabilitation.
2. Child development deviations—Complications.
I. Blackman, James A. II. Infants and young children.
[DNLM: 1. Child Development Disorders—prevention & control—collected works.
2. Child Development Disorders—rehabilitation—collected works.
WS 350.6 M489 1995]
RJ138.M44 1995
618.92—dc20
DNLM/DLC
for Library of Congress
94-38543
CIP

Editorial Resources: Jane Colilla

Library of Congress Catalog Card Number: 94-38543
ISBN: 0-8342-0648-X
Series ISBN: 0-8342-0652-8

Printed in the United States of America

1   2   3   4   5

Table of Contents

Preface

In Dr. Arnold Sameroff's transactional model of development a child's constitutional endowment interacts with the environment continuously over time. Whether that interaction at one point is positive or negative will influence the interaction in the future. This concept provides the crux of early intervention's *raison d'être*. Turning what might have been a negative interaction into a positive one, either by intervening on the constitutional or environmental side, is the goal. A successful intervention in this regard is likely to have a compounding effect, just as investing in a savings account yields continuous dividends which themselves build equity.

As an illustration, consider a substance abusing woman during pregnancy. At interaction point A, the fetus, during a critical period of central nervous system development, is exposed to alcohol and cocaine. The genetically normal child's brain is irrevocably altered by this environmentally noxious exposure. The resulting irritability that the infant displays at two weeks of age, interaction Point B, causes an edgy mother and her companion to abandon her. The child is placed, at interaction point C, with a nurturing foster parent who is tolerant of frequent spitting up.

While resilience in babies and young children is truly remarkable, we know there are limits when adversity is persistent. An appropriate intervention at the earliest possible moment is more likely to be successful than a delayed one when the ill-effects of a negative interaction are magnified. Viewing intervention in this way takes on a preventive orientation. Drug rehabilitation prior to pregnancy would have avoided the ensuing cascade of tragic events. Assistance with parenting a fussy baby may have held the family intact. Although prompted by abandonment, placement with a loving foster family was the first successful intervention that hopefully alleviated the previous stresses.

There is no clearer-cut intervention than a medical one. Unless health is optimized, other child and family supports will be hindered. Furthermore, avoidance of preventable health problems is possible only if caretakers are knowledgeable about how, where, and why to do this. Often, it is an early intervention team member who becomes a strong advocate for a child's health. Knowing that propping a bottle for a child with cerebral palsy in a supine position can lead to ear infections, or that smoking in the home of a child with bronchopulmonary dysplasia exacerbates symptoms, or that vomiting can be a sign of a shunt malfunction enhances the interventionist's ability to serve the child and family.

Ensuring good health should never displace attention to the child's environment. However, ensuring that the constitutional input into a child's development and emotional growth is favorable provides one tangible step everyone can take, regardless of one's primary responsibility. The contributions in this volume comprise a medical information resource not readily available elsewhere. Although not intended to be a comprehensive text, it does give us detailed insights into complex health problems of special populations of young children who typically require early intervention services.

James A. Blackman, MD, MPH
Editor

Neonatal extracorporeal membrane oxygenation: Neurodevelopmental outcome of survivors

Jan G. Hunter, MA, OTR
Pediatric Supervisor
Department of Occupational Therapy
Children's Hospital
Assistant Professor, Clinical Faculty
School of Allied Health
Department of Occupational Therapy
University of Texas Medical Branch

Joseph B. Zwischenberger, MD
Associate Professor
Division of Cardiothoracic Surgery
Department of Surgery
University of Texas Medical Branch
Galveston, Texas

Jatinder Bhatia, MD
Professor of Pediatrics
Medical College of Georgia
Augusta, Georgia

AS MEDICAL technology becomes increasingly sophisticated, an increasing number of infants with conditions or complications previously incompatible with life are now surviving. Their very survival creates a population at increased risk for developmental delay or dysfunction potentially in need of early intervention services by specialized personnel in accordance with Public Law 99-457 (Part H).

Extracorporeal membrane oxygenation (ECMO) provides one example of modern medical technology with developmental implications for survivors. ECMO is a dramatic state-of-the-art life support system that uses a modified heart-lung machine to treat a select group of critically ill neonates with severe respiratory failure unresponsive to conventional medical management. ECMO may also be utilized for perioperative or postoperative support of neonates with correctable congenital heart disease.

Understanding the etiology and pathology of respiratory failure requiring ECMO is necessary to appreciate application of this extreme life support measure. Factors complicating successful postnatal transition to mature cardiopulmonary circulation and subsequent respiratory distress or failure are reviewed. Awareness of potential medical complications during ECMO and developmental implications of ECMO survival will assist in implementation of screening and intervention strategies for this population.

FETAL AND MATURE CIRCULATION

Before birth, the placenta removes waste products and provides oxygen to the blood that is then pumped by the fetal heart throughout the body; only the small amount of blood needed to nourish developing lung tissue flows through the nonaerated fetal lungs.[1-3] Most of the circulating blood bypasses the lungs by diversion into the ductus arteriosus, a short fetal blood vessel connecting the pulmo-

Inf Young Children 1992;4(4):63–76

1

nary artery (artery from the heart to the lungs) with the aorta (artery from the heart that supplies oxygenated blood for the body).[4] Simultaneously, blood within the fetal heart is partially shunted from the right atrium to the left atrium through an opening (foramen ovale) between the two sides of the heart. This pattern of circulation represents a right-to-left shunt that occurs because the fetus has extremely high vascular resistance in the lungs and low vascular resistance in the systemic circuit; therefore, blood flows right to left across the ductus arteriosus and foramen ovale back to the low-resistance placenta.[1]

At birth the infant's own lungs must assume responsibility for blood gas exchange; this change generally occurs normally because clamping of the umbilical cord increases the systemic vascular resistance, and lung inflation with the first postnatal breath begins to decrease pulmonary vascular resistance. Blood flow then follows this new path of lesser resistance and fills the blood vessels in the lungs rather than being diverted through the ductus arteriosus. The direction of blood flow through the ductus arteriosus is reversed (left-to-right shunt) and ultimately ceases during the next few days. Simultaneously, the amount of blood entering the left atrium from the pulmonary veins is greatly increased. The resultant increase in left atrial pressure functionally closes the foramen ovale.[3]

RESPIRATORY DISTRESS

Neonatal respiratory distress is an early symptom of impaired or incomplete transition from fetal to mature circulation and may result from multiple etiologies.[1,5] Neonatal lung function may be compromised by such complications as meconium aspiration, pneumonia, pulmonary air leaks, pulmonary hypoplasia (often secondary to congenital diaphragmatic hernia), and decreased surfactant associated with prematurity. Central nervous system problems negatively affecting ventilation include such diagnoses as apnea of prematurity, seizures, birth asphyxia, hypoxic encephalopathy, and intracranial hemorrhage. Congenital cyanotic heart disease, sepsis, severe metabolic imbalances, airway obstruction or malformation, and neuromuscular disorders are additional potential causes of respiratory distress.

A vicious cycle is established as respiratory distress leads to hypoxia and acidosis, both of which are potent stimuli for pulmonary vasoconstriction. The resultant additional increase in pulmonary vascular resistance and decrease in pulmonary blood flow allow the ductus arteriosus and foramen ovale to remain open; hypoxia then worsens as the fetal pattern of circulation persists.[6] Persistent fetal circulation (PFC) is a known sequela of many of the conditions previously mentioned (perinatal asphyxia, respiratory distress syndrome, bacterial pneumonia, meconium aspiration syndrome, and congenital diaphragmatic hernia), but occasionally there may be no apparent precipitating event or causal etiology. PFC is more widely referred to as persistent pulmonary hypertension of the newborn and is a shared diagnosis of most neonates with severe respiratory failure regardless of the underlying etiology.

CONVENTIONAL MEDICAL MANAGEMENT OF RESPIRATORY FAILURE

Comprehensive medical management of respiratory failure typically involves such measures as maintenance of a neutral thermal environment, assisted ventilation, medications, respiratory therapy, metabolic homeostasis, and treatment of underlying disorders such as infection. Minimal stimulation may also be recommended because pain and agitation contribute to pulmonary vasoconstriction.[7,8] Conventional assisted ventilation for respiratory failure generally requires high oxygen concentrations, rapid ventilatory rates, and high inspiratory pressures to expand and aerate the lungs. If the neonate does not respond quickly, continued use of mechanical ventilation may cause iatrogenic lung damage that soon complicates the original problem. High-frequency ventilation, which provides small volumes of oxygenated air at rapid rates (high frequencies), may be attempted in some hospitals before ECMO. Five percent to 10% of infants with severe pulmonary dysfunction do not respond to aggressive but conventional medical management; historically, there has been an 80% or greater mortality rate for this group of infants. Survivors have an increased risk of developmental problems resulting from perinatal asphyxia, chronic lung disease, and accompanying medical complications.

EXTRACORPOREAL MEMBRANE OXYGENATION

The significant morbidity and late mortality that occur in survivors of respiratory failure unresponsive to conventional treatment have prompted the application of cardiopulmonary bypass techniques for temporary cardiopulmonary support of qualifying newborns.[9] ECMO attempts to reverse high mortality and morbidity for this select group of moribund term or near-term neonates by use of a modified heart-lung machine to provide nearly total rest of the damaged lungs for up to 10 days (or more) to allow time for lung healing to occur.

The first successful use of ECMO in neonatal respiratory failure was reported in 1976.[10] By October of 1991, a cumulative total of nearly 5,500 infants had been treated with ECMO across the nation, with approximately 82% surviving.[11] This observation alone is sufficient to establish ECMO as therapeutically effective because these infants had met criteria predictive of an 80% to 100% mortality rate before ECMO was initiated.[12]

ELIGIBILITY CRITERIA FOR ECMO

Over the past 10 years specific medical criteria have been proposed that are considered predictive of 80% or greater potential mortality from respiratory failure.[12,13] Only those infants who meet these high mortality criteria are considered for ECMO because it is an extreme life support measure used only when all other options have failed. The alveolar-arterial oxygen gradient (a calculation that reflects alveolar efficiency in transporting oxygen to pulmonary capillaries) and the oxygenation index (a measure of respiratory distress that is based on calculations involving ventilator pressures and oxygen factors) are most commonly used as indicators predicting mortality, although astute clinical judgment is crucial because none of the scoring systems works in all cases.[9] Because some infants deteriorate rapidly and severe hypoxic ischemic encephalopathy or death may occur before these more common indicators are met, acute deterioration and failure to respond to medical management are additional entry criteria for ECMO.[14]

Although the respiratory failure must be of sufficient severity to classify the infant as moribund, the lung condition must also be potentially reversible in 10 to 14 days. The most frequent diagnoses appropriate for neonatal ECMO are

- Persistent pulmonary hypertension of the newborn
- Respiratory distress syndrome
- Meconium aspiration syndrome
- Infection (sepsis, pneumonia)
- Perinatal asphyxia
- Barotrauma with air leaks
- Congenital diaphragmatic hernia with air leaks
- Perioperative/postoperative support of neonates with correctable congenital heart disease

Eligibility is likely to be expanded in the future as continued improvements and refinements in ECMO equipment and techniques reduce potential risks.

CONTRAINDICATIONS FOR ECMO

No studies have defined the limitations of ECMO application, although empirically derived guidelines have emerged. ECMO has not been as successful in treatment of preterm infants younger than 35 weeks gestational age or smaller than 2,000 g because the fragility of the immature cerebral vasculature creates a high risk of severe intracranial hemorrhage with subsequent death or poor functional outcome. Relative contraindications to ECMO include cyanotic congenital heart disease, intracranial hemorrhage more severe than a germinal matrix or subependymal (grade I) bleed, bleeding disorders, irreversible lung damage, and any other nonreversible condition incompatible with normal quality of life (ie, severe neurologic damage, some chromosomal abnormalities, and severe uncorrectable congenital anomalies).[12,13,15] Thus the ideal ECMO candidate is a term or near-term infant (older than 34 weeks gestational age and exceeding 2,000 g) who is generally healthy except for critical, but potentially reversible, lung disease.

ECMO currently is a limited resource, and infants with the best chance for survival and a good outcome must be identified. For example, assisted ventilation at high pressures and high oxygen concentrations may cause pulmonary air leaks and barotrauma leading to chronic lung disease (bronchopulmonary dysplasia, BPD).[2,16] Although ECMO minimizes barotrauma and is well suited to the healing of air leaks, an infant who has already been mechanically ventilated for 10 days or more is less responsive to ECMO because chronic lung changes have already occurred.[9,15] Current data indicate that infants without significant barotrauma before ECMO will not develop BPD while they are on ECMO.[9,17]

ECMO PROCEDURE

ECMO provides prolonged extracorporeal cardiopulmonary bypass through use of extrathoracic vascular cannulation and a modified heart-lung machine.[9,12,15,18,19] The ECMO circuit typically consists of polyvinylchloride (PVC) tubing to transport blood to and from the infant's body; a silicone-rubber bladder for collection of venous blood; a bladder box alarm system that acts as a servoregulator for the pump; a roller pump to push the blood in the PVC tubing forward through the circuit; a membrane oxygenator for the exchange of oxygen, carbon dioxide, and water vapor; a heat exchanger to warm the blood; and an infusion pump to infuse continuously a heparinized solution to prevent clot formation within the ECMO circuit (Fig 1).

Blood samples are sent to the blood bank for analysis on a probable ECMO candidate so that blood components necessary for priming the pump will be available when needed; preparation of the infant for bypass and final priming of the circuit are performed simultaneously once the infant meets ECMO criteria.[9] The infant is iatrogenically paralyzed with pancuronium to avoid respiratory movement and to prevent air embolism during cannulation.[13,20] After a loading dose of heparin is administered to reduce blood clotting, a catheter is placed within the right internal jugular vein and advanced to the right atrium; this catheter allows deoxygenated blood to drain from the body by gravity into the distensible bladder reservoir. The internal diameter of the venous catheter determines the maximum flow possible; the catheter must be large enough to allow total cardiopulmonary bypass.[21] The blood is oxygenated, carbon dioxide and water vapor are removed, and the blood is reheated as it moves through the circuit. It is then perfused back into the infant's body via a second cannula placed in the right carotid artery to the entrance of the aortic arch, where the oxygenated blood from the circuit mixes

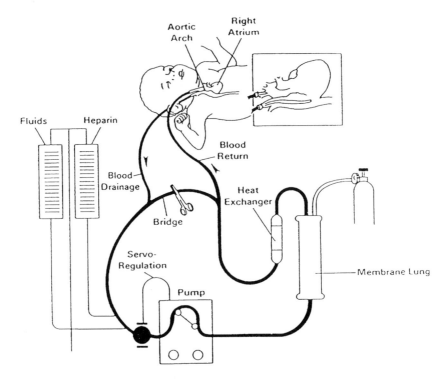

Fig 1. ECMO circuit.

with the poorly oxygenated blood from the ductus arteriosus and left ventricle to yield an oxygen content adequate for the infant's metabolic requirements.[19] Single-cannula venovenous bypass via the jugular or femoral vein is possible and may soon become the ECMO method of choice for most neonates, the advantages being one-site cannulation and elimination of carotid artery ligation after ECMO is completed.[12]

Initiation of ECMO often produces dramatic improvement in oxygenation and color of the moribund infant because the heart and lungs are fully supported; muscle relaxants and vasoactive drugs are generally discontinued, and the infant is maintained awake and alert.[15,19] Lung function begins to recover as the pulmonary vasculature relaxes; the ductus arteriosus usually closes spontaneously as the direction of blood flow reverses but may require ligation during ECMO in about 20% of the patients.[19]

The infant remains intubated on minimal ventilator settings during the course of ECMO, which averages 5 days but may be continued for up to 10 days; ECMO for longer than 10 days is possible but significantly increases mortality and morbidity.[22] Lung healing is demonstrated by improved oxygen transport from the small amount of blood moving through the lungs; the arterial oxygen tension increases, and weaning from the ECMO circuit is gradually begun. The flow rate is decreased in small amounts, thus diverting less blood into the ECMO circuit and allowing more blood to flow through the lungs. Weaning is continued in this fashion over several days until the infant is able to maintain adequate gas exchange at low ventilator settings without ECMO assistance.[10]

Placement of the infant on ECMO requires a surgical procedure that is performed in the neonatal intensive care unit (NICU). A team of highly trained specialists is involved in the care of the infant; a NICU nurse is in constant attendance on the infant, and an ECMO technician is constantly monitoring and adjusting the circuit.

INHERENT RISKS OF ECMO

Although mortality in the group of moribund infants treated with ECMO has been essentially reversed from 80% mortality or greater to 80% survival or greater, morbidity is still under investigation. It has been speculated that this life-saving technology has resulted in a new population of infants who are at increased risk for developmental delay or dysfunction and thus in need of early intervention services.[23–25]

Respiratory failure and asphyxia are potentially damaging to the brain.[26,27] The presence of more severe acidosis, hypercarbia, and hypoxia in the pre-ECMO period has been associated with subsequent development of neurologic injury.[28–30] Potential complications during ECMO include problems such as seizures, intracranial hemorrhage, hypertension, and infection.[11,19,25] Ligation of the right carotid artery and internal jugular vein is currently a consequence of ECMO and may result in altered cerebral perfusion, seizures, and lateralizing brain injury.[31–33]

Major and minor neurodevelopmental sequelae have been identified in this surviving population, although the difficulty in separating effects due to the underlying disease state from potential ECMO factors has been recognized.[14,19] Some of the reported complications and/or sequelae among ECMO survivors have included seizures, air embolus, intracranial hemorrhage, cortical atrophy, persistent respiratory problems, sensorineural hearing loss, muscle tone abnormalities, developmental delay (including cognition, speech, and language as well as motor milestones), lateralizing brain injury, and death.[19,24,25,34–38]

Thus, surviving ECMO infants are potentially at risk for developmental problems from at least three sources: (1) The underlying disease state may impose developmental sequelae, (2) respiratory failure in itself implies some degree of hypoxia in the infant because maximal mechanical ventilatory assistance before

ECMO did not succeed in providing adequate oxygenation, and (3) ECMO carries inherent risks.

OUTCOME OF ECMO SURVIVORS AT THE UNIVERSITY OF TEXAS MEDICAL BRANCH AT GALVESTON

ECMO has been available at the University of Texas Medical Branch (UTMB) since March 1987. Follow-up developmental assessments for all ECMO survivors are scheduled at 3, 6, 12, and 24 months of age. Evaluations during the first year are performed by an occupational therapist; the 2-year examinations are completed by a developmental psychologist.

One of the authors (JGH) frequently noted that subtle neuromotor abnormalities were not reflected by the Bayley Scales of Infant Development (BSID) scores. Therefore, an initial study, approved by the UTMB Internal Review Board, was conducted in 1990 to examine further the developmental status of UTMB ECMO survivors. From the initial population of 35 infants treated with ECMO to that point in time, 26 of the 30 survivors had received some developmental follow-up and formed the sample population for this study. Data were collected by retrospective chart review. Although the available sample population was small, the composite results supported the previously individualized observations.

The Mental Development Index (MDI) and Psychomotor Development Index (PDI) of the BSID were used as the baseline measures of developmental outcome.[39] Because subtle neuromotor findings were not adequately included on any available standardized developmental evaluation, a subjective assessment of components and quality of movement was developed (see Appendix) to detect subtle abnormalities that have significance in the interpretation of developmental status and that may predict future risk for subtle learning disabilities and emotional or behavioral problems.[25,34,40]

The standard BSID classification allows a 1 standard deviation (SD) variability of 16 points, with scores between 84 and 116 being considered in the normal range. We noted that two infants of identical ages (born 2 days apart) scored at opposite ends of this spectrum; both were within normal limits by BSID criteria but demonstrated significantly different developmental abilities. Therefore, we stratified the infants as high normal (MDI and PDI, 109 to 117+), average normal (MDI and PDI, 93 to 108), and low normal (MDI and PDI, <93) to allow for more meaningful interpretations of evaluation results. A similar, more conservative reclassification has been reported by other examiners.[34]

Tables 1 and 2 summarize the distribution of MDI and PDI scores over a 2-year span. It is apparent that, although the proportion of lower scores has increased with age, more than 70% of UTMB survivors functioned at or above a normal developmental level on the BSID with the conservative classification; this number

Table 1. Sequential distribution of MDI scores

	Percentage of patients scoring in range				
MDI scores	*3 months (n = 22)*	*6 months (n = 18)*	*12 months (n = 13)*	*24 months (n = 8)*	*Net change (%)*
117+ to 109	50	56	64	62.5	+12.5
108 to 93	41	22	7	12.5	−28.5
92 to 68	9	22	29	25	+16.0

Table 2. Sequential distribution of PDI scores

	Percentage of patients scoring in range				
PDI scores	*3 months (n = 22)*	*6 months (n = 18)*	*12 months (n = 13)*	*24 months (n = 8)*	*Net change (%)*
117+ to 109	50	59	77	43	−7.0
108 to 93	36	23	0	28.5	−7.5
92 to 68	14	18	23	28.5	+14.5

would increase to more than 86% if traditional standard deviation categories (mean ± 1 SD) had been used to represent the normal range.

Quality of movement scores, however, clearly illustrate the presence of worrisome neuromotor findings that largely resolve by 12 months of age. Sixty-two percent of the infants tested by this researcher (a subset representing 70% of the sample population) demonstrated suspect or abnormal neuromotor signs at 3 months of age; this decreased to 50% at 6 months of age and to 18% at 12 months (Figs 2 to 4). This pattern, which was not evident by BSID scores alone, may identify transient neuromotor abnormalities that have been linked to later school, learning, and emotional problems.[25,34,40,41]

CURRENT CONCERNS FOR ECMO SURVIVORS

Recent ECMO presentations and literature have expressed the following interrelated concerns regarding typical ECMO follow-up:

- Consistent with general infant developmental follow-up, BSID scores on ECMO graduates at 3 and 6 months do not correlate with future outcome.[42,43]
- ECMO follow-up should include long-term follow-up for accurate analysis. Because the proportions of normal, suspect, and abnormal performance on

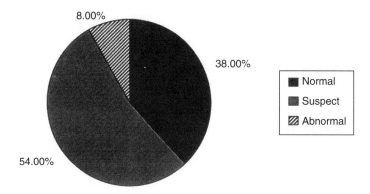

Fig 2. Quality of movement at 3 months.

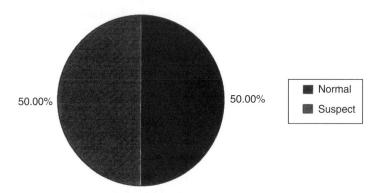

Fig 3. Quality of movement at 6 months.

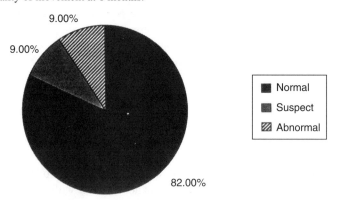

Fig 4. Quality of movement at 12 months.

cognitive and neurodevelopmental measures differ significantly at 1 year and 3 years of age, outcome cannot be reliably predicted from one or two neurodevelopmental assessments.[30]

- Short-term follow-up of 3 years or less is only predictive of major handicaps.[44]
- Outcome reported only as composite psychometric scores may not reflect specific deficits that increase risk for later learning and functional difficulties. Specifically, significant speech and language problems that may affect later learning were demonstrated in an increasing percentage of ECMO survivors at 1, 2, and 3 years of age but were not adequately reflected by psychometric scores.[30]
- Visual-motor integration deficits have been identified in a significant number of otherwise normally functioning 3-year-old ECMO survivors.[25]

Children's National Medical Center in Washington, DC, has initiated a major study to examine 150 5-year-old ECMO survivors and 50 control children because "it is generally accepted that these children are at risk for minor neuromotor and neuropsychological abnormalities such as attention or memory deficits, learning disabilities, or difficulty with motor planning and control."[44] Issues addressed will include general intellectual integrity, learning risk, major neurobehavioral deficits (language, visual, sensorimotor, memory, and emergent executive function), neuromotor dysfunction (tonal abnormalities, impaired motor planning and coordination, poor balance, and articulation errors), and psychosocial adjustment (hyperactivity, maladaptive behavior, and poor social skills). Studies such as this will help clarify the true outcome of ECMO survivors, suggest areas for further study, and assist educators and therapists in planning appropriate assessments and/or interventions.

ECMO has progressed from an experimental option to an accepted life-saving measure for treating severe respiratory failure unresponsive to conventional medical management in term or near-term neonates. Collective data on short-term outcome of infants who received ECMO are compiled at the Extracorporeal Life Support Registry at the University of Michigan; current statistics reveal a national average of 82% survival for infants given less than a 20% chance at life.[11] Subsequent developmental outcome of post-ECMO neonates has generally been favorable, with an overwhelming majority functioning within defined normal limits on standard developmental tests; this is comparable with our study results. Approximately 80% or more of survivors reportedly function within normal limits (generally construed as within 1 SD of the mean on the BSID, or 100 ± 16), about 10% of the ECMO population are classified as abnormal (2 SD or more below the mean on the BSID), and 10% remain suspect.[25,34,41]

There has, however, been increasing concern expressed about subtle deficits in many ECMO survivors that may correlate with later learning and behavior prob-

lems. Resolution of observed neuromotor abnormality in early life does not eliminate risk for related problems in later childhood, as stated by Rapin:

> Plasticity, the capacity for reorganization after an injury, was assumed
> until fairly recently to be so great in the immature brain that full behav-
> ioral recovery was thought to be the rule in young children unless dam-
> age is extensive. We have come to appreciate that plasticity is limited,
> and that recovery without discernible deficit is in fact uncommon.[45(p1)]

It is recommended that routine developmental follow-up of ECMO survivors
provide assessment of subtleties in neuromotor functioning in addition to standard
psychometric scores. Ideally, routine follow-up should be continued into the early
school years to assess true outcome and to minimize subtle or late sequelae; if this
is not feasible by the ECMO center, an assessment by the local early childhood or
kindergarten screening program before school age can be recommended. Although only a small percentage of ECMO graduates may require therapeutic early
intervention services, personnel in these programs should be aware of the benefits
and potential risks of ECMO and the developmental course of ECMO survivors.

REFERENCES

1. Harris TR. Physiological principles. In: Goldsmith J, Karotkin E, eds. *Assisted Ventilation of the Neonate.* 2nd ed. Philadelphia, Pa: Saunders; 1988.

2. Korones SB. *High-Risk Newborn Infants: The Basis for Intensive Nursing Care.* 2nd ed. St Louis, Mo: Mosby; 1986.

3. Williams L, Bullaboy C, King TD. Cardiovascular aspects. In: Goldsmith J, Karotkin E, eds. *Assisted Ventilation of the Neonate.* 2nd ed. Philadelphia, Pa: Saunders; 1988.

4. Harrison H, Kositsky A. *The Premature Baby Book.* Tucson, Ariz: Therapy Skill Builders; 1983.

5. Goldsmith JP, Karotkin EH. Introduction to assisted ventilation. In: Goldsmith J, Karotkin E, eds. *Assisted Ventilation of the Neonate.* 2nd ed. Philadelphia, Pa: Saunders; 1988.

6. Oh W. Respiratory distress syndrome: Diagnosis and management. In: Stern L, ed. *Diagnosis and Management of Respiratory Disorders in the Newborn.* Menlo Park, Ca: Addison-Wesley; 1983.

7. Hazinski MF, Pacetti AS. Nursing care of the infant with respiratory distress. In: Carlo WA, Chatburn RL, eds. *Neonatal Respiratory Care.* 2nd ed. Chicago, Ill: Year Book Medical; 1988.

8. Walsh MC, Carlo WA, Miller MJ. Respiratory diseases of the newborn. In: Carlo WA, Chatburn Rl., eds. *Neonatal Respiratory Care.* 2nd ed. Chicago, Ill: Year Book Medical; 1988.

9. Redmond CR, Loe WA, Bartlett RH, Arensman RM. Extracorporeal membrane oxygenation. In: Goldsmith J, Karotkin E, eds. *Assisted Ventilation of the Neonate.* 2nd ed. Philadelphia, Pa: Saunders; 1988.

10. Bartlett R, Gazzaniga AB, Jeffries MR, et al. Extracorporeal membrane oxygenation (ECMO) cardiopulmonary support in infancy. *Trans Am Soc Artif Intern Organs.* 1976;22:80–88.

11. Extracorporeal Life Support Organization. *Extracorporeal Life Support Organization Registry.* Ann Arbor, Mich: University of Michigan; 1990.

12. Zwischenberger JB, Bartlett R. Extracorporeal circulation for respiratory or cardiac failure. *Semin Thorac Cardiovasc Surg.* 1988;2:320–331.

13. Nugent J. Extracorporeal membrane oxygenation in the neonate. *Neonat Network.* 1986;4:27–38.

14. Redmond CR, Graves ED, Falterman KW, et al. Extracorporeal membrane oxygenation for respiratory and cardiac failure in infants and children. *J Thorac Cardiovasc Surg.* 1987;93:199–204.

15. Nicks JJ, Bartlett RH. Extracorporeal membrane oxygenation and other new modes of gas exchange. In: Carlo WA, Chatburn RL, eds. *Neonatal Respiratory Care.* 2nd ed. Chicago, Ill: Year Book Medical; 1988.

16. Pettett CJ. Medical complications of the premature infant. In: Sweeney J, ed. *The High-Risk Neonate: Developmental Therapy Perspectives.* New York, NY: Haworth; 1986.

17. Kornhauser MS, Cullen JA, Wolfson P, et al. Bronchopulmonary dysplasia after ECMO. Presented at the 6th annual Children's Hospital National Medical Center ECMO symposium, February 1990; Breckenridge, Colo.

18. Short BL, Lotze A. Extracorporeal membrane oxygenator therapy. *Pediatr Ann.* 1988;17:516–523.

19. Zwischenberger JB, Null D, Goldthorn J, Harper N. Neonatal extracorporeal membrane oxygenation (ECMO) in Texas. *Journal of Texas Medicine.* 1990;86:72–79.

20. Arnold JH, Truog RD. Sedation for infants undergoing ECMO. Presented at the 6th annual Children's Hospital National Medical Center ECMO symposium; February 1990; Breckenridge, Colo.

21. Bartlett R. Extracorporeal life support in neonatal respiratory failure. *Surg Rounds.* August 1989:41–48.

22. Mendoza JC, Cook LN. ECMO duration: How long is too long? Presented at the 6th annual Children's Hospital National Medical Center ECMO symposium; February 1990; Breckenridge, Colo.

23. Ramos A, Nield TA, Garg M, et al. Neurodevelopmental outcome of extracorporeal membrane oxygenation (ECMO) patients in relation to cranial computed tomography (CT) findings. *Clin Res.* 1989;37:172A.

24. Whitley SB, Nelson KG, Georgeson KE, Johnson SE. Neuromotor development of ECMO graduates. Presented at the 6th annual Children's Hospital National Medical Center ECMO symposium; February 1990; Breckenridge, Colo.

25. Glass P. Patient outcomes after neonatal ECMO. In: Arensman R, Cornish D, eds. *Extracorporeal Life Support.* Oxford, England: Blackwell Scientific. In press.

26. Dykes FD, Ahman PA, Brann AW. Central nervous system morbidity. In: Goldsmith J, Karotkin E, eds. *Assisted Ventilation of the Neonate.* 2nd ed. Philadelphia, Pa: Saunders; 1988.

27. Bernbaum JC, Russell P, Sheridan P, et al. Long-term follow-up of newborns with persistent pulmonary hypertension. *Crit Care Med.* 1984;12:579–583.

28. Adolph V, Ekelund C, Smith C, et al. Developmental outcome of neonates treated with extracorporeal membrane oxygenation. *J Pediatr Surg.* 1990;25:43–46.

29. Goodwin DA, Clark RH, Schwendeman CA, et al. Neurologic morbidity in term and near-term infants treated for severe respiratory failure. Presented at the 6th annual Children's Hospital National Medical Center ECMO symposium; February 1990; Breckenridge, Colo.

30. Mendoza JC, Wilkerson SA, Reese AH, Vogel R. Outcome of neonates treated with ECMO: Longitudinal follow-up from 1 to 3 years of age. Presented at the 7th annual Children's Hospital National Medical Center ECMO symposium; February 1991; Breckenridge, Colo.

31. Bartlett R, Toomasian J, Roloff D, et al. Extracorporeal membrane oxygenation (ECMO) in neonatal respiratory failure: 100 cases. *Ann Surg.* 1986;204:236–244.

32. Mendoza J, Shearer LT, Cook LN. Lateralization of brain lesions following ECMO. Presented at the 6th annual Children's Hospital National Medical Center ECMO symposium; February 1990; Breckenridge, Colo.

33. Schumacher RE, Barks JD, Johnston MV, et al. Right-sided brain lesions in infants following unilateral carotid ligation for extracorporeal membrane oxygenation. *Pediatrics.* 1988;82:155–161.

34. Glass P, Miller M, Short BL. Morbidity for survivors of extracorporeal membrane oxygenation: Neurodevelopmental outcome at one year of age. *Pediatrics.* 1989;83:72–78.

35. Hofkosh D, Clouse H, Smith-Jones J, Thompson AF. Ten years of ECMO: Neurodevelopmental outcome among survivors. Presented at the 6th annual Children's Hospital National Medical Center ECMO symposium; February 1990; Breckenridge, Colo.

36. Horton EJ, Goldie WD, Lew CD, et al. Risk of neurological sequelae in patients suffering focal seizures while on extracorporeal membrane oxygenation. Presented at the Child Neurology Society symposium; October 1989; San Antonio, Tex.

37. Krummel TM, Greenfield LJ, Kirkpatrick BV, et al. The early evaluation of survivors after extracorporeal membrane oxygenation for neonatal pulmonary failure. *J Pediatr Surg.* 1984;19:585–591.

38. Andrews AF, Nixon CA, Cilley RE, et al. One-to-three year outcome for 14 neonatal survivors of extracorporeal membrane oxygenation. *Pediatrics.* 1986;78:692–698.

39. Bayley N. *Manual for the Bayley Scales of Infant Development.* New York, NY: Psychological Corporation; 1969.

40. Amiel-Tison C, Grenier A. *Neurological Assessment During the First Year of Life.* New York, NY: Oxford University Press; 1986.

41. Wilkerson SA, Stewart DL, Cook LN. Developmental outcome of ECMO patients over a four year span. Presented at the 6th annual Children's Hospital National Medical Center ECMO symposium; February 1990; Breckenridge, Colo.

42. Hunter J. *Neurodevelopmental Outcome of ECMO Survivors During the First Two Years.* Denton, Tex: Texas Woman's University; 1990. Thesis.

43. Steward DL, Wilkerson SA, Cook LN. Developmental outcome of ECMO patients over a five year span. Presented at the 7th annual Children's Hospital National Medical Center ECMO symposium; February 1991; Breckenridge, Colo.

44. Wagner A, Glass P, Papero P, et al. Evaluating the long-term outcome of neonatal ECMO survivors: A progress report. Presented at the 7th annual Children's Hospital National Medical Center ECMO symposium; February 1991; Breckenridge, Colo.

45. Rapin I. *Children with Brain Dysfunction.* New York, NY: Raven; 1982.

46. Bly L. The components of normal movement during the first year of life. In: Slaton D, ed. *Development of Movement in Infancy.* Chapel Hill, NC: Division of Physical Therapy, University of North Carolina at Chapel Hill; 1980.

Appendix

Quality scale

Because this study was a retrospective chart review, the quality rating was determined from detailed clinical observations documented in the evaluation reports. Although a subjective, examiner-specific measure has limited generalization value, it was included in this initial study to detect subtle neuromuscular abnormalities that are not reflected in standard developmental scores.

Only those infants personally evaluated by this investigator (approximately 70% of the sample population) were given quality ratings because interrater reliability for scoring of movement could not be established in a study based on retrospective chart review. Each infant included was assigned a total quality index score on the basis of assigned ratings (normal, 5 points; suspicious, 3 points; abnormal, 1 point) for each of two general categories. The first category (muscle tone) utilized clinical observations, physical handling, and directed movement to determine passive and active normal tone, hypotonia, or hypertonia.[40] The second category (coordination and components of movement) was based on documented observation of general coordination of movements, presence and ease of age-appropriate transitional movements, and performance within Bly's[46] description of components of normal movement during infancy.

The two subscores were added to give a total quality score of normal (10), suspect (6 to 8), or abnormal (below 5). Thus an infant had to be clinically judged as completely normal in neuromotor development with no suspicious findings to achieve a quality score of 10; any unusual or atypical finding that may or may not proceed to clinical significance lowered the score to suspect. Any definitely abnormal neuromotor behavior lowered the quality score to abnormal because an abnormal rating in either muscle tone or coordination/components of movement implied or created suboptimal performance in the other category.

The following excerpts from the 3-month evaluation report of one infant illustrate the type of information utilized for the quality score; the excerpts are verbatim except for the infant's name.

- **Infant A:** ECMO for persistent pulmonary hypertension of unknown etiology. Post-ECMO complications or symptoms of potential neurodevelopmental significance included seizures (tonic-clonic movements of the right upper extremity); initial hypotonia after ECMO decannulation with subsequent development of clonus of all extremities, hyperreflexia, and jitteriness; an initial abnormal electroencephalogram (EEG, generalized slowing and no focal activity) with an improved follow-up EEG; and initially poor oral feeding.

- **Age at follow-up evaluation:** 3 months, 23 days.
- **BSID scores:** MDI, 105; PDI, 117.
- **Neuromuscular:** Muscle tone was significantly increased (flexion in the upper extremities and extension in the trunk and lower extremities), affecting both resting posture (albeit very brief quiet periods) and quality of movement. Infant A was able spontaneously to break through the upper extremity flexion (ie, open fisted hands to grasp, delayed reach into space above chest) but required constant inhibitory handling to break up the trunk and lower extremity extensor tone in upright antigravity positions (ie, sitting). Some primitive reflexes were still present (Galant, palmar grasp, and flexor withdrawal); Moro, head righting, plantar grasp, and lower extremity positive support were also observed and were age-appropriate reflexes except that the positive support was too pronounced and obligatory for age. Hip extension was also more pronounced in ventral suspension than is typical for his age.
- **Gross motor:** Skills were scattered from the 2- to 8-month level, with high muscle tone falsely inflating this upper limit and negatively affecting quality of movement. *Supine* (2 to 4 months): Infant A was able to keep his head in midline, although extraneous side-to-side head movements occurred in conjunction with generally increased body movement. Upper extremities were usually in a W position (shoulders retracted and externally rotated, elbows flexed, and hands fisted), but he was able spontaneously to open his hands on occasion and once reached into space toward a toy. Lower extremities were extended but not stiff, although spontaneous leg movements were decreased in excursion and frequency. *Prone* (3 to 5 months): Infant A raised his head to 90° on extended arms; hands remained fisted, and no attempt was made to reach for a toy. Legs were in line with his trunk, again with decreased movements. He reportedly rolls to supine, which I was unable to elicit but am confident is true because his posture and activity in prone meet the component requirements for rolling prone to supine. *Sitting:* Abnormal quality precludes age-level comparison because his performance in sitting is not normal at any age. Although there was only a fleeting initial head lag in pull-to-sit and arms pull in this maneuver (4-month level), Infant A consistently pulled to stand with knees and hips tight in extension and legs adducted. Sitting was only possible with forced passive hip flexion well beyond 90° to break up the strong extension; even then, supported sitting was brief because Infant A soon thrust backward with extended legs, a posterior pelvic tilt, and back arching. *Standing:* The ability to bear his full weight with minimal support passes as a 7- to 8-month skill but was due to increased extensor tone with components and quality of movement both abnormal. Infant A's legs were adducted and stiff in standing but should be apart for a wide base of support and not stiff at this age.

- Fine **motor, adaptive, language, and personal-social:** Skills tested but not included here.
- **Summary:** Infant A is a 3-month, 3-week-old Black boy seen today per ECMO follow-up protocol. His BSID scores appear inflated secondary to his increased muscle tone and by his missing a higher BSID age bracket—and thus increased developmental expectations—by only 1 day; it is of concern that Infant A is not performing all age-appropriate tasks and that his quality of movement is disturbed. In addition to limb and trunk stiffness, Infant A appeared somewhat "wild" both neuromuscularly and neurobehaviorally throughout the evaluation, as evidenced by such factors as an increased generalized activity level, excessive jerky movements, delayed motor response time to specific test items, significant distractability to extraneous stimuli (ie, voices and people), difficulty in attaining/maintaining a calm (quiet) alert state, and difficulty in smooth sustained ocular tracking.
- **Addendum:** No neuromotor abnormalities were observed or elicited at this infant's 6- to 12-month evaluations; BSID scores remained normal.

The effects of prenatal alcohol exposure on child development

Heather Carmichael Olson, PhD
Research Assistant Professor
Department of Psychiatry and
  Behavioral Sciences
School of Medicine
University of Washington
Seattle, Washington

PRENATAL EXPOSURE to alcohol can be the cause of a growing child's learning and behavior problems. Alcohol is a teratogen: a substance that can produce lasting birth defects by affecting the growth and proper formation of the fetus' body and brain. When a pregnant woman drinks alcohol, it crosses the placenta and circulates in the bloodstream of the developing child. The brain and central nervous system (CNS) of the unborn child are especially sensitive to disruption due to prenatal alcohol exposure.

Researchers have been studying the effects of prenatal alcohol exposure for about the past 20 years. Initial clinical reports noted that children of alcoholic mothers had a unique, characteristic appearance and pattern of behavior.[1-3] Subsequent research strongly confirmed these clinical observations[4-6] and documented that alcohol is indeed a teratogen.[7-12] This research knowledge, along with Native American activism and efforts in community education, spurred interest in fetal alcohol effects. A significant turning point came in 1989, with a surge of media interest in prenatal alcohol exposure and publication of the book *The Broken Cord*. This poignant tale records author Michael Dorris' struggle to understand and deal with his adopted son's serious developmental and behavior problems, which were finally identified as the result of alcohol exposure before birth.[13] With increased awareness has come a growing flood of public and professional concern about prevention of alcohol effects and intervention with children and adults afflicted before birth by exposure to alcohol. Now careful, systematic community and professional education is strongly needed and is beginning to occur. For example, in 1993 the American Academy of Pediatrics published a discussion of fetal alcohol effects, as well as prevention, intervention, and policy recommendations, for pediatricians.[14]

Exposure to large quantities of alcohol before birth can lead to fetal alcohol syndrome (FAS), a medical diagnosis and lasting birth defect. FAS is preventable: If a fetus is not exposed to alcohol before birth, FAS will not occur. But if a child is born with FAS, the damage is permanent. FAS has been called the leading known cause of mental retardation in the western world,[15] and current research

The author wishes to acknowledge the pioneering work of the following Seattle colleagues in the field of fetal alcohol effects, listed in alphabetical order: Donna Burgess, Sterling Clarren, Robin La Due, Sandra Randels, and Marceil Ten Eyck. The author particularly acknowledges the invaluable work and mentorship of Ann Streissguth and the willingness of the families described in this article to share their important life stories. Finally, the author acknowledges the careful editorial assistance of Ninia Ingram, the comments of Kim Shay, and the word processing efforts of Kitti Downing and Tracy Smith.

Inf Young Children 1994;6(3):10–25
© 1994 Aspen Publishers, Inc.

suggests that there are also children diagnosed with FAS who are not defined as mentally retarded.[16] FAS is gradually becoming recognized as a developmental disability that lasts a lifetime, that is characterized by persistent and varied cognitive deficits and a spectrum of behavior problems, and that has a pattern that is distinct from other birth defects.

Not every child affected by prenatal alcohol exposure will show sufficient features for a firm diagnosis of FAS. Based on evidence from animal studies, researchers have suggested that there is a range of "alcohol-related birth defects" (ARBD).[5] Within this continuum some investigators are exploring a clinical and medical research category termed "possible fetal alcohol effects" (FAE). At this point individuals classified with "possible FAE" have a clear history of prenatal alcohol exposure and show a partial expression of the characteristics seen in FAS in cases where there is no strong alternative diagnosis. Alcohol is thought to make a significant contribution, among other factors, to the very real problems of those classified with possible FAE. Use of the term *possible FAE* is still evolving, and while an important category of concern to parents and professionals, it may not be easily recognized.

It is not yet clear why one child exposed to alcohol before birth shows FAS, while another is affected but does not show the full syndrome, and yet another child is apparently unaffected. The developmental impact of alcohol, like that of other teratogens, depends on the amount, timing, and conditions of exposure, as well as on characteristics of the mother (eg, in metabolism of alcohol, chronicity, and severity of alcohol use) and the child's genetic susceptibility to alcohol effects. It is important to note that there is no documented "safe" level of drinking during pregnancy. Though children with full FAS are usually born to women who clearly abused alcohol during pregnancy,[11] intensive research is revealing some developmental consequences of lower doses of alcohol exposure before birth.[8,17–21]

The incidence of FAS has been estimated at 1 to 3 per 1,000 live births.[15,22] But researchers are debating incidence figures for FAS, given how hard it is to establish the frequency of a birth defect that is difficult to identify at birth, can be confused with other medical problems, and must be diagnosed by trained individuals via history and physical examination rather than by a laboratory test. In addition, drinking levels and demographics of populations must be kept in mind when estimating how often FAS occurs. It is even harder to estimate the prevalence of the clinical and research category of possible FAE, which may be two times as common as FAS (or more), depending on how it is defined.

The societal costs of FAS are alarming. Practitioners can help in the important task of preventing fetal alcohol effects by learning about the problem and educating others. Early interventionists, health professionals, teachers, and parents can watch for indications of fetal alcohol effects, finding children at risk and referring them for diagnosis. Of course, information about prenatal alcohol exposure is necessary in the diagnostic process and is important to know in care of the child. Asking families about alcohol and drug use during pregnancy requires care and training and should be done according to agency guidelines by staff members chosen and trained to ask about these issues. The actual identification of FAS or possible FAE requires a trained health professional, such as a specialist in birth defects, or a specially trained nurse or doctor who knows about neurodevelopmental assessment, as well as the effects of prenatal alcohol exposure. Properly used, a diagnosis of FAS or label of possible FAE can be the key to setting up appropriate early (and later) intervention and to helping caregivers to understand an important reason behind a child's misbehavior or slow developmental progress.

Several resources in the list of references at the end of this article will help the reader become more familiar with the diagnostic characteristics and developmental pattern of behavior across time among fetal alcohol-affected individuals, as well as with the referral process and currently suggested intervention strategies.[23,24] One particularly useful reference about school-aged children is *Educating Children Prenatally Exposed to Alcohol and Other Drugs*, by Burgess, Lasswell, and Streissguth.[25]

This article presents a brief overview of the characteristics of fetal alcohol-affected infants and young children and presents a discussion of how this developmental disability compares to other, more familiar childhood disorders. Later sections of this article give histories of several children with FAS, followed by a discussion of intervention ideas.

CHARACTERISTICS OF FETAL ALCOHOL-AFFECTED INDIVIDUALS

In the presence of prenatal alcohol exposure, FAS is uniquely defined by the combination of three characteristics.[5,14] First is a pattern of dysmorphic features and physical anomalies, especially specific craniofacial characteristics (see all photos and Paul's story, later in this article). Second is prenatal or postnatal growth deficiency of height and weight; children with FAS are small, often falling below the 10th percentile, though this may change after puberty. Third are signs of CNS dysfunction, such as microcephaly, developmental delay, hyperactivity, problems in attention or learning, intellectual deficits, or seizures. These signs change in form over the course of development and are expressed among individuals with FAS in many different ways. CNS dysfunction among individuals with FAS is still being carefully studied by researchers, who are learning more all the time. Diagnosis of FAS is easiest between 8 months and 8 years.[26] This is because it is difficult to recognize newborns with FAS and because bodily changes at puberty make the physical features associated with FAS harder to recognize.[11] Yet clinical observations suggest that diagnosis of FAS is currently not often made before the age of 3 years, making it impossible to provide early intervention.

Streissguth and LaDue[27] have described a general behavioral picture of FAS, finding that it is usually characterized by a highly social orientation and childhood hyperactivity, coupled with lasting problems in social judgment and learning. Nanson[28] has described a less common and different behavioral type for children with FAS, one more typical of autistic children. This article presents in detail the characteristics of infants and young children with FAS and possible FAE.

According to current research, about three quarters of FAS infants show irritability as infants, including signs of tremulousness or jitteriness. Many show difficulties with sucking and muscle tone, and some may be considered failure to thrive.[29–33] Problems become more evident as a child ages. While not much data are available, some researchers are beginning to systematically test the abilities of children with FAS/FAE during the years from birth to 3 years and on into the preschool period.[34–38]

In early childhood, about three quarters of those diagnosed with FAS exhibit mild to moderate mental retardation, though a range of intelligence quotient (IQ) levels exists among individuals with FAS. Microcephaly is usually present, indicating smaller brain size. About half of young children with FAS show poor coordination, decreased muscle tone, hyperactivity, and/or attention deficits.[14,29–32] For many children with FAS, there may also be language problems, which are only now being uncovered.[39,40] For a small number of children with FAS, autistic-like behavior may occur.[28]

As they grow, children with FAS often appear to have memory and learning deficits (with sporadic retention of information and uneven developmental progress) and, even for their age and IQ level, often show particular difficulties in relating cause and effect, in making social judgments, and in planning. As children with FAS grow older, there are emerging discrepancies between their apparent ability level, as compared to their actual level of achievement and daily function. For example, clinical observations of many individuals with FAS indicate a discrepancy between their relatively good verbal skills and their relatively poor ability to effectively communicate and function in social situations.[41] The cognitive and linguistic deficits and discrepancies of children with FAS seem related to the troubles they have in handling the complexities of peer interaction and in conforming to social norms and may underlie their behavior problems. For young children with FAS, these problem behaviors often include persistent temper tantrums, difficulty making transitions between activities, and poor relations with peers (which can be a powerful predictor of later psychiatric problems). For somewhat older children with FAS, problem behaviors can include poor peer relations, apparent lying and stealing, inappropriate social behavior, and poor social judgment.

Children with FAS also show characteristics that are quite positive. As Burgess, Lasswell, and Streissguth[25] have pointed out, children with FAS can often be socially engaging, interested in others, talkative, good with animals, and affectionate. It is important to keep a balanced and hopeful view of children with FAS. Many of these children do not show the most severe manifestations of the syndrome, and some can be expected to show improvement given appropriate treatment.

As the term is currently defined, children given the label "possible FAE" may also show these kinds of positive characteristics but are also at increased risk for attentional deficits and other cognitive difficulties, impairment in fine and gross motor skills, and speech/language problems. Their deficits may be similar in type to those seen in children with FAS and may seriously compromise their ability to function day to day. Compared to someone with FAS, it may be harder to recognize that an individual described as having possible FAE has alcohol-related birth defects arising from CNS dysfunction. As a result, the individual's learning and behavior difficulties may be quite debilitating, as they fall short of their own expectations of normal performance and those of the people around them.

Though they may change in form, these deficits and discrepancies seem to persist as fetal alcohol-affected individuals grow older, continuing to affect how they function in daily life. Recent work by Streissguth et al[16] and by LaDue et al[42] following FAS/FAE individuals into adulthood clearly demonstrates their persistent and debilitating problems in cognition, behavior, effective communication and socialization, and daily function. Research is underway to define more clearly the range of neuropsychologic profiles in individuals with FAS and other alcohol-related birth defects and to detail the patterns of their performance on standardized tests. Research is also being conducted to uncover the myriad of mental health problems; substance abuse; educational, vocational, and legal difficulties; and behavior problems of fetal alcohol-affected individuals and to find better strategies for intervention and prevention. The variety of alcohol-related birth defects makes it hard to predict how any one fetal alcohol-affected child will function as an adult and points out the necessity for an individualized, flexible, and realistic approach to intervention.

COMPARING FETAL ALCOHOL EFFECTS AND OTHER CHILDHOOD DISORDERS

A diagnosis of FAS or a label of possible FAE provides etiologic information and implies that prenatal alcohol exposure has led to significant CNS dysfunction that is organic in nature. The FAS diagnosis suggests that prenatal alcohol exposure acts as a primary *cause* of a child's learning and behavioral difficulties, though other causes may affect the child's problems as well. As the term is currently used, a description of "possible FAE" suggests that prenatal alcohol exposure plays a role as a significant *contributor*, among many factors, to the child's learning and behavior problems.

When describing childhood disorders, there are numerous diagnostic labels used in the fields of special education, child psychology and psychiatry, and social work. Many of these labels are descriptive in nature and are given on the basis of the child's behavior and development (or clinical features), as well as on the natural history of the disorder, rather than on the basis of etiology. Depending on the constellation of the child's problems (how the alcohol effects are expressed) and the demands of the intervention setting, diagnostic labels such as mental retardation, attention deficit-hyperactivity disorder, learning disabilities, conduct disorder, and perhaps even autism, attachment disorder, and failure to thrive can co-occur with the medical diagnosis of FAS. For a child described as having possible FAE, some of these other diagnostic labels may apply as well. A diagnosis of FAS may be listed as a physical disorder or condition on Axis III of a DSM-III-R diagnosis[43] and may qualify a child for special education services as health impaired.

Many children with FAS, or those described as having possible FAE, may meet DSM-III-R criteria for mental retardation or specific developmental disorders or may meet special education guidelines for a learning disabilities classroom. Children classified with FAS or possible FAE show a range of intellectual function, with IQ scores reflecting severe impairment through the normal range. Even in the absence of mental retardation, a child with FAS or possible FAE may show evidence of learning problems (especially sporadic memory deficits and cause-effect reasoning problems) and sometimes signs of early developmental delay. Testing often seems to show a relatively greater weakness in adaptive functioning, especially in socialization, compared to the tested IQ level of the fetal alcohol-affected child.

Some children with FAS or possible FAE may also fit the DSM-III-R diagnostic criteria for attention deficit-hyperactivity disorder (ADHD). The definition of ADHD includes behavioral signs such as easily distractible, fidgety, difficulty sustaining attention, and talking excessively. Note that deficits in attention are a final common pathway in many childhood disorders, including FAS and possible FAE. The attentional problems of children with fetal alcohol effects are not surprising, since exposure to alcohol appears to have diffuse effects on the CNS and since the attentional system requires integrated action of widespread parts of the brain.[44]

For children with FAS or seen as having possible FAE, there can often be evidence of social interaction problems. Parents sometimes report having problems in "attachment" or "bonding" to their fetal alcohol-affected child. Particular difficulties in social skills and social judgment are very characteristic of these children, even for their age and IQ level, and they may meet local guidelines for special counseling assistance or placement in a behavior disorders classroom. In rare cases, a child with FAS may show autistic features. More commonly, the descriptive DSM-III-R diagnoses of conduct disorder or oppositional defiant disorder may apply as a fetal alcohol-affected child grows.

RECOGNIZING FETAL ALCOHOL EFFECTS

A diagnosis of FAS or a description of possible FAE provides anticipatory guidance by helping parents and interventionists to reframe a child's difficulties as organically based, long-term, and thus potentially difficult to alter. A diagnosis of FAS can be a key to accessing community services such as adoption support, Social Security Income (SSI) funding, and special education services under the provisions of the Public Law 94-142 and Public Law 99-457. Unfortunately, a label of possible FAE does not yet allow access to many services.

Understanding that a child has fetal alcohol effects can lead to new intervention strategies, suggesting helpful techniques or explaining why some strategies may be ineffective. For instance, if memory deficits are organic in nature (and due to prenatal alcohol exposure), then they are not under the child's control to the extent that they would be if the child were simply stubborn. Such organic deficits must be dealt with through compensatory strategies, rather than with disciplinary techniques to control "stubbornness." Note that when another diagnostic label applies along with a description of FAS or possible FAE, it is very important to mesh the intervention recommendations that arise from the two labels. For example, understanding that a child with conduct disorders also has FAS (and therefore difficulty with abstract thought about cause and effect) means that the common recommendations of talk therapy, contracts and negotiation, and even reasoning and explanation may not prove very effective in changing a child's behavior. Instead, concrete, long-term behavior management techniques and social skills training may be more useful, and the child's violation of social norms may be understood as due more to cognitive deficits than to deliberate rule breaking or manipulation.

The diagnosis of FAS or label of possible FAE is most helpful if it begins needed changes in the network and type of care the child receives. Such change often requires the ongoing support and advocacy of a professional who understands fetal alcohol effects. Physicians, who often make the diagnosis, may be called on to find or to act as an advocate for the family. Such advocacy is challenging but can make a real difference in the lives of fetal alcohol-affected children and their families.

HISTORIES OF CHILDREN WITH FAS

To understand and help children made vulnerable by prenatal exposure to alcohol, parents and professionals should remember that these children have a biologically based disability that potentially has lifelong and very individualized consequences. With this in mind, parents and early interventionists can look ahead and better puzzle out what places each child at risk and what will help protect the child as he or she grows older.

One way to guide thoughts about intervention is through three short case studies of children with FAS, who differ in ethnicity. These histories illustrate the struggles of biologic, adoptive, and foster families adjusting to a developmental disability that could have been prevented. These stories begin in infancy and early childhood, but go beyond the first 3 years of each child's life, highlighting the importance of a long-term view on FAS. Illustrated briefly are the range of these children's developmental difficulties, the process and value of a diagnosis, and the hazards of going without appropriate intervention. These histories show that intervention is needed at the many levels of community, school, family, and the individual child and highlight some keys to successful early intervention, which are also outlined in the box entitled "Intervention Guidelines for Working with Young Fetal Alcohol-Affected Children." Sources of information about intervention strategies are listed at the end of this article.[25,45–49]

Matthew

Matthew is a 7-year-old boy with a diagnosis of FAS. He is also classified as moderately to severely mentally retarded and lives with his biologic parents. While pregnant, Matthew's mother did not drink often but consumed a fairly large amount of beer each time she did drink. After Matthew reached the age 4 years, his mother entered alcohol treatment, stopped drinking, and achieved sobriety. As a result, Matthew's two younger brothers are unaffected and are developing normally.

No one realized the full extent of Matthew's problems while he was very young, and no one asked questions about his mother's alcohol use. But at the age of 2 years, Matthew's doctor referred the family to a center for developmental disabilities. Again, no one inquired about possible prenatal alcohol exposure. Matthew was identified as developmentally delayed, but even with extensive testing (including a genetic workup), no cause was found for his problems. His parents then struggled through the difficult process of adjusting to their son's mental retardation. It was during this time, when Matthew was a toddler, that his mother learned about FAS. Consequently she stopped denying her alcohol abuse and actually informed her doctor of her drinking during pregnancy. Matthew's parents then

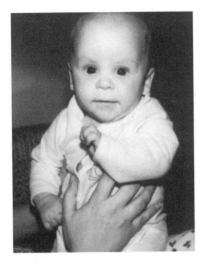 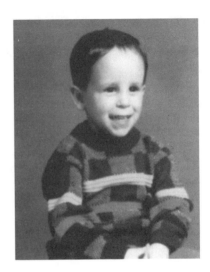

Fig 1. Matthew, born 1986, at 6 months (left) and 4 years (right).

sought out a birth defects specialist who examined Matthew and rendered a diagnosis of FAS. The family was fortunate in being located near a research center on fetal alcohol effects, where a diagnostic clinic was available. Even though they had been the ones to initiate the diagnostic process, coming to terms with the idea that Matthew's problems were the result of FAS was a new struggle. It was tremendously difficult for his parents to adjust to the idea that Matthew had a birth defect that could have been prevented. This knowledge created in them feelings of guilt, shame, loss, and anger.

Matthew's low cognitive test scores and generalized developmental delay qualified him to enter an organized and multilevel early intervention system. He and his family have been well served by that system. From a developmental disabilities center, Matthew moved into special education classes in public schools. His family has been part of the multidisciplinary team assessment process at his school. Matthew's classrooms have been small with predictable classroom routines, careful planning for transitions between activities, and monitoring for signs of overstimulation. A strong partnership has been built between home and school. Educational goals for Matthew have been individualized and realistic, focused on functional skills (such as toilet training) and on enhancing communication (such as training him to use picture cards and new words, since he has limited verbal skill). The school staff and family have even embarked on a campaign to educate others about FAS and its lifelong consequences and on the importance of prevention. This effort has helped Matthew's mother maintain her recovery.

Intervention Guidelines for Working with Young Fetal Alcohol-Affected Children

1. Recognize the fetal alcohol-affected child's diagnosis, and learn what it means. Reframe ideas about problems, as well as treatment, strategies, and outcome goals, in light of the child's diagnosis. Be realistic given the child's underlying organic CNS dysfunction.
2. Respond to the individual child and his or her situation. Let the child teach you what works. Be flexible enough to keep trying new behavior management strategies for a fetal alcohol-affected child and to think about how to set up behavior management past the period of early childhood.
3. Set up an environment that protects the child and facilitates development. To do that:
   - Assess and assist the family. (Examples: Give information about normal child development and fetal alcohol effects. Connect family to FAS/FAE support groups. Help them move beyond denial of substance abuse problems. Set up respite care for parents.)
   - Monitor the child's health and developmental progress. (Examples: Enroll the child in a high-risk follow-up clinic, or make sure the child has ongoing, informed pediatric care. Make sure the child is enrolled in an appropriate early-intervention program, if needed.)
   - Shape the environment to help the child learn to better regulate his or her behavior. (Examples: Set up regular routines at home or at school. Identify signs of overstimulation, and teach child and caregiver strategies to recognize these signs and to alter situations to reduce overstimulation. Set up cues to help a child sequence events.)
   - Teach concrete, functional skills to the child. (Examples: Explicitly teach the child ways to calm himself down. Explicitly teach effective communication. Assess what skills the child needs to function in the community, such as toilet-training or the ability to accompany family to a friend's home, and teach those skills at school as soon as possible.)
   - Let the child know what behaviors are expected of him or her, rather than rely on applying consequences to change the child's behavior. (Examples: When a young fetal alcohol-affected child has a tantrum when asked to put her coat on to go home, consider this alternative to time out: help her calm down, then provide a choice between two acceptable behaviors. Try to understand what message the tantrum might be communicating [eg, transitions are too hard].)
4. Create a partnership between systems serving the child to best accomplish effective child advocacy and continuing care for the child and family.

Matthew is in a fortunate position compared to the children with FAS who have come before him. The cause of his mental retardation is known, so his caregivers are aware that he may show behavior problems that differ from those seen in other forms of mental retardation. His progress is being carefully monitored. He is being served with full awareness that he has FAS accompanied by mental retardation, and much is known about how to serve children who are mentally retarded. His intervention program is individualized, flexible, and multidisciplinary and is intended to give him functional skills. Family members have been acting as advocates ever since Matthew's parents initiated the diagnosis. His care is long-term as systems are set up to serve him at least until he reaches the age of 21 years. Adulthood, however, presents an uncertain picture for Matthew as is often the case for those who are developmentally disabled.

Josie

A bright-eyed energetic little girl, Josie is now 5 years old. Her facial features are characteristic of FAS but do not immediately (or even always) alert an observer to her developmental disability. Her birth defect is more hidden than Matthew's. She has a history of early developmental delay, notable memory deficits, persistent and pronounced temper tantrums, and impulsiveness. Yet, unlike Matthew, her tested IQ is within the average range, and current testing yields an IQ score of 96. She lives with her adoptive family who has cared for her since the age of 7 months. Josie's adoption came about largely because of parental termination of rights due to her mother's polydrug use and her relatives' preference for a stable out-of-home placement.

Because her mother's prenatal drug use was well known, Josie was evaluated at the age of 3 years for fetal alcohol and drug effects, and was given a diagnosis of FAS by a physician specializing in birth defects. Earlier diagnosis might have been helpful but was not really available. Josie's early health problems, including persistent respiratory difficulties and ear infections, were initially thought by parents and teachers to explain her slowed developmental progress.

At the age of 3 years, Josie was placed by her determined and knowledgeable adoptive family in a day treatment program for children with behavior and emotional problems. According to Josie's teacher, she was accepted because of her

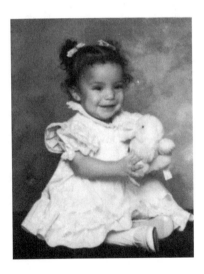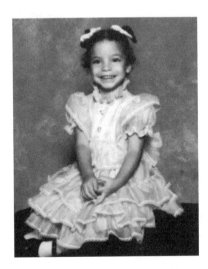

Fig 2. Josie, born 1988, at 7 months (left) and 3 years (right).

history of prenatal drug exposure, possible hyperactivity, and the difficult behavior she was showing in day care. The FAS diagnosis was not yet known, but the treatment was helpful for a youngster with FAS. In the day treatment program, the teacher–child ratio was 1:2, the class size was eight children, and staff were trained in therapeutic child-care techniques (such as a high degree of routine and consistency, well thought-through behavior management, careful transitions between activities, child empowerment, and a policy of providing children with language for their feelings).

Placement in the day treatment program was not without drawbacks. At first Josie imitated many of the deviant behaviors of her classmates, to the dismay of her adoptive family. The staff were uncertain of how to handle Josie's behavior, since she did not seem to learn in altogether predictable ways, often regressed or forgot skills, and showed great scatter in her abilities. Once the FAS diagnosis was known, Josie's adoptive mother provided information about FAS to the staff, which helped a great deal. As time went on, school staff and family had to work together very closely to create a treatment plan that worked but could be changed on short notice to accommodate Josie's inconsistencies. They also had to support each other when dealing with the daily frustrations and unexpected setbacks that are typical of Josie's developmental progress. In addition, information about FAS helped teachers shape the classroom environment to facilitate Josie's development, to avoid overstimulation and behavioral breakdowns, and to set realistic expectations. The teachers learned to let Josie know what was expected of her, rather than to discipline her for misbehavior. The results so far have been hopeful, and Josie's achievements have been impressive. Her ability to participate in group activities and individual work is close to age appropriate. Her temper tantrums have decreased dramatically, and her language skills have increased by leaps and bounds.

Josie is now about to make the transition into the public schools, although she does still qualify for special services based on her history of developmental difficulties, prior day treatment intervention, and, significantly, her FAS diagnosis. Josie's family must start over as advocates for appropriate services, a tiring prospect and one that taxes the family's resources. Her day treatment teachers are very supportive and are helping to plan the transition. It is likely that Josie will encounter setbacks at each life transition and stage in development, and because of her potential, this may be more frustrating for Josie's caregivers than might be true for those caring for Matthew. She has been quite successful so far, demonstrating that hope lies in careful and informed early intervention. But her future is less certain. In a sense, Josie's more "hidden" birth defect, coupled with her earlier success, increases the risk that she will not receive appropriate services and that her problems could worsen in the future.

Paul

Paul has been followed in a long-term child-development research study and so received a "seems to have FAS" diagnosis at birth. He is now 19 years old and lives in a small community with his supportive and caring extended family, who assumed custody of Paul after his birth mother died.

As can be seen from his pictures, taken at ages 1 day and 7 years, Paul showed the characteristic facial features of FAS, though diagnosis (as always) took into account ethnic characteristics. He had a specific cluster of features, including short palpebral fissures (eye slits) so that his eyes appear set widely apart, a flat midface, a thin upper lip, and a somewhat indistinct philtrum (the ridges between the nose and upper lip) After puberty, as is typical, his facial features became less distinctive for an FAS diagnosis. Early in life, Paul showed some growth retardation, as he was called small and frail at 18 months. The growth retardation disappeared by adolescence, when he actually seemed stocky and of average height.

As a baby, Paul was tremulous and showed variable muscle tone: very rigid at times and floppy at others. He was quite active, and it was hard for him to orient visually. In early childhood he showed disrupted sleep in the form of nightmares. As a preschooler, Paul was impulsive and active and showed attentional problems, and his speech was difficult to understand. Yet he was engaging and attractive,

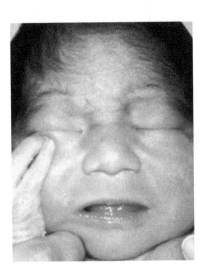 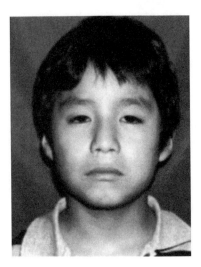

Fig 3. Paul, born 1974, at 1 day (left) and 7 years (right).

and people were hopeful about his future. Testing showed an IQ level typical of the average in the FAS/FAE population: around 70, in the mildly mentally retarded range. Reading was a relative strength, while math was a relative weakness. In school, he repeated first grade and met school guidelines for special education, where he was thought to do less well than his peers. He was rated by his teachers as showing average behavior in many areas (such as cooperation), though he was still considered inattentive, impulsive, and easily frustrated.

In middle school Paul really began to have school problems, and his path through life clearly diverged from that of his peers. As a teenager, Paul's adaptive behavior (ability to function day to day) was at the level of an 8-year-old, a typical discrepancy within the FAS/FAE population. His academic skills remained at about the 3rd- to 4th-grade level. Because of problems in classes and with peers, he was only successful in attending school part of the day. He got into fights with schoolmates. His teachers became extremely frustrated, recommending a change in schools because of behavior problems. A structured academic curriculum did not seem to be the answer. Paul could not consistently function independently at or away from home. Luckily his community was small and his conscientious adoptive parents helped protect him from serious trouble.

As more information about FAS became available over time, there has been greater awareness and acceptance of Paul's diagnosis and his long-term problems. He has been involved in vocational training and in other programs to develop functional skills. Paul's family has remained stalwart advocates for ongoing, appropriate services and have repeatedly sought expert advice on FAS to try to convince each new service system to be flexible and protective of Paul. Crises have occurred, but his family has been learning to "reframe" Paul's problem, to be realistic and concrete, and to not expect that Paul should act his age or behave in typical ways. Even though Paul is now actually reaching adulthood, his family still needs ongoing support and advice. Paul still needs coordinated services, mandated funding given his diagnosis of FAS, and a protective environment.

INTERVENTION FOR CHILDREN WITH FAS AND POSSIBLE FAE: FOUR IMPORTANT GUIDELINES

As is clear from the stories of Matthew, Josie, and Paul, fetal alcohol-affected children have lifelong developmental disabilities. Compensatory strategies are needed to help these children function up to their potential. Their caregivers need support and clear, practical advice to best handle a complex, confusing, and emotional situation. The following four intervention guidelines for young children with fetal alcohol effects can be of value to parents, physicians, nurses, and early interventionists. These guidelines are also outlined in the box entitled "Intervention Guidelines for Working with Young Fetal Alcohol-Affected Children."

One: Recognize and reframe

The first and biggest steps are to recognize the child's diagnosis and learn what it means. Taking these steps yields several benefits. Awareness of FAS or possible FAE in a child can bring help to the biologic mother by uncovering her drinking problems and, perhaps, those of other family members. This can ultimately lead to improvements in the child's home environment and may prevent the birth of future alcohol-affected children. Remember that ongoing substance use, by either or both parents, usually requires referral for alcohol/drug treatment and that asking about substance use requires care and training.

Knowing the diagnosis, parents and practitioners can learn to reframe, or rethink, behaviors they see in their children as manifestations of the organic CNS dysfunction arising from fetal effects. They can also reframe ideas about appropriate treatment goals, strategies, and timeline for expecting change in the child's behavior. Awareness of the long-term impact of fetal alcohol effects can help parents and care providers to build realistic intervention early in the child's life and to understand that intervention may well continue throughout the child's life. Reframing was certainly helpful to Josie's and Matthew's parents and to Paul's teachers and family. Caregivers of fetal alcohol-affected children can learn that it takes different parenting or teaching strategies and perhaps more time than expected for the child to learn better ways of coping with change or overstimulation.

Two: Create individualized, flexible intervention

The next step involves creating interventions that are individualized and flexible, keeping in mind that what is effective with the child may continually change over time. It is important not to become discouraged. Teachers and parents report that it helps to "let the child teach you what works," by carefully watching the child's behavior (and their response to it) and writing down which ideas work to improve the child's behavior and which do not. With fetal alcohol-affected children, the key is to figure out how much of their learning difficulties and misbehavior can be changed and how much may be due to underlying damage to the CNS and simply may not be changeable. For example, if a child has memory and attention deficits because of FAS, it may help to move him out of a preschool that is unpredictable and highly stimulating. But even in a quieter and more consistent preschool setting, the child may still have trouble remembering what he has learned and may eventually begin to misbehave once again. Over and over, new strategies may be needed to keep intervention effective.

Three: Build a protective environment

The next step lies in providing an appropriate environment for the fetal alcohol-affected child, which can facilitate development and offer protection against the consequences of prenatal alcohol effects. As can be seen from the stories of Matthew, Josie, and Paul, a good deal is already known about what constitutes appropriate intervention for the fetal alcohol-affected young child. But we are learning more all the time, and some of our traditional ideas about early intervention will need to be challenged when working with fetal alcohol effects.

Assist the family

To provide an appropriate environment for fetal alcohol-affected children, family assessment and assistance are critical. Family stress and coping strategies and characteristics of the family environment (including ongoing substance abuse and other concerning factors in the child's home environment) should all be assessed. If the problem has been identified early, it is during their children's infant and toddler years that families realize that FAS or possible FAE will present lifelong problems. This means dealing with guilt, anger, and sorrow over past alcohol use and the fact that the children's problems could have been prevented. Assistance should be geared to the different needs of adoptive, foster, or biologic families as each type of family adapts to the idea of raising a child with developmental disabilities. All families can use information about normal development and fetal alcohol effects and help in looking toward the future.[50] Many will want a connection to resources such as respite care and counseling. Long-term support to the family is critical. Parent self-help and FAS support groups can be extremely helpful, as can the personal attention of a professional who thoroughly understands fetal alcohol effects.

Monitor the child

For infants with fetal alcohol effects, the most important initial intervention is enrollment of the baby in a high-risk infant monitoring system that follows the child's developmental progress, home environment, and health. Children with fetal alcohol effects may have particular problems with otitis media and eating difficulties, as well as dental and eye problems.[32] Over time, risks in the child's life should be identified and minimized, such as parental psychiatric dysfunction or chemical dependence or perhaps unrealistic expectations by a teacher or a pediatrician not informed about FAS. Protective factors should be enhanced by helping parents to become aware of and to respond to the sometimes confusing cues of fetal alcohol-affected babies. Infancy is a good time to build a caregiving network, including respite care, that can support parents or be activated if the parent cannot care for the child.

Set up safeguards

In general, it is extremely helpful to find ways to set up safeguards in the environment, rather than focusing only on changing the fetal alcohol-affected child. Shaping the environment, rather than the child's behavior, may be a most effective strategy. For early intervention, well-established principles of therapeutic child care can be useful, as described in the stories of Matthew and Josie. In early childhood, careful behavior management at home and at school, keeping the FAS/FAE labels in mind, is tremendously important. In their 1992 publications, Burgess et al[25] and Burgess and Streissguth[41] offer the important insight that for fetal alcohol-affected children, inappropriate or challenging behaviors can be a form of communication, rather than a simple attention-getting device. This means that problem behaviors can be managed by helping the child find a more appropriate way to communicate the message he or she has tried to express through misbehaviors such as temper tantrums or biting.

Teach functional skills

It is wise to focus on teaching concrete, functional skills to the fetal alcohol-affected child. Burgess et al[25] and Burgess and Streissguth[41] state that caregivers should analyze what the child needs to know to function as independently as possible and should make those skills his or her educational goals. Experiential learning is important so that a child can practice and generalize skills. Matthew, for example, was taught toileting and communication through picture cards and was given many opportunities to practice at home and at school. Paul's family was advised to teach him vocational skills and substance abuse prevention, to give him work practice and experience, and to deemphasize academics, which were not as useful to him. Part of Josie's school and day-care curricula have clearly focused on improving her communication: teaching her to "use her words" to express feelings, needs, and desires, rather than to hit, bite, or throw temper tantrums to express herself. Communication disorders specialists can help teachers to focus on communication in the classroom and to pinpoint and work on specific problems in the children's social language use (eg, not listening to others, not staying on the topic, using routine or formulaic phrases to participate in conversation without really comprehending what is being discussed).

Teach what is expected

As Burgess has emphasized in her work, it can be useful to let the fetal alcohol-affected child know what behaviors are expected of him or her rather than to rely on applying consequences to change the child's behavior. If fetal alcohol-affected children have a particular difficulty in understanding cause and effect, then they may not readily understand why they are being disciplined, placed in time out, or even rewarded or praised. Strategies that one might use with a child too young to thoroughly understand cause–effect connections may actually continue to be the most effective techniques for an older fetal alcohol-affected child. To teach what is expected, caregivers must first define what it is that they expect from the child. This process of definition allows for more realistic and practical expectations for the child, and for more successful behavior management.

A final note

Even though early intervention may not overcome the problems of a child with FAS or possible FAE, it can be a key to reducing the family's stress and to changing the child's early environment, thereby improving later outcome for both the child and his or her family. This was certainly true for Matthew and his family. Informed early intervention professionals may even be able to remove obstacles to the child's future by helping to qualify a child for services later, when he or she is older, such as special education (as was true in Josie's case), even if the child does not have "low enough" test scores at a particular time to meet eligibility requirements.

Four: Form a partnership of services

The final step is to form an ongoing partnership between systems serving the child: home, school, doctor, child care, as well as later possibilities (eg, the correctional system, public health, vocational training, substance abuse treatment). This kind of partnership has been the key to Matthew's, Josie's, and Paul's success so far. The truth is that it takes time and persistence to handle the successive, long-term challenges offered by fetal alcohol-affected children. Perhaps more than with other developmental disabilities, this can be a trying task. Throughout their lives, individuals with fetal alcohol effects will need a series of advocates to bridge and to connect systems and to create the comprehensive services that are needed. Parents can be advocates, as they have been for Matthew, Josie, and Paul. But these children also need professionals who know and understand fetal alcohol effects to help these children along their way.

GOALS: PREVENTION AND EARLY INTERVENTION

Fetal alcohol effects are a *preventable* form of developmental disability. The United States' "Healthy 2000 National Health Strategy" aims to significantly reduce the incidence of FAS by the year 2000, a challenging task.[51] Prevention must occur on many levels. Public awareness is critical and can be most effectively achieved through accurate discussion in the media, organized community activism, and concerted efforts by state governments (especially through creation of state coordinators for FAS prevention). To raise public awareness, several FAS/

FAE newsletters for parents and professionals are currently available, as are several toll-free numbers (see box entitled "Newsletters, Telephone Help Lines, and Information Centers"). Health, educational, social service, and correctional professionals should also be educated about fetal alcohol effects and alcoholism and about how to gather information on these topics from patients. Specialized substance abuse treatment services to pregnant women, in an effort to prevent prenatal alcohol/drug exposure, are also important.

For children born with fetal alcohol effects, however, prevention of the disabilities is no longer possible. Hope then begins with early intervention, carried out with a full awareness of the possible lifelong effects of prenatal alcohol exposure.

Newsletters, Telephone Help Lines, and Information Centers

Iceberg Newsletter. A quarterly educational newsletter for people concerned about FAS and FAE because "the problems readily seen are only the tip of the iceberg." Available from PO Box 4292, Seattle, WA 98104.

Clearinghouse for Drug-Exposed Children, newsletter and information line from the Division of Behavioral and Developmental Pediatrics, University of California, San Francisco, 400 Parnassus Ave, Room A203, San Francisco, CA 94143-0314; (415) 476-9691.

Fetal Alcohol Education Program, Boston University School of Medicine, 7 Kent St, Boston, MA 02146.

Fetal Alcohol and Drug Unit, University of Washington School of Medicine, Department of Psychiatry and Behavioral Sciences, 2707 NE Blakeley St, Seattle, WA 98105.

National Association for Perinatal Addiction Research and Education (NAPARE), 11 E Hubbard St, Suite 200, Chicago, IL 60611; (312) 329-9131.

National Clearinghouse for Alcohol and Drug Information, PO Box 2345, Rockville, MD 20852; (301) 468-2600 or 1-800-729-6686.

National Organization on FAS (NOFAS), 1815 H St NW, Suite 750, Washington, DC 20006; (202) 785-4585.

REFERENCES

1. Jones KL, Smith DW. Recognition of the fetal alcohol syndrome in early infancy. *Lancet.* 1973;2:999–1001.

2. Lemoine P, Harousseau H, Borteyru JP, Menuet JC. Children of alcoholic parents: abnormalities observed in 127 cases. Available from: *National Clearinghouse for Alcohol Information,* Rockville, Md; 1968.

3. Ulleland CN. The offspring of alcoholic mothers. *Ann NY Acad Sci.* 1972;197:167–169.

4. Russell M. Clinical implications of recent research on the fetal alcohol syndrome. *Bull NY Acad Med.* 1991;67(3):207–222.

5. Sokol RJ, Clarren SK. Guidelines for use of terminology describing the impact of prenatal alcohol on the offspring. *Alcoholism.* 1989;13(4):597–598.

6. Streissguth AP. Fetal alcohol syndrome and fetal alcohol effects: a clinical perspective of later developmental consequences. In: Zagon IS, Slotkin TA, eds. *Maternal Substance Abuse and the Developing Nervous System*. San Diego, Calif: Academic Press; 1992.

7. Clarren SK, Astley SJ, Bowden DM, et al. Neuroanatomic and neurochemical abnormalities in nonhuman primates exposed to weekly doses of alcohol during gestation. *Alcoholism.* 1990;14(5):674–683.

8. Day NL, Richardson GA. Prenatal alcohol exposure: a continuum of effects. *Semin Perinatol.* 1991;15(4):271–279.

9. Miller MW. *Development of the Central Nervous System: Effects of Alcohol and Opiates*. New York, NY: Wiley-Liss; 1992.

10. Randall CL. Alcohol as a teratogen: A decade of research in review. *Alcohol Alcohol.* 1987;(suppl 1):125–132.

11. Streissguth AP. Fetal alcohol syndrome and the teratogenicity of alcohol. In: Stefanis CN, Rabavilas AD, Soldatos CR, eds. *Psychiatry: A World Perspective*. Amsterdam: Excerpta; 1990:1.

12. West JR. *Alcohol and Brain Development*. New York, NY: Oxford University Press; 1986.

13. Dorris M. *The Broken Cord: A Family's Ongoing Struggle With Fetal Alcohol Syndrome*. New York, NY: Harper Collins; 1989.

14. Committee on Substance Abuse and Committee on Children With Disabilities. Fetal alcohol syndrome and fetal alcohol effects. *Pediatrics.* 1993;91(5):1004–1006.

15. Abel EL, Sokol RJ. Incidence of fetal alcohol syndrome and economic impact of FAS-related anomalies. *Drug Alcohol Depend.* 1987;19:51–70.

16. Streissguth AP, Aase JM, Clarren SK. Randels SP, LaDue RA, Smith DF. Fetal alcohol syndrome in adolescents and adults. *JAMA.* 1991;265(15):1961–1967.

17. Carmichael Olson H, Sampson PD, Barr H, Streissguth AP, Bookstein FL. Prenatal exposure to alcohol and school problems in late childhood: a longitudinal prospective study. *Dev Psychopathol.* 1992;4:341–359.

18. Coles CD, Brown RT, Smith IE, Platzman KA, Erickson S, Falek A. Effects of prenatal alcohol exposure at school age, I. Physical and cognitive development. *Neurotoxicol Teratol.* 1991;13(4):357–367.

19. Fried PA, Watkinson B. 36- and 48-month neurobehavioral follow-up of children prenatally exposed to marijuana, cigarettes and alcohol. *J Dev Behav Pediatr.* 1990;11(2):49–58.

20. Greene TH, Ernhart CB, Ager J, Sokol RJ, Martier S, Boyd TA. Prenatal exposure to alcohol and cognitive development. *Neurotoxicol Teratol.* 1990;13(1):57–68.

21. Russell M, Czarnecki DM, Cowan R, McPherson E, Mudar PJ. Measures of maternal alcohol use as predictors of development in early childhood. *Alcoholism.* 1991;15(6):991–1000.

22. National Institute for Alcoholism and Alcohol Abuse. *Seventh Special Report to the US Congress; Alcohol and Health*. Washington, DC: US Department of Health and Human Services; 1990.

23. Carmichael Olson H, Burgess DM, Streissguth AP. Fetal alcohol syndrome (FAS) and fetal alcohol effects (FAE): a lifespan view, with implications for early intervention. *Zero To Three.* 1992;13(1):24–29.

24. Giunta CT, Streissguth AP. Patients with fetal alcohol syndrome and their caretakers. *Soc Casework: J Contemp Soc Work.* 1988;September:453–459.

25. Burgess D, Lasswell SL, Streissguth AP. *Educating children prenatally exposed to alcohol and other drugs*. A booklet published for the Planning for Learning Project, Olympia, Wash; 1992.

26. Carmichael Olson H. Fetal alcohol syndrome. *Encyclopedia of Intelligence.* 1994. In press.

27. Streissguth AP, LaDue RA. Teratogenic causes of developmental disabilities. In: Schroeder SR, ed. *Toxic Substances and Mental Retardation.* AAMD Monographs 8; 1987:1–32.

28. Nanson JL. Autism in fetal alcohol syndrome: a report of six cases. *Alcoholism.* 1992;16(3):558–565.

29. Clarren SK, Smith DW. The fetal alcohol syndrome. *N Engl J Med.* 1978;298:1063–1067.

30. Jones KL. Fetal alcohol syndrome. *Pediatr Rev.* 1986;8:122–126.

31. Streissguth AP. The behavioral teratology of alcohol: performance, behavioral, and intellectual deficits in prenatally exposed children. In: West JR, ed. *Alcohol and Brain Development.* New York, NY: Oxford University Press; 1986.

32. Streissguth AP, Giunta CT. Mental health and health needs of infants and preschool children with Fetal Alcohol Syndrome. *Int J Fam Psychiatry.* 1988;9(1):29–47.

33. Randels SP, Streissguth AP. Fetal alcohol syndrome and nutrition issues. *Nutrition Focus.* 1992;7(3):1–6.

34. Aronson M, Olegard R. Fetal alcohol effects in pediatric and child psychology. In: Ryberg U, Alling C, Engel J, Pernow LA, Rossner S, eds. *Alcohol and the Developing Brain.* New York, NY: Raven; 1985.

35. Autti-Ramo I, Granstrom ML. The psychomotor development during the first year of life of infants exposed to intrauterine alcohol of various duration. Fetal alcohol exposure and development. *Neuropediatrics.* 1991;22(2):59–64.

36. Autti-Ramo I, Korkman M, Hilakivi-Clarke L, Lehtonen M, Halmesmaki E, Granstrom ML. Mental development of 2-year-old children exposed to alcohol in utero. *J Pediatr.* 1992;120(5):740–746.

37. Janzen L, Nanson J. *Neuropsychological evaluation of preschoolers with fetal alcohol syndrome.* Paper presented at the Society for Research in Child Development; March 25–28, 1993; New Orleans, La.

38. Spohr HL, Steinhausen HC. Clinical, psychopathological and developmental aspects in children with fetal alcohol syndrome: a four-year follow-up study. In CIBA Foundation Symposium 105: *Mechanisms of Alcohol Damage In Utero.* London, England: Pitman; 1984.

39. Becker M, Warr-Leeper GA, Leeper HA. Fetal alcohol syndrome: a description of oral motor, articulatory, short-term memory, grammatical, and semantic abilities. *J Commun Dis.* 1990;23(2):97–124.

40. Carney LJ, Chermak GD. Performance of American Indian children with fetal alcohol syndrome on the test of language development. *J Commun Dis.* 1991;24(2):123–134.

41. Burgess D, Streissguth AP. Fetal alcohol syndrome and fetal alcohol effects: principles for educators. *Phi Delta Kappan.* 1992;September:24–29.

42. LaDue RA, Streissguth AP, Randels SP. Clinical considerations pertaining to adolescents and adults with fetal alcohol syndrome. In: Sonderegger TB, ed. *Perinatal Substance Abuse: Research Findings and Clinical Implications.* Baltimore, Md: Johns Hopkins University Press; 1992.

43. American Psychiatric Association. *Diagnostic and Statistical Manual of Mental Disorders.* 3rd ed. rev. Washington DC: American Psychiatric Association; 1987.

44. Mirsky AF, Anthony BJ, Duncan CC, Ahearn MB, Kellam SG. Analysis of the elements of attention: a neuropsychological approach. *Neuropsychol Rev.* 1991;2(2):109–145.

45. Los Angeles Unified School District, Division of Special Education, Prenatally Exposed to Drugs (PED) Program. *Today's challenge: Teaching strategies for working with young children at risk*

due to prenatal substance exposure. Los Angeles, Calif: Los Angeles Unified School District; 1990.

46. Morse BA, Weiner L. *FAS: Parent and Child.* Brookline, Mass: Massachusetts Health Research Institute; 1992.

47. Smith IE, Coles CD. Multilevel intervention for prevention of fetal alcohol syndrome and effects of prenatal alcohol exposure. *Recent Dev Alcohol.* 1991;9:165–180.

48. Sparks SN. *Children of Prenatal Substance Abuse.* San Diego, Calif: Singular Publishing Group, Inc; 1993.

49. Villarreal SF, McKinney L, Quackenbush M. *Handle with Care: Helping Children Prenatally Exposed to Drugs and Alcohol.* Santa Cruz, Calif: ETR Associates; 1992.

50. Randels S. *The needs of families with FAS/FAE children.* Snohomish County Health District Conference on Fetal Alcohol Syndrome and Fetal Alcohol Effects. Snohomish, Wash, May 1992.

51. US Department of Health and Human Services. *Healthy People 2000: National Health Promotion and Disease Prevention Objectives.* DHHS Publication No. (PHS) 91-50213; 1990.

Integrated services for children who are medically fragile and technology dependent

Lisa Richter Beck, MSN, RN
Director of Home Care and Discharge
  Planning
Children's Hospital, San Diego
San Diego, California

Mary Hammond-Cordero, MA
Project Director
Outreach and Early Intervention
  Project
San Diego and Imperial Counties
  Developmental Services, Inc.
Chula Vista, California

Jennifer Poole, RN, BSN
Director of Professional Services
Special Care Corporation
San Diego, California

COMMUNITY agencies in any large urban or urban/suburban setting must plan to meet a diversity of technologic needs for infants and young children. The last four decades have seen a tremendous growth in technology that has forever changed outcomes and long-term care needs for the pediatric population. Specialized equipment and procedures, such as ventilators designed for infants, and extracorporeal membrane oxygenation (ECMO) have increased the overall survival rate of neonates. On the other hand, advanced technology has created a new population of children now termed medically fragile or technology dependent. These children are characterized by the use of a particular medical device that compensates for the loss of the use of a body function and who require substantial and complex daily care to avert death or further disability.[1]

For many of these children, pediatric units have become their long-term home. As the length of stay at the hospital has increased, family visits often consistently decrease as the demands of siblings, employment, and a variety of day-to-day tasks take their toll. As a result, creative approaches to care must be developed to meet the needs of patients and families in the community.

Over the last 10 years a variety of programs that provide support to the families of children who are medically fragile/technology dependent have been developed in San Diego. Parents and professionals collaborate closely through participation on committees and advisory boards. Although administered individually, there is a great effort to coordinate services at the child/family level.[2]

This article focuses on three key programs that designate at least one specific employee to coordinate referrals to other appropriate programs, to keep the agency informed regarding updates and changes in community programs, and to participate in individual case conferences, on committees, and on advisory boards. The first program is the Public Health In-Home Monitoring Program. It is one of 21 high-risk infant follow-up programs in the State of California. These programs are funded by the Department of Health Services, Maternal and Child Health Divi-

Inf Young Children 1994;6(3):75–83
© 1994 Aspen Publishers, Inc.

sion, under Title V. The second program is provided by Children's Hospital, San Diego. It is a decentralized-collaborative model of discharge planning for children who are medically fragile or technology dependent. The third program that will be described is a reverse-mainstreamed pediatric-day health care facility. This facility is operated by Special Care Corporation, a home health agency, and provides nursing care, therapy services, and an educational curriculum in a typical preschool environment. Through coordination and collaboration, these three agencies exemplify the efforts being made in many communities to foster integrated family-focused services for infants and young children as promoted/mandated by federal legislation.

In recognition of the importance and the value of collaborative early intervention services, Congress passed amendments to the Individuals with Disabilities Education Act in 1986. This is known as Public Law 99-457. Part H of Public Law 99-457 provides funds for states to plan for implementation of a statewide, comprehensive, multidisciplinary, interagency program of early intervention services.[3] In applying for these funds, California formalized the collaborative efforts already in existence.

PUBLIC HEALTH IN-HOME MONITORING

The Public Health In-Home Monitoring Program is known in the San Diego area as the Outreach and Early Intervention Program (OEIP). OEIP is designed to identify and provide services for infants at risk of developing handicapping conditions. The program ensures that all infants at risk receive basic public health services and appropriate community referrals.

Identification of infants who are at risk occurs through attendance by an OEIP representative at discharge conferences and weekly medical rounds at 10 neonatal intensive and intermediate care units in San Diego County. Structured identification criteria is used by the OEIP staff (Table 1). Appropriate candidates for OEIP Monitoring Services include infants who require basic care or supportive medical intervention, such as tube feedings, apnea monitoring, and positioning to prevent gastroesophageal reflux and aspiration.[4,5]

Once an infant is identified as a candidate for OEIP, a public health nurse (PHN) under contract with the San Diego County Department of Public Health, begins home visits to the infant and caregivers. Although the program has established a protocol for home visits, the actual intensity of visits and duration of follow-up is determined by the family needs and preferences (Table 2).

Home visits include a basic health assessment of the infant as well as instruction in the areas of growth, development, nutrition, well-baby care, and medications or treatments. The PHN will also assess for bonding and interaction between infant and caregiver. Special attention is given to the caregiver's impression of the

Table 1. Criteria for entry and severity levels for OEIP/high risk infants

Criteria/Problem	Severity Level 1	Level 2	Level 3
Birth weight	<1000 grams	1001–1500	1501–1750
SGA/IOGR		severe, below 2 percentile	moderate, 5 percentile
Mechanical ventilation (for PFC/PPH, RDS, BPD, CLD)			
• regular ventilatory support	>14 days	40 hrs–13 days	
• ECMO treatment	all		
• high frequency ventilation	all		
Length of hospitalization	>45 days	31–45 days	24–30 days
Infections	congenital	acquired with CNS component	
Hypoglycemia			Symptomatic or prolonged
Hyperbilirubinemia		over 26	21–25 mg%
Neurologic difficulties			
• Neonatal seizures	all		
• Hydrocephaly (congenital or acquired)	all		
• CNS hemorrhage	grades III–IV	grades I–II	
• Periventricular leukomalacia (PVL) documented on ultrasound	all		
Asphyxia, hyporemia	severe	moderate	
Congenital defects/anomalies (severe or multiple minor)	with CNS involvement	without CNS involvement	
Neonatal drug exposure	+ tox infant in NICU	+ tox mother – tox infant in NICU	
Other high risk factors	level to be determined		

infant's progress. OEIP maintains written communication of each home visit with pediatric care providers.

OEIP collaborates closely with several other community agencies to maximize the services available to support the infant and family while avoiding duplication of services, which may overwhelm the family and deplete funding sources unnecessarily. Other community agencies include home health agencies that provide intermittent or continuous care nursing services to children with complex medical needs. Collaboration is achieved through communication between the home health nurse and the PHN, which results in an overall plan of concurrent home visits or initial visits by the home health nurse with transition to the PHN as the infant's medical status improves.[6]

Table 2. Outreach and early intervention project high risk infant follow-up service level for families—PHN follow-up process

Protocol	PRE D/C visit	10 day post d/c	3 mos. post d/c	6 mos. post d/c	9 mos. post d/c	12 mos. post d/c	15 mos. post d/c	18 mos. post d/c	21 mos. post d/c	24 mos. post d/c
Level 1	PRN	H.V.	H.V. & dev. cklst	H.V.	H.V. & dev. cklst	H.V.	T.C.	H.V. & dev. cklst	T.C.	H.V. & dev. cklst (refer &/or close)
Level 2	PRN	H.V.	H.V. & dev. cklst	H.V.	T.C.	H.V. & dev. cklst	T.C. (refer &/or close)			
Level 3	PRN	H.V. within 1 month post d/c	H.V. & dev. cklst			H.V. & dev. cklst (refer &/or close)				

NICU Follow-up for Developmental (spanning 6–9 mos.)

NICU Follow-up for Developmental (spanning 12–15 mos.)

Note: Additional, intermediate or more extensive visits may be made at the PHN's discretion. The family folder may be closed per the PHN's judgment at times other than those indicated.

Abbreviations: D/C = discharge from hospital; H.V. = home visit; PRN = as necessary; T.C. = telephone call; Dev. cklst = developmental checklist (a modified version of the Denver Developmental Screening Test)

Collaboration also occurs with neurodevelopmental follow-up programs in which services for monitoring and intervention are carefully coordinated between the clinic and PHN to maximize the developmental potential. This occurs through the ability of the PHN to reinforce the interventions of the neurodevelopmental program at each home visit.

Infants with developmental disabilities are referred by the PHN to the local Regional Center for Developmental Disabilities. The Regional Center Program is funded by the State Department of Developmental Disabilities and provides case management and direct services to individuals who have or who are at risk for developmental disabilities. A social worker is assigned to assist the family in obtaining medical evaluations and purchased services, such as therapy and respite care, which may not be available through other funding sources. The PHN will maintain contact with the family until a social worker is assigned. This program has been instrumental in ensuring early intervention for neonates at high risk of long-term developmental disabilities.

DISCHARGE FROM HOSPITAL TO HOME

Pediatric tertiary care facilities with a neonatal intensive care unit (NICU) or an acute pediatric program must be fully equipped with staff to meet the needs of children who are medically fragile. A knowledgeable multidisciplinary team, which includes the physician, is required to prepare and to educate patients and families as they transition from hospital to home. Facility linkages to community service organizations and agencies greatly enhance the patient and family integration into the community once discharge occurs.

The multidisciplinary team (Fig 1) involved in the discharge plan consists of the following members:

- Family
- Physician
- Hospital staff
- Home health agency
- School nurse/infant educator
- Home medical equipment vendor
- Insurance case manager
- Community agencies/public health services

It is imperative that the family members be the central focus of the team operations. Without clear input and direction from the family, a successful discharge plan cannot be developed and implemented. Early identification of needs and referrals to appropriate community agencies will also ensure timely services once discharge has occurred.[7,8]

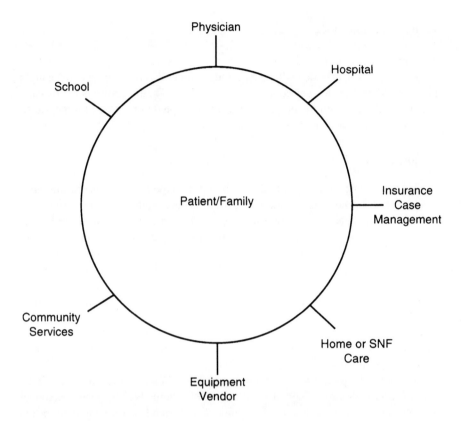

Fig 1. The multidisciplinary team involved in the discharge plan.

Discharge planning meetings should occur on a regular basis to delineate and refine the discharge plan. The role and goals of each team member, including the family members, should be clearly defined. Staff members need to be familiar with state and locally funded programs as well as community agencies that provide services to the medically fragile population.[9,10]

TRANSITIONAL DISCHARGE PLANNING MODELS

Decentralized-collaborative model

In this model the child remains on the unit, where care has been provided up to the point of preparation for discharge. The multidisciplinary team continues to work with the child and family in this familiar environment.

Parent care unit model

Some pediatric tertiary hospitals have a unit devoted to preparing parents to learn all aspects of care that will be required at home. Parents often spend the night in the child's room to feel comfortable with the 24-hour requirements of care. Multidisciplinary team members provide uninterrupted preparation for the transition from hospital to home.

Facility model

This is a free-standing facility that is, by mission, dedicated to preparing families for care at home. Once a child is identified as being stable in the tertiary setting and the family is ready to begin discharge teaching, the child is transferred to the facility. This type of facility, where parents can stay, generally has a more "home-like" atmosphere with traditional furnishings. In this model the multidisciplinary team members provide uninterrupted preparation for the transition from hospital to home.

Children's Hospital, San Diego, a 212-bed tertiary hospital, uses the Decentralized-Collaborative Model with excellent results. The multidisciplinary team is led by the physician discharge planner and primary nurse. Home passes are used to increase the family's comfort level in providing care at home and in operating medical equipment prior to the final discharge.

Children's Hospital, San Diego, has found it beneficial to videotape specialized care of certain children. The video can be used for home health agency personnel as well as parents, extended family members, and friends learning to care for the child with special needs at home.

Careful discharge planning allows an uninterrupted flow of health care services. Infants and young children who are medically fragile or technology dependent need every opportunity to achieve their highest level of functioning. A well-thought-out and well-implemented discharge plan that includes education and community services provides the foundation for a broad scope of care and developmental intervention in the most nurturing environment, the home.[11]

PEDIATRIC DAY HEALTH CARE

Special Care Corporation is an independent, community-based home health agency established in 1980 that provides specialized home health services in San Diego County for children who are medically fragile/technology dependent. As discharge to home has become more commonplace over the past 10 years for this population, communities have slowly responded to their presence outside the acute care setting. As the result, two distinct phenomena have occurred: (1) children with involved medical and developmental needs were often discharged without adequate support; (2) as children grow older, the support systems provided early after discharge have begun to fail, leaving the family to cope largely unassisted by the community. As these children reach the age of 3 years, local school districts are mandated to provide a special education program. Although this can often be a welcome relief for parents, there are inherent problems. Unlike children with disabilities who are basically healthy, the medically fragile/technology dependent children often require a nurse attendant to manage their medical treatment at school. This one-to-one care severely restricts the potential for optimum growth and development in this particular group of children. The dilemma becomes one of availability of a learning environment geared toward the special needs of children who are medically fragile/technology dependent with an emphasis on preparation for mainstreaming. The answer to this dilemma developed in the form of the Pediatric Day Health Care Center.

Also known as "medically fragile child care," the concept of pediatric day health care was first introduced by the Prescribed Pediatric Extended Care Model (PPEC). PPEC was originally designed as an alternative to extended hospital stays. It involves nonresidential, family-centered care prescribed by a physician.

Variation: The key to success

Several companies have since developed similar models throughout the nation. The success or failure of each of these models lies in the corporation's ability to closely analyze the needs, business climate, population, and level of readiness of each particular community. This makes each model unique and irreplicable in its focus on serving the needs of a given community in a predesignated geographic area. Some models are nonprofit, while others choose for-profit status. Most models provide nursing care to children who are medically fragile/technology dependent in a center-based environment; others take the multidisciplinary approach. Some centers provide a development program; others a traditional preschool curriculum; while still others integrate the traditional curriculum with a special education curriculum. Each has developed unique admission criteria based on a particular focus, as dictated by the community needs assessment.

The licensure dilemma

The advent of pediatric extended care centers has presented a unique challenge to licensing bodies. Currently Missouri centers can license under the Division of Family Services—Day Care Licensing regulations. Florida passed model legislation establishing a separate licensure category, as have Kentucky and Delaware. States such as California have only been able to pass interim regulations reminiscent of adult skilled-nursing facility regulations. New Jersey provides licensure under the Department of Human Services.

Authors' experience

Special Care Center, based in San Diego, California, is a reverse-mainstreamed pediatric day health care facility developed by Special Care Corporation. It was born out of the frustration of families and professionals alike over the need for out-of-home respite day care to enable parents to return to work and for a preschool that could prepare children with special needs to go to public schools. This is the Special Care Center, a place where children with heart, lung, muscle, and other conditions, as well as tracheostomies, gastrostomies, ventilators, medications, and treatments are just kids. In a typical preschool environment, both children who are medically fragile and children who are healthy learn respect for the differences that make each child special, unique, and valuable to their community. The goal is to prepare these children for the challenges they will face when mainstreamed into the public school system through a supportive environment staffed by special education teachers, early childhood educators, therapists, and pediatric nurses. The program is designed to provide these children with the tools they need to succeed in public school. Through that success, children who are medically fragile/technology dependent will go on to the ultimate success of integrating into the community as valuable, productive members. Their families, through the alternatives provided by the Center, succeed in reducing the stress created by a child with special needs and thus are able to return their household to more typical lifestyle.

The Special Care Center epitomizes the concept of collaboration. Its success, as with similar centers, is based on the ability to access community resources for both technical support and funding. The local and surrounding school districts can provide expertise in coordinating and integrating special education with early childhood education curriculum. Under special waiver programs, Department of Health Services and Medicaid can provide funding in addition to the Department of Developmental Disabilities. Private insurance and HMOs can also be a source of funding with an understanding of the potential, lifelong benefits provided by the program. A variety of grants are currently available. The Special Care Center also prepares the children who are healthy for mainstreaming into the public school system. They will leave Special Care Center with the certainty that all children are special and unique, each with their strengths and weaknesses, each deserving of care and respect, and each able to contribute to the world throughout their lifetime, be it short or long, to the best of their individual capability.

CONCLUSION

Benefits to families

Collaboration between agencies, as discussed within this article, offers service alternatives and site-of-care options to families otherwise not possible. In San

Diego, integrated services provide a continuum of care that allows families the ability to receive services initially in the supportive environment of the hospital. As the status of the child improves and the family is ready, the transition to home occurs. In-home services are then implemented. The public health nurse, home health agency, and infant education specialist all work with the family, providing specialized care and an individualized education/stimulation program. As the child and family become ready, a referral can be made for center-based care.

Benefits to community agencies and health professionals

Since medically fragile/technology dependent children return to the hospital for acute admissions and outpatient care from the home setting, it is important that collaboration between agencies continues on an ongoing basis. This collaboration provides health professionals with updated information regarding status of the child and any newly identified needs. Duplication of services can, therefore, be markedly reduced. This type of networking also allows each professional within an agency to develop a very focused high level of expertise.

Benefit to payers

Health care cost-effectiveness is an identified priority in every community. Payers are interested in managing health care utilization and promote or dictate transitioning a child from a higher level of care to a less expensive level.[12] When skilled care or private duty is no longer necessary, a transition to a public health or center-based day health care program can be made. Close monitoring by physicians in each setting through interagency collaboration, or case management, can, at times, avert hospitalization. A well-developed network of agencies prepared to transition the medically-fragile child from one level of care to the next can prove to be cost-effective.

•   •   •

As growth in technology changes patient outcomes, the manner in which community agencies structure long-term health and educational services for children also requires change. The community of San Diego began implementing the concept of collaboration through basic networking among professionals in the early 1980s. As the needs of children who are medically fragile/technology dependent grew, the community responded by creating new programs and services, such as those described herein. This small network of pediatric professionals was called to participate on each other's advisory committees to provide the unique perspective of each agency, as well as individual discipline. Over time the small group expanded to include physicians; nurses; physical, occupational, and speech therapists; educators; developmental specialists; social workers; discharge planners; and, most recently, equipment vendors. Today representation has been obtained from all community agencies, clinics, and hospitals, as well as third party payers, home health agencies, and equipment vendors. Each entity commits a representative to serve on an advisory committee or a community group, such as the Pediatric Continuity of Care Coalition, the Regional Network Team, and the Cooperative Council for Services for Young and Handicapped Children. Although each group has a specific focus, each has the same primary goal: more comprehensive, more accessible, more coordinated services for children.

These working committees and agency/facility models are examples of one community's successful attempt to meet the changing needs of the pediatric population. Such an approach to integrated care can be applied or replicated in other communities, settings, or regions of the country.

REFERENCES

1. Office of Technology Assistance. *Technology-Dependent Children.* Washington, DC: US Government Printing Office; 1987.

2. Commission for Cooperative Services for Young Handicapped Children and Their Families in San Diego County. *Getting Started: A Guidebook for Interagency Collaboration.* San Diego, Calif: 1988.

3. Department of Developmental Services. *California's Early Intervention Program. Public Law 99-457, Title 1, Part H.* State of California, Amendments of 1986.

4. Taeusch HW, Yogman MW. *Follow-Up Management of the High-Risk Infant.* Boston, Mass: Little, Brown; 1987.

5. Blackman J. *Warning Signals: Basic Criteria for Tracking At-Risk Infants and Toddlers.* Washington, DC: National Center for Clinical Infant Programs; 1986.

6. Davis BD, Steele S. Case management for young children with special health care needs. *Pediatr Nurs.* 1991;17(1):15–19.

7. Monahan C, Manago R. Technology in pediatric home care: issues in monitoring for quality. *J Home Health Care Pract.* 1992;5(1):1–11.

8. Hamilton B, Vessey J. Pediatric discharge planning. *Pediatr Nurs.* 1992;18(5):475–478.

9. Quality life deserves quality care: pediatric homecare the other side of the story. *Caring.* 1986;5(11):27–29.

10. Ahman ED, ed. *Home Care of the High-Risk Infant: A Holistic Guide to Using Technology.* Rockville, Md: Aspen; 1986.

11. Corkey E. Discharge planning and home health care: what every staff nurse should know. *Orthopaedic Nurs.* 1986;8(6):27–29.

12. Ferren EA. Effects of early discharge planning on length of hospital stay. *Nursing Econ.* 1991;9(1):25–30.

Diagnosis and developmental issues for young children with fragile X syndrome

Lisa S. Freund, PhD
The Kennedy Kreiger Institute
Department of Behavioral Genetics
  and Neuroimaging and Department
  of Psychiatry
Division of Child and Adolescent
  Psychiatry
Johns Hopkins School of Medicine
Baltimore, Maryland

FRAGILE X syndrome is a hereditary condition that can cause mental retardation or learning problems in both males and females. It is the most common inherited form of mental retardation, with a prevalence rate estimated at 0.5 to 1.0 per 1,000 live male births and 0.2 to 0.6 per 1,000 females.[1] The spectrum of developmental disabilities associated with fragile X ranges from subtle learning disabilities and normal intelligence quotient (IQ) to severe mental retardation and autism. In addition to cognitive impairment, fragile X syndrome includes physical and behavioral characteristics and speech and language delay. Identifying this condition in the infant or young child can be difficult. Some of the common characteristics can be quite subtle, especially in the very young. Typically it is not until the child grows older and may be delayed in walking or talking that parents and clinicians become concerned. This genetic syndrome can be passed on in a family whose members show no signs of the condition, yet other families may show numerous individuals affected through the generations.

It is only in the last 15 years that studies of the characteristics of the fragile X syndrome began to be published. Much of what is known about fragile X syndrome comes from studies of older children and adults, primarily males, since they are typically much more affected than females. Literature regarding the very young child with fragile X is just beginning to emerge. The goal of this article is to review some initial findings regarding the key physical, behavioral, medical, and family history features that occur with some frequency among young children with fragile X and that can be useful for deciding when one should suspect the disorder. Specific developmental issues relevant to the child with fragile X will also be discussed. Background information regarding the major characteristics of the syndrome in older children and adults as well as the main features of the genetics of the syndrome will be presented first.

FRAGILE X SYNDROME: MAJOR CHARACTERISTICS

Males

Affected males are usually diagnosed in early childhood with mental retardation, typically in the mild to moderate range. Some physical features thought to be asso-

Supported in part by Grant MH19677 from the National Institute of Mental Health.

Inf Young Children 1994;6(3):34–45

ciated with fragile X in the older child or adolescent include elongated face and jaw, prominent and large ears, high arched palate with malocclusion, hyperextensibility of the joints, flat feet, and macroorchidism (abnormally large testicles).[2] The occurrence of these physical features is variable, and diagnosis can never be made on the basis of physical characteristics alone. Studies of males with fragile X suggest there is enough consistency in the quality of dysfunction associated with the syndrome to characterize a fragile X behavioral phenotype. This behavioral phenotype consists of social deficits with peers, qualitative abnormalities in communication, unusual responses to sensory stimuli, stereotypic behaviors, and hyperactivity.[3-6] The behavioral characteristics of the male with fragile X are often consistent with the diagnosis of autism. Studies of fragile X males in the autistic population range from 6.5% to 15.7%, and studies of fragile X males show that from 16% to 55% meet criteria for autism or its less severe form, pervasive developmental disorder.[7] In terms of cognitive features, there is evidence of a plateau in intellectual abilities resulting in a decline in IQ beginning in prepuberty.[8-10] Males with fragile X show greatest cognitive deficits in visual short-term memory and visual-motor coordination and have difficulty with impulsiveness and with maintaining attention.[11-14]

Females

Approximately two thirds of females with fragile X have IQs in the normal ranges. Those females with mental retardation are usually less affected than males, functioning in the mild mental retardation or borderline IQ ranges. Although the majority of fragile X females have normal IQs, initial reports have indicated that they too are vulnerable to a range of developmental and psychiatric disabilities. For example, fragile X females with normal IQs are reportedly at risk for learning disabilities, including significant problems in math and auditory linguistic processing deficits,[15] short-term memory deficits,[12] and frontal lobe deficits.[16] Behavioral descriptions of female adults and children with the fragile X mutation have suggested that depressed, hyperactive, and socially withdrawn behaviors severe enough to interfere with normal functioning are common for this group.[17-19]

Genetics

To discuss how the fragile X syndrome is diagnosed and how it can be passed on in families, it is helpful to begin with a basic genetics review. Fragile X is an X-linked disorder because its gene is located on the X chromosome. The X chromosome is a member of one of 23 pairs of chromosomes in humans that carry a combination of genetic instructions from both parents. The pair to which the X chromosome belongs is called the sex chromosomes because these two chromosomes determine whether an individual is male or female. In females, both sex chromosomes are similar and are called X chromosomes. Males have one X and one Y chromosome. Females can only pass on an X chromosome to their progeny, while males can pass on a Y (resulting in a son) or an X (resulting in a daughter).

The fragile X syndrome received its name from the identification of a fragile site on the far end of one of the long arms of the X chromosome of mentally retarded individuals with the condition. A fragile site is a variation in chromosome structure that is observable by microscope and is characterized by a nonstaining gap or constriction when cells are subjected to specific culture conditions. This gap makes the X chromosome look as if a piece of it is "fragile" and might break off (Fig 1).

A female who has the fragile X chromosome abnormality is referred to as a carrier female. Carrier females usually do not experience the more severe effects

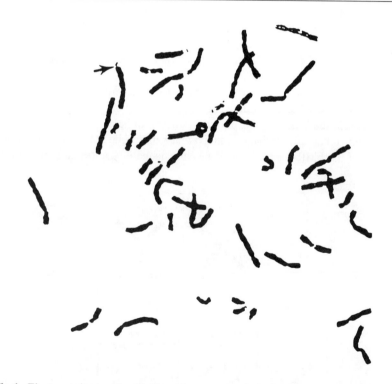

Fig 1. Electron micrograph of human chromosomes from lymphocytes. Arrow points to fragile X site on X chromosome. Reprinted with permission from Elsevier Science Publishing Co. Reiss AL and Freund L. Fragile X syndrome. *Biol Psychiatry.* 1990;27:223–240. Copyright © 1990 by The Society of Biological Psychiatry.

of the syndrome because they have a second X chromosome that can compensate for the affected chromosome with the fragile X gene. However, as noted above, approximately 30% of females with fragile X do have mental retardation, and some normal IQ females appear to suffer more subtle learning and behavior effects. When a female carries the fragile X abnormality on one of her X chromosomes, there is a 50/50 chance that she will pass it on to either a daughter or son (Fig 2). A male with the fragile X gene will pass it on to all of his daughters but to none of his sons (Fig 3). Most males with the fragile X abnormality are affected to the degree that they do not have children. However, approximately 20% of males with fragile X are completely unaffected. This latter group of males is called nonpenetrant, or transmitting, males.

The genetic transmission of the fragile X syndrome appears to be similar to recessive X-linked disorders such as hemophilia. In hemophilia, for example, females who carry the gene are rarely affected by this blood-clotting deficiency disease. Males who receive the gene from their mother via the X chromosome will manifest the disease. In the case of fragile X, however, the variability in the degree to which females are affected and the existence of males who are not affected but pass on the fragile X gene to their daughters indicates a much more complex picture of heredity.

Fortunately, how fragile X is inherited has become clearer since the identification of the gene responsible for the syndrome.[20,21] The gene is called FMR-1. All humans possess the FMR-1 gene, and it is believed to be crucial in normal brain development. What differentiates an individual with fragile X from those without is the size of the FMR-1 gene. This gene can change in size (mutate) when it is

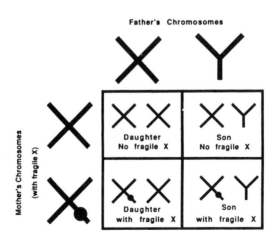

Fig 2. Inheritance of X chromosome with fragile site from mother.

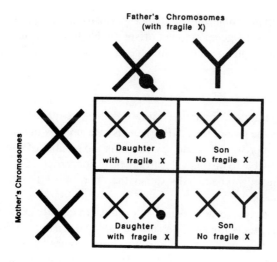

Fig 3. Inheritance of X chromosome with fragile site from father.

passed from generation to generation. If the gene changes enough, the individual receiving the gene will be intellectually impaired. The actual change in the gene involves the amplification of the sequence of chemical base pairs that make up the gene. This sequence is called a CGG repeat, referring to the sequence, cytosine (C), guanine (G), guanine (G). The size of the CGG repeat varies from individual to individual. The normal functioning human being without fragile X has an FMR-1 gene of about 6 to 50 CGG repeats. Among individuals with fragile X, two categories of amplification have been identified:

1. Amplification of the FMR-1 gene of approximately 50 to 600 repeats. Individuals with this mutation of the gene have normal IQs and are generally unaffected. This category is referred to as a premutation.

2. Amplification of the FMR-1 gene that exceeds 600 repeats. This is called a full mutation. When the gene mutates to this point, the FMR-1 gene basically turns off, resulting in mental impairment in the individual carrying this gene.

Permutations are unstable and may increase in size when passed from a female to her children. Specifically, the children of a female with the premutation can end up with a full mutation. This is one reason why individuals in a family carrying the fragile X gene can be more affected through the generations (Fig 4). Premutation status also accounts for the existence of the nonpenetrant male who is not affected but who can pass on the premutation FMR-1 gene to his daughters. When the gene is passed from a male to a daughter, it does not appear to increase in size, that is, a girl receiving the premutation from her father will also carry the premutation. It is only when she passes the gene on to her offspring that the gene changes into the full mutation. An example of such a family pedigree is shown in Figure 5.

Diagnosis

Diagnosis of the fragile X syndrome is now possible through direct DNA analysis. In this analysis the size of the FMR-1 gene is measured by the actual number of CGG repeats comprising the gene. By checking the number of CGG repeats a person has, it is possible to distinguish carriers from noncarriers. The direct DNA test can be conducted prenatally by either the chorionic villus technique or through amniocentesis.

Although DNA analysis is now available, the most frequently used test to identify fragile X in a mentally impaired person is a karyotype analysis of the person's blood. Karyotype analysis involves observing chromosomes by microscope and looking for evidence of fragile sites. Affected males with fragile X usually show the fragile site in between 5% to 50% of their cells. It is considered very accurate when testing for fragile X in individuals with mental retardation but will miss carriers who are intellectually normal and who must be tested through DNA analysis.

WHEN TO SUSPECT THE FRAGILE X SYNDROME

It would not be prudent to recommend cytogenetic or DNA studies for fragile X for all children with developmental delay, behavior disorders, or learning disabilities. Instead, the clinician and other professionals working with young children should focus on certain key physical, behavioral, and family history features that have been identified as common among children with fragile X.

Physical examination

Many of the physical features most often associated with the fragile X condition do not appear until the child with fragile X grows older. For example, enlarged testicles, or macroorchidism, is not easily detectable until puberty, and the characteristic elongated, prominent jaw is not usually noted until after puberty.[2] Simko et al[22] report that the most frequent physical finding for young boys and girls with fragile X in their sample was long, wide, or protruding ears (75% of their sample showed this feature). Three other features were reported with elevated frequency: long face (70%), flattened nasal bridge (50%), and high arched palate (50%). Figures 6 and 7 show a young male at 24 and 53 months and a young female at 6 and 36 months. An increased head circumference has been reported with incidence as

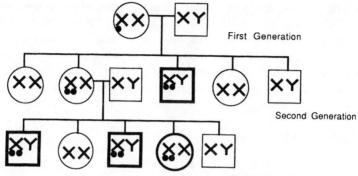

Fig 4. Pedigree of three generations of a family with first-generation mother carrying the fragile X permutation.

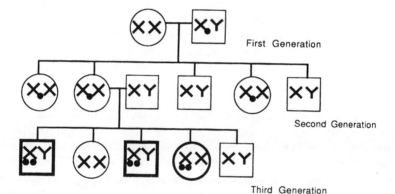

Fig 5. Pedigree of three generations of a family with first-generation nonpenetrant father carrying the fragile X permutation.

high as 40% of young fragile X children displaying head circumferences greater than the 90th percentile.[22–24] Other features that occur with somewhat less frequency are epicanthal folds, hypotonia, and skull asymmetry.[24] Since all of these abnormalities occur in the general population of young children, it is not reasonable to suspect fragile X based on these physical features alone. Only in combination with the other characteristics listed below would the physical features lead to suspicion of fragile X.

Behavioral/cognitive features

Cognitive

Although the majority of older males with full mutation fragile X have moderate to severe mental retardation, the very young fragile X male typically scores in the moderate to mild mental retardation or even borderline ranges of intellectual function. Early cognitive testing of the young fragile X male may be particularly unstable, since decline in intellectual function, especially during the early puberty period, has been reported for males with fragile X.[8–10] Among those young females with fragile X and mental retardation, the severity of intellectual impairment is generally less than that of males, and there is no evidence of intellectual decline.[19]

Motor milestones

Prouty et al[25] report that among 25 fragile X male infants, the mean age for sitting alone was 10 months (range 6 to 12 months), and walking unassisted was 20.6 months (range 11 to 33 months). Only 4 of the 25 children walked before 15 months, the upper limit of the normal range of walking. Data on 27 young fragile X males seen at the author's clinic show similar results: mean age for sitting was 8.50 months (range 5 to 13 months), and walking unassisted was 18.46 months, with only 7 of the 27 walking before 15 months (Reiss & Freund, 1993, unpublished data). This delay is moderately severe with fragile X males, who require nearly twice as long as expected to sit alone and walk unassisted. Among 14 females with fragile X (7 of whom had moderate to mild mental retardation), mean age for sitting and walking milestones were within normal limits, at 6.0 and 13.7 months respectively. Eighty percent of these fragile X girls walked unassisted before 15 months.

Language

Language delay is very common in fragile X children, especially males. Simko et al[22] reported that 95% of their sample of young fragile X children, most of whom were males, presented with language delay. Fragile X boys can show delays of between 18 and 29 months for first clearly spoken words, delays of 45 to 56 months for coupling of words into phrases, and delays of up to 60 months for use

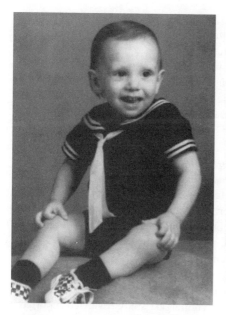
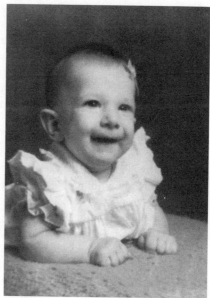

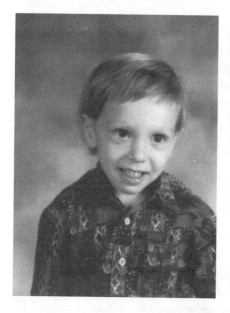
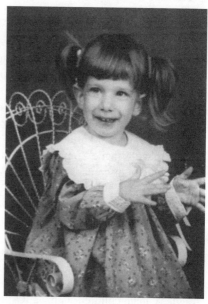

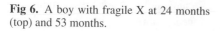

Fig 6. A boy with fragile X at 24 months (top) and 53 months.

Fig 7. A girl with fragile X at 6 months (top) and at 26 months.

of sentences[25,26] (Reiss and Freund, 1993, unpublished data). The speech of boys with fragile X can have an unusual rhythm, with bursts of staccato-like speech. Repetition of words or phrases (perseverative speech) is a frequent speech abnormality observed in the fragile X male but is generally not apparent until the child is school-aged or older. Higher functioning young girls with fragile X may show some of the same speech qualities as males with fragile X but typically show deficits at an older age in higher level aspects of communication such as pragmatics.[27]

Autistic behaviors

Autism or autistic-like behaviors have often been associated with fragile X in males. Autism has been reported in fragile X females with mental retardation, but it is not a common finding.[28,29] General features of the disorder of autism include poor ability to relate to other people normally, abnormal development of verbal and nonverbal communication and imaginative ability, and repetitive or restricted activities. Autism is usually diagnosed on the basis of criteria specified in the Diagnostic and Statistical Manual of Mental Disorders (DSM-III[30] and DSM-III-Revised[31]). In reviewing screening studies of autistic males for fragile X syndrome, Hagerman and Cronister Silverman[24] found a mean reported prevalence of 6.5% fragile X in the autistic population. The largest study reviewed reported a prevalence as high as 15.7%. Reports of the prevalence of autism among males with fragile X vary in estimates from 14% or less[23] to 47%.[32] These variable estimates have led to controversy as to whether autistic behavior is common in fragile X males. One of the few studies using a nonfragile X comparison group reported no differences in the proportion of fragile X males and females meeting overall diagnostic criteria for autism when compared to a group of fragile X-negative, developmentally disabled males.[33] Alternatively, Hagerman and Cronister Silverman[24] point out in their review that studies with larger samples are fairly consistent in reporting that between 16% and 18% of fragile X males meet criteria for autism when DSM criteria are used. Although studies investigating the relation of autism with fragile X appear to be inconsistent, some of this inconsistency may be the result of discrepancies among investigators in diagnostic protocol or subject characteristics. There may well be an overlap between autism and fragile X, but a precise estimate of the degree of overlap has not been ascertained thus far. In clinical practice, the possibility of an association between autism and fragile X is strong enough to warrant diagnostic testing for all children displaying autistic behaviors.

An important clinical issue is the consistency and specificity with which certain autistic features are seen among fragile X males. Reiss and Freund[6] compared 34 fragile X male children with 32 IQ- and age-matched, nonfragile X controls for presence of each of the DSM-III-R criteria for autism. In the area of social interactions, over 50% of the fragile X males showed abnormality in peer social play beginning between 3 and 4 years of age compared to 30% of controls. Importantly, most of the fragile X males did not show a significant impairment in reciprocal interactions with caregivers either at the time of evaluation or in the past. Thus the young fragile X male is not likely to exhibit the pervasive impairment in social relatedness usually associated with the autistic disorder. Fragile X infants and toddlers are no different from controls in terms of their development of attachment behavior to caregivers. Not until the establishment of peer relationships becomes developmentally important do the fragile X boy's social impairments become apparent.

Within the communication sphere, Reiss and Freund[6] reported that boys with fragile X met many of the communication abnormalities associated with autism to a greater degree than controls. Approximately 80% met criteria for nonverbal abnormalities because of gaze aversion while communicating, compared to 30% of controls. This behavior was first noticed by parents when their fragile X child was between 19 and 42 months. Poor eye contact has also been reported to be specific to fragile X males when compared to nonfragile X autistic males.[34] Other areas of abnormal communication in the Reiss and Freund[6] sample involved abnormal gestures and unusual rate, volume, and repetition of speech (82% usually first noticeable by 4 years of age). Repetitive motor behaviors were also observed in approximately 90% of the fragile X boys (30% controls). These behaviors typically involved hand flapping, rocking, or hand biting that started during early preschool years. Overall, this study suggests that fragile X males manifest a specific subset of behaviors from the autistic spectrum that begin during early childhood.

Hyperactivity

Hyperactivity is a prominent problem associated with fragile X, especially in the very young child with the syndrome. This behavior disorder involves extreme distractibility, inattention, impulsiveness, and difficulty focusing on goal-directed activity for any length of time. The research literature is consistent in reporting significant problems with attention, hyperactivity, and impulsiveness among boys with fragile X.[35] Estimates of the percentage of fragile X males with hyperactivity range from 65% to 93%.[22,24,36] Similar to the course of hyperactivity in nonfragile X populations, the onset of this behavior disorder in fragile X males is typical by the age of 2 years and usually decreases significantly by puberty. Attentional problems may change, depending upon the age of the fragile X male. Motoric overactivity, impulsiveness, and aggressive symptoms may be more problematic among very young fragile X boys, while distractibility and poor attention maintenance may be more problematic among older fragile X males.[37] Although hyperactivity in developmentally delayed children is common, comparisons with nonfragile X mentally retarded boys showed twice the incidence of hyperactivity in fragile X boys.[26] Attention problems with or without overactivity can occur with some frequency even in normal IQ girls with fragile X,[17-19] but not with the same severity as that of boys with fragile X.

Other behavior problems

Other behavior problems have been associated with the fragile X syndrome. Simko et al[22] report that 60% of their sample of fragile X children displayed mouthing of objects beyond the age expected, 55% had excessive temper tantrums, and 40% engaged in self-abusive behaviors such as head banging or hand biting. Since there was no comparison group, it is not clear whether these particular behaviors occur with more frequency among fragile X children than among nonfragile X developmentally delayed children.

Family history

Family history can be a primary indicator for suspicion of fragile X in a developmentally delayed child. The presence of mental retardation in the child's immediate family or among maternal relatives was reported in 65% of the young fragile X children in the Simko et al[22] study. For 90% of the boys in this study, family members had mental retardation, or learning disabilities, or hyperactivity, or a combination thereof.

Medical history

Recurrent otitis media (middle ear infections) is a common childhood ailment, but there is some evidence that it occurs more frequently than expected among young fragile X children. Hagerman et al[38] found that 63% of fragile X boys had recurrent otitis compared to 38% of developmentally disabled, nonfragile X children. Simko et al[22] report that 45% of their sample of young fragile X children had a history of frequent otitis media. An early history of colic or vomiting during infancy was also reported in 45% of these fragile X children.

Although increased birth weights of children with fragile X have been reported, results across studies are conflicting. Turner et al[39] found a mean birth weight of fragile X males at the 70th percentile, and Simko et al[22] report that 78% of their fragile X sample had birth weights greater than the 75th percentile. However, two other studies have not found increased birth weights and conclude that fetal and postnatal growth appears normal among fragile X children.[25,40]

Developmental issues

The typical child diagnosed with fragile X is developmentally delayed. No unique or specific interventions for young fragile X children have been identified through research. Most often the established methods of infant and preschool enrichment, language and speech therapy, behavioral management, occupational therapy, and sometimes even psychopharmacologic interventions are recommended. In addition, the facilitation of two important behavioral areas, temperament and social skills, can significantly affect the young fragile X child's development.

Temperament

The fragile X child, particularly the young male, can often have a temperament described as "difficult." The difficult child is one who reacts with fussing and turmoil when faced with new foods, new people, and new places and whose hunger, sleep, and elimination patterns can be unpredictable. In general the difficult child with fragile X reacts too intensely, and the child may only require a very low intensity of stimulation for a response to be evoked. In our evaluations of 18 preschool-aged fragile X children that included the Infant Characteristics Questionnaire, 90% of mothers reported that their child was moderately to extremely difficult to parent, displayed extreme reactions, and was moderately unpredictable in mood and biologic functions (Reiss and Freund, 1993, unpublished data). It is important for parents and professionals working with families to acknowledge the stress and frustrations that can occur when attempting to manage the behaviors that can be exhibited by the fragile X child. The difficult young child can lead a parent to respond inconsistently to his or her child's behaviors and thus increase the child's noncompliant behaviors. As a result, the frustration of both parents and child can reach high levels. Family interventions stressing behavior management techniques can be useful. This is particularly important if the primary caregiver of the young child (usually the mother) has fragile X and experiences cognitive or behavioral symptoms associated with the syndrome that might interfere with effective parenting.

Social development

Much of the behavior difficulties described for the young child with fragile X can interfere with adaptive social development. This is probably the single-most important issue of development for the developmentally delayed fragile X child, since these children have much greater success academically and adaptively when they are socially appropriate. Intervention is important early on for fostering appropriate social behaviors, such as getting along in small groups and making and maintaining friendships with peers, and for eliminating behaviors that lead to rejection by others. Language therapy for the young fragile X child should address not only speech and articulation problems but also appropriate verbal and nonverbal social communication skills. Social development issues are important for normal IQ girls with fragile X as well. In a study comparing fragile X females with nonfragile X female controls matched on age and IQ, 65% of fragile X girls versus 12% of controls were found to show shyness and social avoidance to the degree of interfering with social functioning with peers.[18] Parents of the fragile X girls indicated that the avoidant behaviors were noticeable very early on during preschool years. Thus shyness, social awkwardness, and socially inappropriate behaviors in young fragile X children should not be dismissed as something they will grow out of but should be addressed early in development.

•   •   •

Because identification of the characteristics of the fragile X disorder has been relatively recent, there are undoubtedly many families who have the syndrome and have not been diagnosed. As more medical, social work, psychology, and education professionals become familiar with fragile X, recommended testing of young children with autistic behaviors or mental retardation or a combination of the other key features of the disorder will become more routine. As a result, more families with the fragile X syndrome can receive genetic counseling about inheritance risks in future generations. Identification of the disorder in children at younger ages will allow for the medical, behavioral, and educational interventions that can facilitate the young fragile X child's maximum potential for development.

REFERENCES

1. Sherman S. Epidemiology. In: Hagerman RJ, Cronister Silverman A, eds. *The Fragile X Syndrome*. Baltimore, Md: Johns Hopkins University Press; 1991.

2. Chudley AE, Hagerman RJ. Fragile X syndrome. *Pediatrics.* 1987;110:821–831.

3. Freund L, Abrams M, Reiss A. Brain and behavior correlates of the fragile X syndrome. *Curr Opin Psychiatry.* 1991;4:667–673.

4. Hagerman R, Amiri K, Cronister A. Fragile X checklist. *J Med Genet.* 1991;38:283–287.

5. Reiss A, Freund L. Neuropsychiatric aspects of fragile X syndrome. *Brain Dysf.* 1990;3:9–22 .

6. Reiss A, Freund L. The behavioral phenotype of fragile X syndrome: DSM-III-R autistic behavior in male children. *Am J Med Genet.* 1992;43:35–46.

7. Simon V, Abrams M, Freund L, Reiss A. The fragile X phenotype: cognitive, behavioral and neurobiological profiles. *Curr Opin Psychiatry.* 1990;3:581–586.

8. Hodapp R, Dykens E, Ort S, Zelinsky D, Leckman J. Changing patterns of intellectual strengths and weaknesses in males with fragile X syndrome. *J Autism Dev Disord.* 1991;21:503–516.

9. Lachiewicz A, Gullian C, Spiridigliozzi G, Aylsworth A. Declining IQs of young males with the fragile X syndrome. *Am J Ment Retard.* 1987;92:272–278.

10. Dykens E, Hodapp R, Ort S, Finucane B, Shapiro L, Leckman J. The trajectory of cognitive development in males with fragile X syndrome. *J Am Acad Child Adolesc Psychiatry.* 1989;28:422–426.

11. Crowe S, Hay D. Neuropsychological dimensions of the fragile X syndrome: support for a nondominant hemisphere dysfunction hypothesis. *Neuropsychologia.* 1990;28:9–16.

12. Freund L, Reiss A. Cognitive profiles associated with fragile X syndrome in males and females. *Am J Med Genet.* 1991;38:542–547.

13. Kemper MB, Hagerman RJ, Altshui-Stark D. Cognitive profile of boys with the fragile X syndrome. *Am J Hum Genet.* 1988;30:191–200.

14. Theobald T, Hay D, Judge C. Individual variation and specific cognitive deficits in the fra(X) syndrome. *Am J Med Genet.* 1987;28:1–11.

15. Wolff P, Gardner J, Lappen J, Paccia J, Meryash D. Variable expression of the fragile X syndrome in heterozygous females of normal intelligence. *Am J Med Genet.* 1988;30:213–225.

16. Mazzocco M, Hagerman R, Cronister Silverman A, Pennington B. Specific frontal lobe deficits among women with the fragile X gene. *J Am Acad Child Adolesc Psychiatry.* 1993;31:1141–1148.

17. Lachiewicz A. Abnormal behaviors of young girls with fragile X syndrome. *Am J Med Genet.* 1992;43:72–77.

18. Freund L, Reiss A, Abrams M. Psychiatric disorders associated with fragile X in the young female. *Pediatrics.* 1993;91:321–329.

19. Hagerman R, Jackson C, Amiri K, Cronister Silverman A, O'Connor R, Sobesky W. Girls with fragile X syndrome: physical and neurocognitive status and outcome. *Pediatrics.* 1992;89:395–400.

20. Oberle I, Rousseau F, Heitz D, et al. Instability of a 550-base pair DNA segment and abnormal methylation in fragile X syndrome. *Science.* 1991;252:1179–1181.

21. Yu S, Pritchard M, Kremer E, et al. Fragile X genotype characterized by an unstable region of DNA. *Science.* 1991;252:1179–1181.

22. Simko A, Hornstein L, Soukup S, Bagamery N. Fragile X syndrome: recognition in young children. *Pediatrics.* 1989;83:547–552.

23. Fryns JP. The fragile X syndrome. *Clin Genet.* 1984;26:497–528.

24. Hagerman RJ, Cronister Silverman A. *Fragile X Syndrome: Diagnosis, Treatment, and Research.* Baltimore, Md: Johns Hopkins University Press; 1991.

25. Prouty LA, Rogers RC, Stevenson RE, et al. Fragile X syndrome: growth, development, and intellectual function. *Am J Med Genet.* 1988;30:123–142.

26. Borghgraef M, Fryns JP, Dyck K, Van den Berghe H. Fragile (X) syndrome: a study of the psychological profile in 23 prepubertal patients. *Clin Genet.* 1988;32:179–186.

27. Pennington B, Schreiner R, Sudhalter V. Towards a neuropsychology of fragile X syndrome. In: Hagerman RJ, Cronister Silverman A, eds. *The Fragile X Syndrome.* Baltimore, Md: Johns Hopkins University Press; 1991.

28. Bolton P, Rutter M, Butler L, Summers D. Females with autism and the fragile X. *J Aut Dev Disord.* 1989;19:473–476.

29. Hagerman RJ, Chudley AE, Knoll JH, Jackson AW, Kemper M, Ahmad R. Autism in fragile X females. *Am J Med Genet.* 1986;23:375–380.

30. American Psychiatric Association. *Diagnostic and Statistical Manual of Mental Disorders (DSM III).* Washington, DC: American Psychiatric Association; 1980.

31. American Psychiatric Association. *Diagnostic and Statistical Manual of Mental Disorders.* 3rd ed. Washington, DC: American Psychiatric Association; 1987.

32. Hagerman R, Jackson A, Levitas A, Rimland B, Braden M. An analysis of autism in 50 males with fragile X syndrome. *Am J Med Genet.* 1986;23:359–374.

33. Einfeld S, Molony H, Hall W. Autism not associated with the fragile X syndrome. *Am J Med Genet.* 1989;38:498–502.

34. Cohen I, Vietze P, Sudhalter V, Jenkins E, Brown W. Parent-child dyadic gaze patterns in fragile X males and in non-fragile X males with autistic disorder. *J Child Psychol Psychiatry.* 1989;30:845–856.

35. Hagerman RJ, Murphy M. Wittenberger M. A controlled trial of stimulant medication in children with the fragile X syndrome. Paper presented at First National Fragile X Conference; June 1987; Denver, Colo.

36. Bregman J, Leckman J, Ort S. Fragile X syndrome: a model of genetic predisposition to psychopathology. *J Autism Dev Disord.* 1988;18:343–354.

37. Dykens E, Hodapp R, Leckman J. Adaptive and maladaptive functioning of institutionalized and noninstitutionalized fragile X males. *J Am Acad Child Adolesc Psychiatry.* 1989;28:427–430.

38. Hgerman RJ, Altshui SD, McBogg P. Recurrent otitis media in boys with the fragile X syndrome. *Am J Dis Child.* 1987;141:184–187.

39. Turner G, Daniel A, Fronst M. X-linked mental retardation, macroorchidism and the Xq27 fragile site. *Pediatrics.* 1980;96:837–841.

40. Partington MW. The fragile X syndrome: preliminary data on growth and development in males. *Am J Med Genet.* 1984;17:175–194.

Universal precautions in early intervention and child care

Mary Rathlev, MSN
Program Manager
Project CHAMP (Children's HIV and
AIDS Model Program)
Children's National Medical Center
Washington, DC

RISKS from exposure to bloodborne pathogens, such as the human immunodeficiency virus (HIV) and hepatitis B virus (HBV), have recently become a concern to professionals serving young children with chronic health and developmental conditions. According to Occupational Safety and Health Administration (OSHA) estimates, "more than 5.6 million workers in health care and related occupations could be potentially exposed to these viruses."[1(p1)] This article will help caregivers take the first steps toward understanding these infections and protecting themselves in the workplace by exploring the epidemiology of bloodborne pathogens in children, learning the facts about transmission, calculating personal risks in any situation, and committing to universal precautions at all times.

EPIDEMIOLOGY OF BLOODBORNE PATHOGENS

According to the Centers for Disease Control (CDC), "public health officials rely on health providers, laboratories, and other public health personnel to report the occurrence of notifiable diseases to state and local health departments. Without such data, monitoring trends or evaluating the effectiveness of interventions would be difficult."[2(p1)] Acquired immune deficiency syndrome (AIDS) and HBV are two infections included in the National Notifiable Infection Surveillance System.[2]

HIV epidemic

Today the number of HIV infections in the United States is increasing dramatically among women of childbearing age, adolescents, and infants. While all infants born to women with HIV infection carry maternally transferred antibodies and thus will test positive by routine methods for up to 18 months of age, two thirds to three quarters are not infected. In addition, the physical health of infected children can remain intact for months to years.

For every child reported with AIDS, another two to three have HIV infection; projections indicate that 6,000 to 30,000 children are infected in the United States.[3]

The author acknowledges Dr Robert Parrott for his review and comments and the staff of Project CHAMP for their efforts in preparing community caregivers to respond sensitively, compassionately, and competently to HIV-affected children and their families.

Inf Young Children 1994;6(3):54–64

HBV endemic

Among children in the United States, HBV infection is most common in populations of high endemicity (eg, Alaskan Natives, Pacific Islanders, immigrants from HBV-endemic areas, particularly eastern Asia and Africa) and among residents of institutions for the developmentally disabled.[4] HBV infection produces typical illness in only 5% to 15% of young children, whereas 35% to 50% of adults develop symptoms.[5]

The American Academy of Pediatrics (AAP) now recommends universal HBV immunization of all infants to protect them when they are young and as adolescents and adults. Because over one third of HBV infections occurs when there is no apparent exposure, the following caregivers may also consider immunization: health care workers exposed to blood or blood products; staff of institutions for the developmentally disabled; and staff of nonresidential day-care programs and programs for the developmentally disabled.[4]

TRANSMISSION OF BLOODBORNE PATHOGENS

Transmission of germs depends partly on the following characteristics: infective dose; survival in the environment; unrecognized, asymptomatic infection or carrier state; immunity to the pathogen; and mode of spread.[6] Direct person-to-person contact is the major mode of spread of most organisms among children. This occurs by hand-to-mouth transmission or by inhalation of oral secretions from the cough or sneeze of another person. Indirect transmission occurs via the hands of caregivers or from fomites on environmental surfaces.[5]

The good news about bloodborne pathogens such as HIV and HBV is that they are not as easily transmitted as other common germs encountered with small children, such as shigella, rotavirus, hepatitis A, and H influenza. Moreover, HIV and HBV have heightened caregiver awareness about infection control practices.

According to OSHA, bloodborne pathogens are found in "human blood, blood products, or components."[1(p1)] The book also lists other locations:

> Other potentially infectious materials include human body fluids such as semen; vaginal secretions; cerebrospinal, synovial, pleural, pericardial, peritoneal, and amniotic fluids; saliva in dental procedures; body fluids visibly contaminated with blood; unfixed tissues or organs; HIV-containing cell or tissue cultures; and HIV or HBV-containing culture medium or other solutions.[1(p1)]

Caregivers outside of the hospital will primarily be concerned about contact with human blood.

HIV transmission

Medical science has not yet produced a cure for HIV infection or developed a vaccine. However, researchers do know that for the virus to spread from one person to the next it must be in a body fluid; it must get inside an uninfected person's body; and there must be a sufficient quantity as a result of adequate volume or repeated exposures. Although HIV can be found in many different body fluids, transmission occurs only with the following four: blood, semen, vaginal and cervical secretions, and breast milk.[7]

Among adolescents and adults, the most common mode of transmission is anal or vaginal, unprotected sexual intercourse that allows for the exchange of blood, semen, or vaginal and cervical secretions across mucous membranes or through tears in tissue lining. Few data exist on how frequently children have been infected through sexual abuse.[3]

Transmission by blood injection activities typically occurs in one of three ways: (1) sharing drug injection equipment; (2) through transfusions of blood and blood products between 1979 and 1985 in the United States; and (3) through health care accidents. Approximately three dozen health care workers have become infected through accidents in hospitals or laboratory settings, predominantly unintentional needlesticks.[7] The virus can also transmit across the placenta during pregnancy, at delivery, or, in rare cases, through breastfeeding.[7]

Of these three documented routes of transmission, only exposure to infected blood poses a potential risk to uninfected children and caregivers. Studies of household members thus far show that HIV transmission has not occurred in the homes of over 200,000 AIDS cases reported to the CDC because of casual contact. No transmission occurred in an intensive study of over 700 family members, including 100 children living in households with HIV-infected children and adults or with 89 members of households living with 25 HIV-infected children.[5,8] Researchers learned that household members regularly shared items such as toothbrushes, nail clippers, eating utensils, toilets, baths, combs, towels, toys, and beds. They regularly had close physical contact, including sleeping, bathing, hugging, and kissing.[8]

HBV transmission

Possible transmission of HBV is of increasing concern to caregivers due to the escalating number of children known to be HBV carriers, particularly international adoptees from HBV-endemic areas.[9] The major mode of HBV transmission is unprotected sexual intercourse. HBV can also spread through blood products and by percutaneous exposure to blood. Although person-to-person transmission of HBV has been documented in some situations of close personal contact, public health surveillance data and epidemiologic investigations suggest that transmission of HBV is possible but rare from child to child or child to caregiver.[10]

If HBV transmission is to occur from child to child or child to caregiver, it is most likely from direct exposure to blood or body secretions from an HBV carrier that enter the body of the uninfected person through bites or scratches that break the skin or through open wounds.[9] This is because, in addition to blood, semen, and cervical secretions, HBV is also found in wound exudate and saliva. Saliva contains only small quantities of the virus and is not thought to be an effective vehicle for transmission. Infectivity of saliva has been demonstrated only when inoculated through the skin of gibbons and chimpanzees.[6]

Risk assessment

Even with this information concerning the transmission of bloodborne pathogens, especially HIV, caregivers' fears still persist. Some have said: "The facts about transmission are not all in. There is no cure. If you get it you are dead, and no one wants to die"[7(pB2-1)]; or "They told me there is no possibility by just a bite. No one knows for sure; all they say is we have no cases to date. Bite me and I'll be the first case."[7(pB2-3)] Those who are in daily contact with children are afraid of engaging in these activities: changing diapers, cleaning up vomit, wiping noses, feeding food, attempting therapies, stimulating the oral mucosa, and performing first aid.

Factors that influence HIV transmission—body fluid, route of entry, and fluid dose—are listed across the top of Table 1. Items within each category of factors carry a different level of risk—high, moderate, low, no proven risk, and no risk—and are listed down the left-hand column of Table 1. Caregivers can determine the level of risk of HIV transmission by following several steps. First, ask three questions: (1) What body fluid am I being exposed to? (2) How is that body fluid getting inside my body? (3) Is there a sufficient quantity of the body fluid or are there repeated exposures to it? Second, circle the level of risk—high, moderate, low, no proven risk or no risk—in response to each of these questions. Third, add up the circled items, then average the level of risk. If any circled item is of no proven risk or of no risk, the others—route of entry and fluid dose—cannot contribute. The risk of transmission in that particular situation does not exist. Caregivers can follow this procedure, outlined more specifically in the box entitled "Risk Assessment Procedure," to calculate the level of risk in any situation they may encounter with children.[7]

Human bites

In children, bites are seen most often in 2- to 5-year-olds and may be inflicted at any location. The incidence of infection, frequently streptococcus or staphylococ-

Table 1. Risk assessment chart

	Transmission factors		
Level of risk	*Body fluid*	*Route of entry*	*Fluid dose*
High	Blood Semen	Injection Rectum Vagina Placenta	Large volume Repeated exposures
Moderate	Vaginal/cervical secretions	Break in skin Penis Mouth	Occasional exposures
Low	Breast milk	Newly inflicted wound Eyes Nose	Small volume One exposure
No proven risk	Saliva Tears Urine Vomit Nasal secretions		
No risk	Feces Sweat	Intact skin Clothing	No contact

Reprinted with permission from Project CHAMP, Children's Hospital/Children's National Medical Center, Washington, DC. Rathlev MC, Riley MR, Jones SJ. *Caring in the Community for Children with HIV: A Guide for Child Care Providers, Foster Families, Home Health Aides and Volunteers.* Washington, DC: Children's Hospital/Child Welfare League of America; 1992.

cus, following human bites ranges from 10% to 30%. One factor influencing the incidence of infection is delay in seeking medical attention.[11]

Rogers et al[8] reported biting in 11 households with HIV-infected children. No seroconversions occurred in the 9 uninfected contacts bitten by HIV-infected children or in the 7 uninfected children who bit HIV-infected contacts.[8] For transmission to occur, positive blood must enter the oral cavity of the biter under circumstances of manipulation or infection, such as toothbrushing or herpes stomatitis. Based on Table 1, the risk of transmission is greater (moderate risk) when the uninfected biter breaks the skin of the HIV-infected contact and gets blood into his or her traumatized or infected mouth than (no proven risk) when the HIV-infected biter breaks the skin of the uninfected contact and gets saliva into that open wound.

Existing data in humans suggest a small risk of HBV transmission from a bite of an HBV carrier that breaks the skin. The risk of transmission from a bite, however, has not been quantified. The risk of HBV acquisition when an uninfected child

Risk Assessment Procedure[7]

Transmission risk factors have been organized on the preceding chart to show:
The type of factor, across the top of the chart:
- Body fluid
- Route of entry
- Dose

The risk associated with each individual factor, down the left side of the chart:
- High—consistently leads to infection with HIV
- Moderate—can lead to transmission but less consistently than high factors
- Low—not very efficient transmission factors
- No proven risk—largely theoretic risks
- No risk—cannot contribute to transmission

Human body fluids are organized according to how much HIV they can contain:
- Blood and semen: high risk—They contain a sufficient number of the cells for HIV to live.
- Vaginal and cervical secretions: moderate risk—They contain a lesser number of cells for HIV to live.
- Breast milk: low risk—Epidemiologically it has been implicated only in a few cases.
- Saliva, tears, urine, vomit, nasal secretions: no proven risk—Small amounts of the virus have been isolated from them; however, they do not contain enough cells for HIV to live.
- Feces and sweat: no risk—They do not contain even small amounts of the virus.

Routes of entry are organized according to how efficiently they lead to the bloodstream:
- Injection (by means of syringe or transfusion): high risk—This is the most efficient route to the bloodstream, followed by mucous membranes, such as rectal and vaginal tissues, which due to their fragility permit absorption by blood vessels.
- The penis and mouth: moderate risk—The outer skin and mucous membranes offer protection, but a break in the skin or mucous membranes allows ready access to a blood vessel.
- Newly inflicted wound, eyes, and nose: low risk—All provide protection through mechanisms of bleeding, tearing, and sneezing.
- Intact skin: no risk—The body's first line of defense against germs and an effective barrier between HIV and the bloodstream

Dose is a factor more dependent on the other two:
- Large volume (of blood) or repeated exposures (frequent injections): high risk—This is equally effective in transmitting HIV.
- Occasional exposures: moderate risk—The incidence of heterosexual transmission to women is increasing dramatically.
- Small volume and one exposure: low risk—The incidence of transmission after accidental needlesticks by health care workers is 4 per 1,000.

Ask the following questions to determine transmission risk factors in any situation:
- To what body fluid is the uninfected person being exposed?
- How is the body fluid getting inside his or her body?
- How often does this happen?
- Example: If a woman is having unprotected sexual intercourse with an infected man two to three times a week, she is being exposed to semen; the semen is getting into her body through her vagina; this is happening often.
  —Since all are high risk factors, she is at high risk for becoming infected with HIV.
- Example: If a caregiver with open sores on her hands provides first aid for a child

continues

with HIV infection without gloves one time, she is being exposed to blood; the blood is getting into her body through open sores; this is one exposure.

—Since one is a high-risk factor, one is a moderate risk factor, and one is a low-risk factor, she is at moderate risk for becoming infected with HIV.

If a transmission factor falls within the "No Proven Risk" or "No Risk" category, then there is no need to proceed any further. While transmission may be theoretically possible, it has not happened based on "No Proven Risk" or "No Risk" factors.

Reprinted with permission from Project CHAMP, Children's Hospital/Children's National Medical Center, Washington, DC.

bites an HBV carrier is unknown. A theoretic risk exists if positive blood enters the traumatized or infected oral cavity of the biter, but transmission by this route has not been reported.[6,9]

BASIC INFECTION CONTROL

Transmission of germs is also affected by the ages of the children that come together, the hygienic aspects of child handling, and environmental sanitation practices.[6] Basic infection control practices rely on the following principles: (1) prevent contact with germs by avoiding persons, behaviors, and situations that are likely to spread germs; (2) create barriers, that is, put something between yourself and the source of infection that the germs cannot penetrate; (3) kill germs with friction, heat, or chemicals.[7]

The risk of illness can be reduced by following these principles and by enforcing the following common-sense practices: immunization compliance; exclusion policies from group care; appropriate diapering and food handling procedures; and personal and environmental hygienic standards.[6,9]

Prevent contact—Exclusion

Exclusion of ill children from group care is highly controversial. It necessitates that parents find alternative means of child care. For many infections, highest risk of transmission occurs prior to clinical illness; once illness ensues, many other children as well as caregivers have already been exposed to the infectious organism. Exclusion policies must strike a balance between reducing infection risks to others and affording the sick child necessary services.[5,6,9]

Illness is very common in young children, and most should not be excluded from their usual source of care for respiratory and gastrointestinal (GI) symptoms of mild severity. The following are reasons for exclusion: the illness prevents the child from participating comfortably in activities; the illness results in greater care than the staff can provide; the illness is known to be transmitted among, by, and to children.[6,9] Fever, unusual lethargy, persistent crying, difficult breathing, and other signs of severe illness are reasons for exclusion. Table 2 reflects a synopsis of the AAP recommendations for exclusion.[6]

The following conditions do not justify exclusion: asymptomatic excretion of germs in stool; pink conjunctiva with a clear, watery eye discharge and without fever; rash without fever and behavior change; cytomegalovirus infection; HBV carrier state and HIV infection.[6,9]

The AAP makes the following recommendations about children with HIV infection:

> There is no reason to restrict foster care or adoptive placement of children who have HIV infection to protect the health of other family members because the risk of transmission of HIV infection in family environments is negligible.[12(p682)]

> There is no need to restrict the placement of HIV-infected children in child care settings to protect child care personnel or other children in these settings, because the risk of transmission of HIV infection in family environments is negligible.[12(p682)]
> All children with HIV infection should receive an appropriate education that is adapted to their evolving special need.[13(p647)]

> Athletes infected with HIV should be allowed to participate in all competitive sports.[14(p640)]

The AAP also states that "the risk of disease transmission from an HBV carrier child or staff with normal behavior and without generalized dermatitis or bleeding problems is negligible. This extremely low risk does not justify exclusion of an HBV carrier child from day care or hepatitis B vaccination of day-care contacts."[4(p77)]

Create barriers—Diapering

Frequent contamination of the environment with feces is common in programs providing services for infants and toddlers who require diapering or assistance with toileting, explore the environment with their mouth, and are careless about their secretions. In studies conducted in child care centers in Houston and Phoenix, between 12% and 15% of objects and surfaces had detectable coliforms found in feces. Routine samples of hands in both children and caregivers were found to be positive between 17% and 73% of the time. Caregivers were frequently found to be positive, especially those caring for infants and toddlers. A significantly lower rate of infection was found when the children wore paper diapers.[5]

Diaper changing surfaces should be away from food handling areas, should be nonporous, and should be sanitized between uses. Alternatively, the diaper changing surface should be covered with paper and discarded after each use.[6]

Table 2. Recommendations for exclusion[6]

Condition	Signs and symptoms	Remarks
Diarrhea	Increased number of stools, increased stool water, or decreased form—not contained in diaper or by toilet use	
Vomiting	Two or more times in the previous 24 hours	Unless determined to be due to a noncommunicable condition and the child is not in danger of dehydration
Mouth sores	Associated with inability to control saliva	Unless determined the child is noninfectious
Rash	With fever or behavior change	Until determined the illness is a noncommunicable disease
Purulent conjunctivitis	Pink or red conjunctiva with white or yellow eye discharge, often with matted eyelids after sleep and eye pain or redness of the eyelids or surrounding skin	Until examined and approved for readmission
Tuberculosis		Until determined the child is noninfectious
Impetigo		Until 24 hours after treatment is initiated
Streptococcal pharyngitis		Until 24 hours after treatment is initiated or until the child has been afebrile for 24 hours
Head lice		Until the morning after the first treatment
Scabies		Until after treatment has been completed
Varicella		Until the sixth day after the onset of rash or sooner if all lesions have dried and crusted
Pertussis	Confirmed by laboratory or suspected based on symptoms or because of cough onset within 14 days of face-to-face contact with a person in the home/classroom with confirmed pertussis	Until 5 days after appropriate antibiotic therapy has been initiated
Mumps		Until 9 days after onset of parotid gland swelling
Hepatitis A virus infection		Until 1 week after onset of illness and jaundice, if present, has disappeared or until passive immunoprophylaxis has been administered to appropriate children and staff

Diapers should be able to contain urine and feces with an outer cover-barrier made of waterproof materials. The diaper changing procedure includes the following steps: wrap the used wipes within the soiled disposable diaper; seal the soiled diaper with the self-stick adhesive tabs; and discard it in a tightly covered, foot-activated, plastic-lined container that is inaccessible to children.

Kill germs—Personal hygiene

The fundamental principle of infection prevention when working with small children is to kill or to eliminate germs through hand washing. Deficiencies in hand washing have contributed to many outbreaks of diarrhea among children and caregivers.[5]

In child care centers that have implemented a hand-washing training program, rates of diarrheal illness have decreased by 50%. Even more important than training, however, is the need for effective monitoring and enforcement of good practices.[10]

Standards of hand washing described in the box entitled "Handwashing Procedure" emphasize timing (ie, before initiating contact, feeding, or giving a medication; after coughing, sneezing, changing a diaper, and using the bathroom) and technique (ie, use of warm running water, soap, friction, disposable towels, and a foot-activated, plastic-lined container).[5] In addition to personal hygiene standards, written sanitation policies and procedures should reflect care of the environment, special equipment, and toys. Following column 1 in Table 3, caregivers can review other basic practices grouped according to the three principles of infection control.

UNIVERSAL PRECAUTIONS

Since HBV- or HIV-infected children whose status is unknown may be attending child care or seeking therapeutic interventions, basic infection control practices must now extend beyond the careful handling of children's excretions and secretions to include their blood. Preventive measures such as HBV vaccination and universal precautions (ie, treating all blood and potentially infectious materials as if they contained HIV and HBV) will help reduce occupational exposure to blood. According to OSHA, an exposure incident is defined as "a specific eye, mouth, or other mucous membrane, nonintact skin, or parenteral contact with blood or other potentially infectious materials that results from the performance of an employee's duties."[1(p14)]

Specifically, universal precautions mean treating all blood as if it is infected with the bloodborne pathogens HBV and HIV based on the principles of infection control already described: avoid or prevent contact with blood; find a barrier when

Handwashing Procedure

Why   Handwashing is the single-most important procedure for child care providers in preventing the spread of infections to themselves, their families, their coworkers, and the children in their care. Teach children to do the same.

When   Wash hands:
- when visibly contaminated or soiled;
- before eating, feeding or giving a medicine;
- after using the toilet or changing a diaper;
- after drying tears, wiping noses, cleaning up vomit, or performing first aid;
- after caring for a sick child; and
- after removing gloves.

How   For routine handwashing:
- Wet hands.
- Apply liquid soap.
- Rub vigorously, lathering all surfaces for 15 seconds.
- Rinse thoroughly under running water.
- Dry completely with paper towels.
- Turn off the faucet with the same toweling and discard.

Reprinted with permission from Project CHAMP, Children's Hospital/Children's National Medical Center, Washington, DC.

blood contact is anticipated; and kill blood germs correctly.[7]

Prevent contact with blood

Caregivers can prevent contact with blood by not allowing children to share toothbrushes, nail clippers, or pierced earrings. If toothbrushes are kept at a central location, each should be stored in a separate container or cap. After a child is sick, the toothbrush should be discarded and replaced with a new one. One can discourage children from engaging in blood-brother sharing activities or, at the very least, should encourage children to mix blood together on a surface in the presence of an adult who can help clean up afterwards.

Most importantly, if a child gets a bloody nose or cut, caregivers should not touch the blood. They can also use this opportunity to teach children the following: Never touch someone else's blood; blood can have germs; get an adult to help.

Create barriers: Gloves, paper towels, and clothing

When a child is bleeding, caregivers should take a moment to locate appropriate barriers. While latex gloves are excellent, they are not always accessible or available. Sometimes the amount of blood is so small that it can easily be contained by other materials. One need not despair. Be resourceful. Tissues, paper towels, the child's own clothing, a clean diaper, or even the newspaper can serve as an effective barrier. In the event of a nose bleed, the child can be instructed to pinch off the bridge of his or her own nose.

After controlling the bleeding, caregivers can follow these steps for wound care: (1) wash hands; (2) wear latex gloves if bleeding is profuse (or use a thick gauze if it is not profuse), and wash the cut with soap and water; (3) apply a disinfectant; (4) place a bandaid over the cut (bandaids, like scabs, are practical barriers), keeping blood in and other germs out and minimizing the chance for local infection; (5) place disposable blood-soiled items in a plastic bag and tie securely, then discard in a covered, foot-activated, plastic-lined container. If plastic bags and ties are not available, wrap up the soiled items in a diaper or newspaper, both economical and practical barriers. Caregivers and children should keep all open wounds covered; they can provide a route of entry for bloodborne pathogens into the body.

Kill germs: Soap, water, and bleach

Finally, using soap and water, caregivers should wash hands contaminated with blood and after removing gloves. Soap and water kill HIV because the virus is fragile and does not live in the air or in a dried-out state. In places where there are no hand-washing facilities, CDC recommends using antiseptic hand cleaner in conjunction with paper towels or antiseptic towelettes. When antiseptic hand cleaners or towelettes are used, it is still important to wash hands with soap and water as soon as feasible.[1]

If blood contaminates a surface, toys, or communal objects, caregivers can follow these steps: wear gloves and clean up the spill with paper towels; discard the soiled materials in a covered, foot-activated, plastic-lined container; wash the area with a cleansing agent; rinse with a 1:10 bleach-to-water solution; and air dry.

While wearing gloves, one can rinse blood out of the carpet, clothing, or upholstered furniture with cold water or hydrogen peroxide; wash personal clothing when convenient; and bag a child's soiled clothing and send home. Following column 2 in Table 3, caregivers can review other universal precautions practices grouped according to the three principles of infection control.

TAKING THE NEXT STEPS

Once caregivers resolve their uncertainty about what to do in any situation involving blood, they can then address the concerns of their own families, friends, and colleagues. In the workplace they can consider some of the following activi-

Table 3. Infection control chart

Basic precautions	*Universal Precautions*
Prevent contact	
Keep immunizations up to date.	Do not touch blood.
Stay home when sick.	Discourage "blood brother" activities.
Isolate children who become sick.	
Notify parents about exposure to communicable diseases.	
Leave nonwashable toys at home.	
Turn away when someone coughs/sneezes.	
Do not share cups, bottles, plates, utensils, food, drinks, bedding, or mattresses.	Do not share toothbrushes, toothpaste, pierced earrings, nail clippers, or razors.
Do not kiss babies on the mouth.	
Do not use fingers as a pacifier.	
Discard unused refrigerated formula after 24 hours.	
Change diapers away from food preparation areas.	
Dispose of trash daily.	Store toothbrushes/toothpaste separately.
Create barriers	
Cover mouth when coughing or sneezing.	Leave scabs alone.
Cover unused food/formula and refrigerate.	Cover cuts with bandaids.
Cover sand boxes when not in use.	
Wear gloves when changing diapers with loose stool.	Use barriers (gloves, tissues, towels) when caring for blood injuries/noses.
Fold soiled diapers inward and tab to contain urine and stool.	
Discard diapers, disposable soiled materials, and those used for cleaning in a tightly covered, foot-activated, plastic-lined container.	Bag blood-soiled disposable items and discard in a tightly covered, foot-activated, plastic-lined container.
Kill germs	
Wash hands routinely.	Wash hands after touching blood.
Wipe secretions, stool, and urine from the child's skin.	Apply disinfectants to cuts.
Clean/disinfect contaminated surfaces, toys, toilet training equipment, food preparation, sleeping, diaper changing, and bathroom areas.	Remove blood from surfaces, wash with a cleansing agent, rinse with a bleach solution, and air dry.
Wash soiled clothing/bedding.	
	Rinse blood-soiled clothing with cold water or hydrogen peroxide.
Follow routine housekeeping procedures (sweeping, vacuuming, dusting, etc).	

Reprinted with permission from Project CHAMP, Children's Hospital/Children's National Medical Center, Washington, DC.

ties: conduct staff meetings to discuss bloodborne pathogen transmission and basic infection control principles, including universal precautions; emphasize the usefulness of hand washing in preventing the spread of all germs; develop procedures for managing an occupational exposure to blood; and designate a staff member to monitor the workplace for adherence to basic infection control practices, universal precautions, and the continuous availability of supplies.[3]

When confronted with concerns of family members and friends, caregivers may first acknowledge the emotional basis of them and then use facts selectively following basic communication principles. For example, "You seem worried that I am caring for HIV-infected children. Is it because you think I will 'catch it'? I was scared too, until I began to consistently practice universal precautions with all blood." By sharing current knowledge and committing to universal precautions, caregivers can dispel the myths and irrational fears surrounding children with bloodborne pathogens.

REFERENCES

1. *Bloodborne Pathogens and Long-Term Care Workers.* Washington, DC: US Department of Labor, Occupational Safety and Health Administration; 1992.
2. Centers for Disease Control. Case definitions for public health surveillance. *MMWR.* 1990;39(RR13):1–43.
3. Parrott RH, Rathlev MC. *Access to Primary Health Care for Children with HIV: A Guide for Pediatricians, Family Physicians, and Nurse Practitioners.* Washington, DC: Children's National Medical Center; 1993.
4. Committee on Infectious Diseases, American Academy of Pediatrics. Hepatitis B. *Report of the Committee on Infectious Diseases.* Elk Grove Village, Ill: American Academy of Pediatrics; 1991.
5. Pickering LK, Hadler SC. Management and prevention in day care. In: Feigin RD, Cherry JD, eds. *Textbook of Pediatric Infectious Diseases.* 3rd. ed. Philadelphia, Pa: WB Saunders; 1992.
6. Committee on Infectious Diseases, American Academy of Pediatrics. Children in day care. *Report of the Committee on Infectious Diseases.* Elk Grove Village, Ill: American Academy of Pediatrics; 1991.
7. Rathlev MC, Riley MW, Jones SJ. *Caring in the Community for Children with HIV: A Guide for Child Care Providers, Foster Families, Home Health Aides, and Volunteers.* Washington, DC: Children's Hospital/Child Welfare League of America; 1992.
8. Rogers MF, White CR, Sanders R, et al. Lack of transmission of human immunodeficiency virus from infected children to their household contacts. *Pediatrics.* 1990;85(2):210–214.
9. Giebink GS. Controlling childhood infections in day care: the role of the pediatrician. *Rep Pediatr Infect Dis.* 1993;3(4):14-16.
10. Thacker SB, Addiss DG, Goodman RA, Holloway BR Spencer HC. Infectious diseases and injuries in child day care. *J Am Med Assoc.* 1992;268(13):1720–1726.
11. Edwards MJ. Infections due to human and animal bites. In: Feigin RD, Cherry JD, eds. *Textbook of Pediatric Infectious Diseases.* 3rd ed. Philadelphia, Pa: WB Saunders; 1992.

12. Task Force on Pediatric AIDS, American Academy of Pediatrics. Guidelines for human immuno-deficiency virus (HIV)-infected children and their foster families. *Pediatrics.* 1992;89(4):681-683.

13. Task Force on Pediatric AIDS, American Academy of Pediatrics. Education of children with human immunodeficiency virus infection. *Pediatrics.* 1991;88(3): 645–648.

14. Committee on Sports Medicine and Fitness, American Academy of Pediatrics. Human immunodeficiency virus [Acquired Immunodeficiency Syndrome (AIDS) Virus] in the athletic setting. *Pediatrics.* 1991;88(3): 640–641.

The neurologic complications of AIDS in infants and young children

James F. Bale, Jr, MD
Associate Professor
Departments of Pediatrics and
  Neurology
The University of Iowa College of
  Medicine
Iowa City, Iowa

WHEN A NOVEL, lethal disease (ultimately called acquired immunodeficiency syndrome [AIDS]) first appeared among homosexual men in San Francisco, California, and New York City,[1] few envisioned the impact that the disorder would eventually have on medicine and society worldwide. AIDS has permanently altered hygienic and sexual practices, has heightened human awareness regarding infectious diseases and cancer, and, perhaps most important, has reemphasized the fragile balance between microbes and humans. At the outset of the epidemic, few persons suspected that the disorder also would ultimately affect thousands of children. This article summarizes the history, immunology, virology, and clinical features of pediatric AIDS and focuses on the adverse effects of AIDS on the nervous system of the young child.

HISTORICAL BACKGROUND

Although cases of AIDS existed prior to 1980, the disorder was first recognized in 1981 when the U.S. Centers for Disease Control (CDC) began to receive reports of an unusual association of a parasite-induced pneumonia (*Pneumocystis carinii* pneumonia [PCP]) and a skin cancer (Kaposi's sarcoma) in young homosexual men.[1] Initial papers by Gottlieb et al,[2] Masur et al,[3] and Siegal et al[4] described 19 patients and began to define the clinical features of the disorder. Factors common to all patients were unexplained immune system abnormalities and infections with several different opportunistic pathogens (viruses, parasites, or fungi). By early 1983, the CDC had received reports of more than 1,000 cases in the United States and abroad.[5]

The epidemiologic characteristics of the disorder intrigued researchers from the very start of the epidemic. Although many hypotheses were proposed (including exposure to unidentified toxins), several factors, notably sexual contact or intravenous drug use (needle sharing) among AIDS victims, suggested that AIDS was caused by an infectious agent (most probably a virus). Ultimately, researchers in the United States and France linked AIDS in 1983 to infection with a novel human virus,[6,7] now known as the human immunodeficiency virus type 1 (HIV-1).

Inf Young Children 1990;3(2):15–23

VIROLOGY AND IMMUNOLOGY

HIV-1 belongs to the retrovirus family.[8] Retroviruses contain RNA as their genetic material and multiply via a DNA intermediary (this is the reverse of the usual progression from DNA to RNA; hence the name retroviruses). In infected cells, the retroviruses induce the synthesis of viral genetic material (provirus) that becomes incorporated into the host cell genes. Infection can thus be hidden (latent) and may reappear (reactivate) at a much later date. The events that trigger reactivation of latent HIV-1 infections and lead to symptomatic infection (AIDS or AIDS-related conditions) have not been completely determined.

To infect human cells, viruses rely on receptor molecules present on the cell surface. Thus, viruses have a relatively restricted interaction with host cells, a feature that largely determines the signs or symptoms of a particular viral infection. HIV-1 requires the CD-4 molecule found on the human white blood cells called helper T (thymus-dependent)-lymphocytes and monocytes. The latter cells play a critical role in AIDS by harboring latent HIV-1 and disseminating HIV-1 to many body tissues, including the brain.

Understanding AIDS requires a basic knowledge of the human immune system. Human immunity can be categorized into two major components, the humoral (involving production of antibodies) and the cell-mediated (involving cells such as monocytes and T-lymphocytes). Persons with AIDS display several major alterations in their immune function, particularly of the cell-mediated component.[9,10] Because HIV-1 infection leads to the death of helper T cells, patients with AIDS typically have reduced numbers of circulating helper T cells (as well as reduced numbers of total white blood cells) and exhibit a disturbed ratio among the subtypes of T cells (called the helper-to-suppressor T-cell ratio). In addition, HIV-1-infected helper T cells do not function normally and fail to respond when confronted with foreign material (ie, antigens).

Patients (children or adults) with AIDS also exhibit abnormalities in the humoral arm of the immune system. Blood antibody levels are usually elevated in symptomatic AIDS patients, yet such patients may paradoxically fail to produce normal quantities of specific antibodies after challenge with vaccines or infectious pathogens. Children with AIDS, for example, do not respond normally to immunizations for common childhood illnesses.

As a consequence of HIV-1-induced immune dysfunction, persons with AIDS are at extremely high risk for secondary infection with many different microbes, known as opportunistic infections. Abnormalities in cell-mediated immunity (the predominant defense against viruses, parasites and fungi) lead to infections with many different viruses, parasites, or fungi. As a result of defects in humoral immunity (the predominant early defense against bacteria), patients with AIDS are also at increased risk for serious bacterial diseases. By contrast, these infectious agents pose little or no risk to humans with normal immune systems.

EPIDEMIOLOGY

As additional cases of AIDS were identified in the United States and other regions of the world, the CDC was able to determine more precisely the patterns of HIV-1 transmission.[11,12] In North America and Western Europe, most AIDS cases resulted from male-to-male sexual contact or intravenous drug use via shared, contaminated needles. Although transfusions of HIV-1-infected blood products accounted for an important number of early cases, mass screening of blood products for HIV-1 infection eliminated this mode of transmission in developed nations.

By contrast, most cases of AIDS in Africa or in Caribbean countries have been linked to heterosexual (male-to-female) contact. Blood products constitute a potential source of infection, as a result of the absence of widespread serologic screening in many countries. In certain regions, such as Asia, Eastern Europe, or the Middle East, AIDS remains infrequent. However, as recent events in Eastern Europe illustrate, AIDS poses a threat even in nations with a low prevalence of HIV-1 infection among the general population. There, the reuse of HIV-1-contaminated needles in hospitals caused an epidemic of AIDS among young children.

In the initial surveys,[10,13] infants and young children constituted a very minor proportion of AIDS patients. Early cases were linked to blood transfusions, the administration of HIV-1-contaminated factor therapy for hemophilia, or prenatal transmission of HIV-1. As the AIDS epidemic has grown and more women have been infected via intravenous drug use or heterosexual contact with HIV-1-infected men, prenatal or perinatal transmission of HIV-1 has become the principal cause of AIDS among infants and young children.

During a 12-month interval beginning in October 1982, the CDC identified 35 children who met strict criteria for the diagnosis of AIDS.[14] By mid-1988, that number had ballooned to more than 1,000.[10] The numbers of infants born with evidence of HIV-1 infection varies greatly among geographic regions and socioeconomic groups. Although the nationwide seroprevalence rate (the percentage of newborns showing serologic evidence of HIV-1 exposure) is probably less than 0.01%, rates as high as 0.8% have been observed in some inner-city areas.[11] Even though children with AIDS currently represent only 1% to 2% of all AIDS victims, recent estimates suggest that AIDS will affect more than 3,000 children in the United States alone by 1991.[10]

CLINICAL FEATURES

The general clinical features of AIDS in infants and young children have been summarized in several comprehensive articles.[10,14–17] The first report prepared by the CDC in 1984[14] described 35 children who developed illnesses compatible with

AIDS at a mean age of 5 months. Common symptoms among these children included failure to thrive and unexplained enlargement of the liver and lymph nodes. Several infants were premature or small for their gestational age. Nearly all (33 of 35) had opportunistic infections, especially PCP, and 24 of the infants died at ages ranging from 3 months to 4.5 years. Twenty of these 35 infants had parents with risk factors for AIDS, such as intravenous drug use or Haitian background. Among the 15 children who had no parental risk factors, 6 had received blood transfusions during the first month of life.

As the numbers of patients with AIDS increased, several investigators began to recognize that AIDS victims, both adults and children, not only had opportunistic infections and systemic cancers, but also experienced neurologic complications. In 1983, Snider et al[18] described neurologic disorders among 50 male AIDS victims who ranged in age from 23 to 56 years. These complications, most of which were attributed to AIDS-related immunologic defects, included central nervous system infections with many different organisms (especially *Toxoplasma gondii*), primary lymphomas of the brain, strokes, meningitis, and abnormalities of the peripheral nerves.

A substantial proportion of these 50 adults had a primary neurologic condition, which Snider and colleagues called subacute encephalitis, that was characterized by apathy, lethargy, loss of sexual drive, and a decline in mental abilities.[18] The early symptoms of this disorder mimicked psychological depression, which could be attributed to the severe, incurable nature of AIDS. However, such patients experienced an inexorable decline in mental and physical functions and became completely debilitated over a period of weeks or months. The cause of this neurologic disorder was not obvious at first, but by 1985, researchers accumulated sufficient evidence to implicate direct HIV-1 involvement of the brain.[19,20] This disorder, now known as the AIDS dementia complex, remains a serious, devastating complication of AIDS.[21]

Soon after neurologic disorders were recognized in adult AIDS victims, physicians in New Jersey and New York who treated the growing numbers of children with AIDS observed that such children also experienced neurologic complications. Epstein and colleagues[22] and Belman and coworkers[23] initially reported neurologic symptoms in 10 children ranging in age from 6 months to 11 years. The neurologic disorder affecting these children strongly resembled the AIDS dementia complex of adults.

The clinical features of this pediatric neurologic syndrome, labeled progressive encephalopathy, were remarkably constant. All children lost motor skills and experienced progressive declines (ie, regression) in developmental or intellectual abilities. The children exhibited variable combinations of muscle weakness, hypotonia, spasticity, loss of balance (ataxia), abnormalities of deep tendon reflexes, and poor head growth (acquired microcephaly). An occasional child had seizures or cortical blindness.

When evaluated by neurodiagnostic studies, the children had similar findings. Computed tomography (CT) scans of the head disclosed atrophy, or loss of brain substance (Fig 1), an abnormality that progressed in many children and was correlated with microcephaly. Other children had a characteristic pattern of brain calcification that involved the deep nuclear areas (basal ganglia) and frontal white matter.[24] Electroencephalograms frequently revealed diffuse slowing, a nonspecific sign of brain dysfunction, and occasionally showed seizure discharges.[22,23]

Brain calcifications occur quite frequently in pediatric AIDS patients with progressive encephalopathy.[24] These calcifications seem to reflect an underlying disorder of blood vessels that allows the deposition of calcium within the brain substance. Although calcifications are common in pediatric AIDS, there does not appear to be a direct relationship between the extent of calcifications and the severity of neurologic symptoms.[24] Similar brain calcifications have been identified in conditions associated with defects in calcium homeostasis or in rare metabolic disorders.

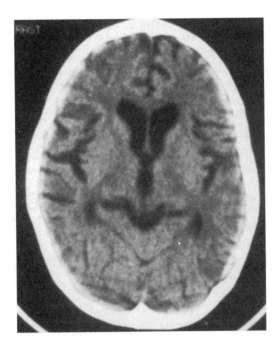

Fig 1. A CT scan of a child with HIV-1 encephalopathy shows diffuse cortical atrophy, as indicated by enlarged cerebrospinal fluid spaces.

Subsequent reports have characterized more completely the clinical spectrum of the neurologic syndromes associated with childhood AIDS (Box). Epstein and colleagues[25] reviewed a group of 36 children, 20 of whom had progressive encephalopathy. The neurologic features comprised loss of milestones, loss of prior intellectual skills (dementia), weakness, spasticity, rigidity, loss of balance (ataxia), and seizures. Children in whom progressive encephalopathy developed had an ominous prognosis. Thirteen of 20 died, whereas there were no deaths among the 16 children who were neurologically normal.

In a report of 61 HIV-1-infected children with neurologic complications, Belman et al[26] described variable patterns of neurologic deterioration. Approximately one half of the children had a slowly progressive course that was heralded by a developmental plateau. Others had a more rapidly deteriorating course, whereas several had static (nonprogressive) encephalopathies with variable degrees of intellectual or motor deficit. Again, mortality was highest in patients with progressive courses. These important observations indicate that AIDS-related neurologic conditions have several variations and can mimic other pediatric neurologic disorders (including metabolic conditions, degenerative disorders and nonprogressive neurologic conditions).

The decline in motor and intellectual skills observed in children with HIV-1-induced progressive encephalopathy can precede the appearance of opportunistic infections or can occur in the absence of any infectious complications. For example, a young HIV-1-infected hemophilic child evaluated at the University of Iowa experienced a regression in school performance, including a deterioration in handwriting (Fig 2), and somnolence. This progressed over a 4-month period to the point that the child performed all tasks slowly and had incontinence of stool. During the fourth month of neurologic symptoms, oral thrush developed. When

---

Neurologic Features in Infants and Young Children with HIV-1 Infection

Progressive loss of milestones (motor, social, language skills)
Static encephalopathy (developmental delay)
Dementia (loss of intellectual skills)
Acquired microcephaly
Ataxia (loss of balance)
Spasticity
Rigidity
Paralysis
Seizures (not common)
Cortical atrophy (identified by CT or magnetic resonance imaging)
Calcifications of basal ganglia and white matter (identified best by CT)
Slowing of brain electrical activity, seizure discharges (identified by electroencephalography)
Occasional abnormalities of cerebrospinal fluid

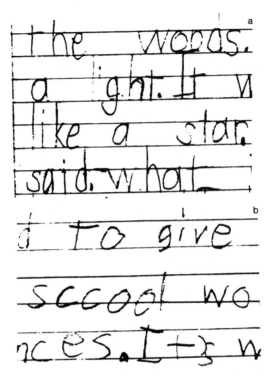

Fig 2. Deteriorating handwriting in a child with HIV-1 encephalopathy. a. Baseline handwriting. b. Handwriting sample approximately 1 year later, coincident with a decline in school performance.

evaluated shortly thereafter, the child was unable to perform age-appropriate calculations and had abnormal muscle tone and gait. A CT scan showed cortical atrophy (Fig 1), and no cause other than HIV-1 infection was identified. The child ultimately died from complications of AIDS.

Most pediatric AIDS cases now reflect congenital or perinatal infection with HIV-1, a consequence of maternal HIV-1 infection. The virus crosses the placenta and appears to infect approximately 50% of the offspring of infected mothers.[10] Infection of the developing fetus can occur even when the mother has asymptomatic HIV-1 infection. Some investigators suggest that congenitally infected infants have a characteristic pattern of birth defects (growth failure, boxlike head, blue sclera, and hypertelorism),[27] although this association has been disputed.[28] HIV-1 infection in infants can have an extremely long incubation period, and several months or years may lapse before the child begins to exhibit neurologic symptoms or other signs of AIDS.[10]

Although the clinical features of HIV-1 encephalopathy in children have now been well characterized, several questions regarding the genesis of the neurologic complications remain unanswered. Abundant evidence (detection of infectious HIV-1 or HIV-1 genes within brain cells) supports the conclusion that HIV-1 directly infects the brain. Nonetheless, the number of brain cells, particularly neurons, that are infected by HIV-1 seems insufficient to account for such severe neurologic dysfunction. Consequently, other mechanisms, such as alterations in the blood-brain barrier or production of neurotoxic substances by infected cells (possibly monocytes), may be operative.[29]

DIAGNOSIS

AIDS was initially diagnosed solely on clinical grounds as a disease "at least moderately predictive of a defect in cell-mediated immunity, occurring in persons with no known cause of diminished resistance to disease."[30(p508)] Once the etiologic agent, HIV-1, was identified, laboratory tests were devised to confirm the diagnosis of AIDS. Currently, AIDS can be defined according to the presence of indicator diseases and on the basis of the results of HIV-1 testing[15]:

- Without laboratory evidence for HIV infection[1]
  1. Candidiasis of the esophagus, trachea, bronchi, or lungs
  2. Crytococcosis, extrapulmonary
  3. Crytosporidiosis with diarrhea persisting >1 month
  4. Cytomegalovirus disease of an organ other than liver, spleen, or lymph nodes in a patient >1 month of age
  5. Herpes simplex infection causing a mucocutaneous ulcer that persists >1 month; or bronchitis, pneumonitis, or esophagitis in a patient >1 month of age
  6. Kaposi's sarcoma affecting a patient <60 years of age
  7. Primary lymphoma of the brain in a patient <60 years of age
  8. *Mycobacterium avium* complex or *M. kansaii* disease
  9. *Pneumocystis carinii* pneumonia
  10. Progressive multifocal leukoencephalopathy
  11. Toxoplasmosis of the brain in a patient >1 month of age
- With laboratory evidence of HIV infection[1]
  1. Any of the above
  2. Multiple or recurrent bacterial infections in a child <13 years of age
  3. Coccidioidomycosis, disseminated
  4. HIV encephalopathy
  5. Histoplasmosis, disseminated
  6. Isosporiasis with diarrhea lasting >1 month
  7. Kaposi's sarcoma at any age

8. Primary lymphoma of the brain at any age
9. Mycobacterial disease other than *M. tuberculosis*
10. Non-Hodgkin's lymphomas of B-cell or unknown phenotype
11. *M. tuberculosis*, extrapulmonary
12. Salmonella septicemia, recurrent

AIDS must be considered in the differential diagnosis of declining motor or intellectual performance in infants or young children, particularly when risk factors are identified either in the child (eg, an HIV-1-infected hemophilic) or parent (eg, an intravenous drug user). The diagnosis can be supported by detection of antibodies to HIV-1 via an enzyme-linked immunosorbent assay (ELISA). Western blot methods can then be used to detect specific antibodies directed against proteins of HIV.[10] Other characteristic laboratory findings include low white blood cell count, disturbed ratios of T-lymphocytes, and elevations of serum immunoglobulins.

The diagnosis of HIV-1 infection in young infants poses several challenges.[10] Because maternal antibodies can cross the placenta and persist for months in the infant's serum in the absence of infection, serial antibody testing is required. In addition, false-negative antibody tests have been observed. Consequently, considerable effort has been expended to devise laboratory methods that have greater sensitivity and can distinguish passive transfer of maternal antibody from true infection. Such methods include the detection of HIV-1 antigens (proteins produced by the virus) or the detection of HIV-1 genetic material using the polymerase chain reaction, a powerful molecular technique that can detect minute quantities of DNA or RNA. The latter method has not, as yet, been adapted for widespread use in diagnostic laboratories.

TREATMENT AND PROGNOSIS

AIDS remains an incurable disease. However, therapy with an antiviral drug, zidovudine (azidothymidine [AZT], Burroughs-Wellcome, Research Triangle Park, N.C.), has been associated with prolonged survival and improved neurologic function.[31,32] This drug interferes with HIV-1 multiplication by altering the production of HIV-1 genes, thus rendering HIV-1 noninfectious. In a large study[31] of adults with AIDS, AZT significantly reduced short-term mortality and the frequency of opportunistic infections. During the study interval (8 to 24 weeks), only one AZT-treated patient died, whereas 19 patients receiving placebo died.

Preliminary studies[33] also suggest that the drug may improve the neurologic functions of young HIV-1-infected children. In certain instances, the improvement may be dramatic. Pizzo and colleagues[34] described their observations during continuous intravenous AZT therapy in 21 HIV-1 infected children. Among 13 children who were evaluated after 6 months of therapy, 12 showed substantial improvement in IQ scores (mean increase, 15.3 points). Serial CT scans in a 3-year-old boy participating in this study demonstrated reversal of cortical atrophy.

Although these results are encouraging, AIDS in children remains a therapeutic challenge. Substantial toxicity (particularly to the bone marrow) may limit the long-term intravenous use of AZT. In addition, 5 of the 21 children studied by Pizzo et al died, usually of infectious complications. Overall, at least 60% of the children with AIDS in the United States have died.[10] Studies are currently in progress to determine the optimum dosage schedules for AZT in children.[35] In October 1989, the manufacturer of the drug and the National Institute of Allergy and Infectious Diseases initiated an open trial of AZT use in children. A toll-free number, 1-800-829-7337, can be used to enroll children in this treatment program.

Other strategies that might treat or prevent AIDS in children are currently being investigated. At present, the incidence of pediatric AIDS is strongly linked to the factors that determine transmission of AIDS among adult women (eg, drug abuse and sexual contact with HIV-1-infected men). Whether HIV-1 transmission can be interrupted among high-risk groups is uncertain. Vaccine trials are currently underway, but many problems must be addressed before vaccines will become widely available.[36]

Children with AIDS pose numerous issues for society. Because their parents frequently cannot care for them (as a result of their own AIDS, drug abuse, or poor socioeconomic conditions), HIV-1-infected children often require long-term placement in foster care environments. As these children reach school-age, educators will have to develop methods to maximize the skills of the children, to minimize the stigma associated with AIDS, and to provide safe environments for children with impaired immunity. Finally, the cost of medical care necessary to treat patients with AIDS is staggering. Whether nations—even the United States with its vast resources—can cope effectively with large numbers of HIV-1-infected children is unknown.

•   •   •

AIDS, the disease of the century, presents several stiff challenges. Medical scientists must unravel the mysteries of how HIV-1 damages the brain and must eventually devise a cure or effective strategies to prevent AIDS. Social scientists must cope with the immense burdens placed on society by AIDS and must deal with behaviors (eg, drug abuse) that place persons at risk for AIDS. Health care professionals who work with young HIV-1-infected children also confront numerous challenges. As recently summarized by Falloon and colleagues, children with AIDS require a "well-organized multidisciplinary team . . . of social workers, psychologists, dieticians, teachers, clergy and occupational, physical and recreation therapists."[10(p22)] Without such a comprehensive approach, the medical community will not be able to cope effectively with AIDS and its devastating effects on the developing nervous system.

REFERENCES

1. Centers for Disease Control. Kaposi's sarcoma and pneumocystis pneumonia among homosexual men—New York City and California. *MMWR.* 1981;30:305–308.
2. Gottlieb MS, Schroff R, Schanker HM, et al. Pneumocystis carinii pneumonia and mucosal candidiasis in previously healthy homosexual men. *N Engl J Med.* 1981;305:1425–1431.
3. Masur H, Michelis MA, Greene JB, et al. An outbreak of community-acquired pneumocystis carinii pneumonia. *N Engl J Med.* 1981;305:1431–1438.
4. Siegal FP, Lopez C, Hammer GS, et al. Severe acquired immunodeficiency in male homosexuals, manifested by chronic perianal ulcerative herpes simplex lesions. *N Engl J Med.* 1981;305:1439–1444.
5. Selik RM, Haverkos HW, Curran JW. Acquired immune deficiency syndrome (AIDS) trends in the United States, 1978–1982. *Am J Med.* 1983;76:493–500.
6. Gallo RC, Sarin PS, Gelmann EP, et al. Isolation of human T-cell leukemia virus in acquired immune deficiency syndrome (AIDS). *Science.* 1983;220:865–867.
7. Barre-Sinoussi F, Chermann JC, Rey F, et al. Isolation of a T-lymphotropic retrovirus from a patient at risk for acquired immune deficiency syndrome (AIDS). *Science.* 1983;220:868–871.
8. Varmus H. Retroviruses. *Science.* 1988;240:1427–1436.
9. Fauci AS, Macher AM, Longo DL, et al. Acquired immunodeficiency syndrome: Epidemiologic, clinical, immunologic, and therapeutic considerations. *Ann Intern Med.* 1984;100:92–106.
10. Falloon J, Eddy J, Wiener L, Pizzo PA. Human immunodeficiency virus infection in children. *J Pediatr.* 1989;114:1–30.
11. Centers for Disease Control. Human immunodeficiency virus infection in the United States: A review of current knowledge. *MMWR.* 1987;36:1–48.
12. Centers for Disease Control. Update: Acquired immunodeficiency syndrome (AIDS)—worldwide. *MMWR.* 1988;37:286–295.
13. Centers for Disease Control. Update: Acquired immunodeficiency syndrome—United States. *MMWR.* 1986;35:17–31.
14. Thomas PA, Jaffe HW, Spira TJ, Reiss R, Guerro IC, Auerbach D. Unexplained immunodeficiency in children: A surveillance report. *JAMA.* 1984;252:639–644.
15. Centers for Disease Control. Revision of the CDC surveillance case definition for acquired immunodeficiency syndrome. *MMWR.* 1987;36:1S–15S.
16. Scott GB, Buck BE, Letterman JG, Bloom FL, Parks WP. Acquired immunodeficiency syndrome in infants. *N Engl J Med.* 1984;310:76–81.
17. Shannon KM, Ammann AJ. Acquired immune deficiency syndrome in childhood. *J Pediatr.* 1985;106:332–342.
18. Snider WD, Simpson DM, Nielsen S, Gold JWM, Metroka CE, Posner JB. Neurological complications of acquired immune deficiency syndrome: Analysis of 50 patients. *Ann Neurol.* 1983;14:403–418.
19. Ho DD, Rota TR, Schooley RT, et al. Isolation of HTLV-III from cerebrospinal fluid and neural tissues of patients with neurologic syndromes related to the acquired immunodeficiency syndrome. *N Engl J Med.* 1985;313:1493–1497.
20. Resnick L, DiMarzo-Veronese F, Schupbach J, et al. Intra-blood-brain-barrier synthesis of HTLV-III-specific IgG in patients with neurologic symptoms associated with AIDS or AIDS-related complex. *N Engl J Med.* 1985;313:1498–1504.

21. Navia BA, Jordan BD, Price RW. The AIDS dementia complex: I. Clinical features. *Ann Neurol.* 1986;19:517–524.

22. Epstein LG, Sharer LR, Joshi VV, Fojas MM, Koenigsberger MR, Oleske JM. Progressive encephalopathy in children with acquired immune deficiency syndrome. *Ann Neurol.* 1985;17:488–496.

23. Belman AL, Ultmann MH, Horoupian D, et al. Neurological complications in infants and children with acquired immune deficiency syndrome. *Ann Neurol.* 1985;18:560–566.

24. Belman AL, Lantos G, Horoupian D, et al. AIDS: Calcification of the basal ganglia in infants and children. *Neurology.* 1986;36:1192–1199.

25. Epstein LG, Sharer LR, Oleske JM, et al. Neurologic manifestations of human immunodeficiency virus infection in children. *Pediatrics.* 1986;78:678–687.

26. Belman AL, Diamond G, Dickson D, et al. Pediatric acquired immunodeficiency syndrome. *Am J Dis Child.* 1988;142:29–35.

27. Marion RW, Wiznia AA, Hutcheon RG, Rubinstein A. Human T-cell lymphotropic virus type III (HTLV-III) embryopathy: A new dysmorphic syndrome associated with intrauterine HTLV-III infection. *Am J Dis Child.* 1986;140:638–640.

28. Qazi QH, Sheikh TM, Fikrig S, Menikoff H. Lack of evidence for craniofacial dysmorphism in perinatal human immunodeficiency virus infection. *J Pediatr.* 1988;112:7–11.

29. Ho DD, Pomerantz RJ, Kaplan JC. Pathogenesis of infection with human immunodeficiency virus. *N Engl J Med.* 1987;317:278–286.

30. Centers for Disease Control. Update on acquired immune deficiency syndrome. *MMWR.* 1982;31:507–514.

31. Fischl MA, Richman DD, Grieco MH, et al. The efficacy of azidothymidine (AZT) in the treatment of patients with AIDS and AIDS-related complex. *N Engl J Med.* 1987;317:185–191.

32. Creagh-Kirk T, Doi P, Andrews E, et al. Survival experience among patients with AIDS receiving zidovudine. *JAMA.* 1988;260:3009–3015.

33. Cullition BJ. AZT reverses AIDS dementia in children. *Science.* 1989;246:21–23.

34. Pizzo PA, Eddy J, Falloon J, et al. Effect of continuous intravenous infusion of zidovudine (AZT) in children with symptomatic HIV infection. *N Engl J Med.* 1988;319:889–96.

35. Koff WC, Hoth DF. Development and testing of AIDS vaccines. *Science.* 1988;241:426–32.

36. Ballis FM, Pizzo PA, Eddy J, et al. Pharmacokinetics of zidovudine administered intravenously and orally in children with human immunodeficiency virus infection. *J Pediatr.* 1989;114:880–884.

Oral care for developmentally disabled children: The primary dentition stage

David J. Kenny, DDS, PhD
Dentist-in-Chief
The Hospital for Sick Children
Associate Professor
Faculty of Dentistry
University of Toronto
Toronto, Canada

Peter L. Judd, DDS, MSc
Staff Pediatric Dentist
The Hospital for Sick Children
Dental Consultant
The Hugh MacMillan Medical Centre
Toronto, Canada

THE FIRST THREE years are often chaotic for a child with developmental disabilities, as well as for his or her family. Pediatricians and family physicians are concerned for the child's medical needs, and the family must cope with the emotional and social aspects of the child's development. During these years, the primary dentition erupts, enabling the child to incise, chop, and, to some extent, shear foodstuffs. In many cases, medical demands and family issues completely override the most basic requirements of dental care. It is during this time that dentists rely on parents and health care professionals to observe and report dental conditions or to seek advice on the management of the child's dental needs.

Advancements in dental care for the developmentally disabled child, who may also be chronically ill, have made early intervention both possible and desirable. Furthermore, it has become obvious that serious consequences can arise from lack of early dental consultation. This article outlines the impact of developmental disabilities and chronic illness on the oral health of children in the preeruptive and primary dentition stages.

Young children with brain damage and seizure disorders are two populations with developmental delay that require special oral care.[1] Developmental delay produced by mental retardation and by learning disabilities has only a minor impact on the dental health of children under the age of 4. Autism, another condition that produces developmental delay, is often associated with brain damage and with some chronic illnesses, yet poses few special dental problems during the early years.[2] The medical problems of stabilization, rehabilitation, and development are the prime focus for these infants and toddlers. The major dental concern continues to be prevention and treatment of dental caries. Children who are taking certain seizure medications may have associated gingival manifestations, or they may be more prone to dental trauma. Management of the structural aspects of the oral cavity is the traditional role of pediatric dentists, as is treatment of children with congenital anomalies and chronic illness. However, management of some of the functional aspects of oral facial disorders is also undertaken by dentists with special training or with interest in children who have developmental disorders. Some oral facial functional issues that affect children with cerebral palsy and sei-

Inf Young Children 1988;1(2):11–19
© 1988 Aspen Publishers, Inc.

zure disorders are sucking, swallowing, mastication, extraoral feeding, and factitial injuries.

Dental care for children with cerebral palsy and seizure disorders are reviewed and suggestions for involvement of health care workers and parents during the first four years are presented. The traditional structural aspects of pediatric dental care are updated first and then the functional issues are subsequently outlined.

PREVENTION AND MANAGEMENT OF DENTAL CARIES

Poor sleep habits, repeated hospitalizations, parental concern for the child's comfort, and a number of similar factors may lead to prolonged bottle feeding or bottle "snacking" during daytime naps and evening sleep. This can lead to caries of the primary dentition before 18 months.[3] In some cases, dental conditions deteriorate to such an extent that extensive dental caries and infection are present and must be treated. Furthermore, a general anesthetic may be required to complete restorative treatment.

In addition, developmentally delayed children often require a range of medications to control their seizures, to counteract repeated infections, or to facilitate ventilation. They take most medication in the form of oral syrup or drops because they are so young. These liquid medications contain 30% to 50% sugar to add sweetness and bulk.[4] Such children may consume over 19 pounds of additional sugar from oral liquid medication alone during the first three years.[3]

Many of these children are not capable of clearing the oral cavity with their cheeks and tongues and do not initiate swallows at the same rate as healthy children.[5] As a consequence, sugars from both medications and snacks, whether from bottles or solids, are slow to clear the mouth.[6] This prolonged retention of sugar extends the period that fermentable carbohydrates are metabolized by oral plaque bacteria. These bacteria convert carbohydrates to acid, which in turn decalcifies or inhibits the normal cyclic recalcification of teeth.[7]

Parents of chronically ill or developmentally delayed children often squeeze oral liquid medications into the mouths of their sleeping children rather than disturb them. This is a perfectly reasonable means of supplying the medication at designated times, but it too serves to deliver fermentable carbohydrates when salivary clearance and acid buffering is minimized by the sleep state.[8] It is this combination of conditions and the fact that, during waking hours, children are probably encouraged to snack continuously from a bottle to reduce the threat of dehydration that predisposes them to rampant caries of the primary dentition.

Home-care suggestions

Diagnostic screening for dental caries can be performed by any interested adult. The inside of the upper incisor teeth is usually the first place that "snacking caries" can be observed. Any brown stain or milky white discoloration of this area should initiate a dental consultation. The flat (chewing) surfaces of the primary molar teeth may also be affected. Once again, any brown stain is reason for a dental consultation. Sometimes stain on the outside of the teeth is caused by medication and can be removed by a dentist. The best way to examine the teeth of a very young or disabled child is to lay the child on his or her back and look directly down into the mouth.

If a child is on an oral, liquid medication regimen, try to find a sugar-free alternative medication, brush the child's teeth *before* dispensing medication, and follow the medication with water. Try to time medication so that it is not dispensed just before or during a nap or bedtime. If this is necessary, it is desirable to brush the teeth more frequently.

GINGIVAL CHANGES

Phenytoin (Dilantin), a commonly used drug to control seizures, produces hypertrophy of the gingiva as a dose-related side effect.[9] The hypertrophy is much less exuberant in the primary dentition than in the permanent teeth and usually amounts to an excessive roll of tissue around the tooth-gingival interface. Careful brushing is thought to decrease the growth of gingival tissue. The hypertrophy is rarely serious enough to justify surgery in the primary dentition, but surgery may be required at the time the permanent teeth are due to erupt. Recent changes in the medical management of seizures has led to increased use of carbamazepine (Tegretol), which does not cause gingival hyperplasia.

Home-care suggestions

Oral hygiene measures for the child on Dilantin therapy should include daily brushing by an adult. This may be difficult because of the oral hypersensitivity that accompanies some neural conditions. The toothbrush is a good instrument to use in desensitizing exercises. Toothpaste is not necessary and may not even be desirable as the taste may provide excessive stimulation. A scrubbing action at the tooth-gingival margin will help remove plaque from this area.

If the gingival hyperplasia is sufficiently pronounced that a rolled border appears at the gingival margin, it may funnel food debris into the trough produced between the tooth and the gingiva. This can lead to inflammation and perhaps to more hyperplasia. Signs of excess gingival tissue at the tooth margin is a good reason to have the child examined by a dentist.

TRAUMA TO THE PRIMARY DENTITION

As soon as children are able to stand, they begin to fall and bump their teeth. Before that, they bang into crib rails, tip out of walkers, and chip their teeth on highchairs. The elastic nature of the supporting bone and the nature of most falls from short distances favor a certain type of injury.[10] That is, the primary teeth are usually moved bodily through the bone, either by intrusion or by being moved laterally (luxated). Traumatic movement can also lead to extrusion or actual loss of teeth (avulsion). Primary teeth should never be replanted. The very low chances of successful reattachment must be weighed against the risk of the tooth coming loose and being aspirated into a lung. Another sequela of primary-tooth trauma is a dental abscess with pain and the subsequent risk of a white or brown spot on the permanent tooth. Ankylosis (root-to-bone fusion) can delay normal shedding of the primary teeth and, in turn, deflection or lack of eruption of the permanent successors. Whether an intruded tooth should be removed or allowed to remain in place is more controversial. A crown that is intruded 4 to 6 mm may not appear to be a serious matter. However, one must consider that the apex of the root has moved 4 to 6 mm closer to the developing permanent tooth; may have touched the unerupted, permanent tooth; or may have pierced the thin plate of bone above the primary tooth. All of these factors are part of the information used to determine if the extraction of a traumatized tooth is in the patient's best interest.

A primary tooth that becomes darkened after a bump or fall simply indicates a "bruise" has occurred in the pulpal tissue. The tooth may actually change color to a light brown or yellow and remain useful.[10] Primary teeth that abscess or exhibit radiographic signs of necrosis may be removed or the pulp may be treated, and the tooth restored and retained until time for it to be shed.[11] There is no reason that the full range of pulp treatments cannot be provided for the developmentally disabled child. The presence of healthy teeth improves appearance, function, and the way the child is perceived by his or her caretakers.

Home-care suggestions

If there is a history of previous trauma, caregivers and parents should examine the gingiva periodically before brushing the child's teeth. It is possible for a primary anterior tooth to abscess and form a fistula without the child experiencing pain. If a gumboil is observed, a dental consultation is required.

CONGENITAL ANOMALIES AND CHRONIC ILLNESS

Two congenital conditions that affect dental health and may be found in the developmentally delayed child are craniofacial anomalies and heart disease. Congenital heart disease is a common chronic illness of children with developmental delay, and it directly affects their dental management.

Unilateral and bilateral cleft lip and palate are common congenital facial anomalies that are found in association with a number of different syndromes.[12]

Children with bilateral cleft lips and palates are more difficult to feed because of their larger anatomic defects. Other, rarer, craniofacial abnormalities alter facial morphology in such a way that feeding, ventilation, speech, hearing, and vision may be affected.[13] Healthy, cleft-palate patients generally manage feeding tasks quite well, so the use of passive feeding plates[14] for cleft-palate children is controversial. It is only when other conditions, such as congenital heart disease, brain damage, or lung disease, are associated with a craniofacial anomaly that significant problems with feeding arise. In such cases, the feeding disorder is sufficiently complicated by neurologic factors that nonoral feeding techniques may be elected by the physician.

Congenital heart disease poses dental problems only if there is dental disease. Infected primary teeth can produce blood-borne bacterial showers that can, in turn, produce inflammation of the heart (endocarditis). Treatment of the primary dentition requires protective antibiotic coverage to reduce the risk of infective endocarditis in many patients with congenital heart disease.[15] Conditions that produce the most risk are those where the blood vascular system is most disrupted from an even flow of blood. Table 1 illustrates congenital cardiac conditions that carry a high, intermediate, and negligible risk of endocarditis.[16]

Table 1. Congenital cardiac conditions with risk for endocarditis in children under 5 years

High risk, antibiotic prophylaxis required
    Cyanotic congenital heart disease
    Aortic valve disease, including bicuspid aortic valve
    Previous infective endocarditis
    Mitral insufficiency
    Patent ductus arteriosus
    Ventricular septal defect
    Coarctation of the aorta
Intermediate risk, antibiotic prophylaxis required
    Tetralogy of Fallot
    Tricuspid valve disease
    Pulmonary valve disease
    Asymmetric septal hypertrophy
    Intravenous catheters
    Alimentation catheters in right heart or pulmonary artery
    Pressure-monitoring catheters in right heart or pulmonary artery
    Nonvalvular intracardiac prosthetic implants (patch)
Very low or negligible risk, antibiotic prophylaxis either not required or optional
    Atrial septal defect
    Mitral valve prolapse
    Cardiac pacemaker
    Surgically corrected cardiac lesion (without prosthetic implants and more than 6 months after surgery)

Home-care suggestions

All preventive measures mentioned previously are particularly important for these children. The pediatrician, nutritionist, dietitian, or nurses involved in the early intervention of these children should arrange for a consultation with an appropriate dentist to establish a preventive program from the time the first primary teeth erupt.

SUCKING, SWALLOWING, AND MASTICATION

By age 3, children are usually capable of a combination of up-down and rotatory chewing, have their full complement of teeth, have passed through the risk years for choking and asphyxia,[17] have no problems initiating voluntary or unconscious swallows, and can control their airways. On the other hand, feeding may pose a multitude of problems for the developmentally disabled child. These problems may be structural, such as malocclusion, high-arched palate, missing teeth caused by trauma or caries, or, more often, functional and neural-based, such as airway management and control during feeding.

Certain foods, such as nuts and beans, are more apt to be aspirated because of their shape and nature. The practice of allowing youngsters to use raw carrot sticks for teething should be discouraged. Once the primary incisors have erupted, young children can incise or nibble away at the raw carrot and produce a mush that is prone to aspiration. In one study,[18] seven of nine cases where children were admitted to a hospital because of accidental aspiration (and choking) from carrot required removal of vegetal matter from the lung by bronchoscopy. This procedure is both complicated and risky in young children. Other foods pose mechanical problems. Fish is a favorite food for youngsters who have not yet developed the masticatory efficiency to chew meats. In the same study,[18] 73 fish bones accounted for 36% of all accidental food swallowings significant enough to prompt an emergency department visit. The fish bones were usually lodged in the pharynx or tonsillar pillars.

Although rare, the most serious danger is asphyxia. Wieners are a dietary staple of many young children, both healthy and disabled, because of their ease of mastication. Unfortunately, the size and shape of this meat product matches the hypopharynx of 1- to 2-year olds.[17] Once again, the child is able to incise a portion of a wiener but does not have the molars or the neuromuscular ability to masticate efficiently. The obvious solution to this purely mechanical problem is to cut wieners lengthwise before cutting them crosswise.

Parents and caretakers should be aware that the development of mastication, bolus, and airway control may be delayed along with other aspects of a child's development. The hypotonic musculature of some children with Down Syndrome and the oral hypersensitivity of some spastic children pose quite different problems during feeding. The complex acts of sucking, swallowing, and later mastication require millisecond timing of a number of sensory, motor, and integrative mechanisms. Lip closure, bolus transport, airway management, initiation of swallow, and development of mastication are separate but related tasks that need to be considered in the context of the nature of the specific developmental disability.[5,19,20] Such clinical problems are best managed in a multidisciplinary milieu, but many children with feeding problems are managed without dental expertise simply because of a lack of consultation.

Home-care suggestions

All children should be fed in a distraction-controlled situation, in the sitting position while attended by an adult.[21] The standard foods that are prone to aspiration should be avoided, as well as raw carrots used for teething. Weiners should be cut lengthwise for all young children and for all children with problems of food and airway control. Feeding problems should be discussed with the pediatrician or family physician at each stage of development.

EXTRAORALLY FED PATIENTS

Disorders of mastication, dysphagia, and chronic lung disease can affect children with a wide range of developmental disabilities and chronic illnesses. Over the past few years, it has become increasingly more acceptable to feed certain children extraorally through a tube directly to the stomach (gastrostomy) or upper bowel (jejunostomy), through the nose (nasogastric), or intravenously (total parenteral nutrition). Some of these techniques are short term; others, long term. They provide controlled nutrition, freedom from long hours of feeding, and safety from aspiration of foodstuffs during swallowing. However, the return to normal feeding practices is often complicated and creates a number of problems of its own.[22,23]

Although the mouth care of such children can be managed by regular examinations by a pediatric dentist and prophylactic cleaning of the teeth by a dental hygienist, little is known of the effects of eliminating oral feeding. Reduced oral feeding decreases the amount of fermentable carbohydrates in the mouth, and reduced mastication alters sensory input from receptors in the periodontal ligament that supports the teeth.[19] Calculus, rarely observed in the primary dentition, is increased because of decreased masticatory function. The importance of intraoral stimulation to a child whose extraoral feeding technique precludes normal development of taste, management of the airway, and leads to altered salivary and mechanoreceptive function is not known. There are considerable knowledge gaps about the effects of decreased oral function in extraorally fed children.

FACTITIAL INJURIES

Although healthy children may produce factitial (self-inflicted) injuries by activities such as scratching at the gingiva with a fingernail or lip biting, developmentally delayed children with brain disorders produce the most serious factitial injuries to the mouth. Cyclic jaw movements have been demonstrated in animals and are thought to be caused by rhythm generators of the neural chewing center that have been released from cortical inhibition.[24] Similar movements may appear in the comatose child, the child with acute meningitis, the child on large quantities of central nervous system (CNS) drugs, or the child with cerebral palsy. Some of these rhythmic chewing habits are destructive to tongue, lips, and buccal mucosa.

The clinical problem is protecting the soft tissue from the teeth that abrade or incise it. The problem is often transitory, but can be chronic in some developmentally disabled children. Management of the child with a protrusive tongue that is damaged by rhythmic chewing movements is the most difficult to manage. This saggital open-close movement is most often transitory, as it is usually observed in comatose patients in the intensive care unit. One approach is to attempt to maintain the jaw in an open position with a fixed, acrylic custom splint attached to the teeth with dental cement. In cases where the tongue is abraded by protrusive-retrusive movement against the lower incisors, a dentist might cement an acrylic custom splint to the lower incisors.

If the patient chews the lower lip, a wire and acrylic appliance could be cemented to the lower primary molars to hold the lower lip forward of the incisors. The buccal mucosa may also be held out of the way of molar teeth with a range of custom splints. Unfortunately, such splints are only marginally successful, and none is esthetically pleasing. The major problem is maintaining the screen or shield in place without impeding the airway.[25] Splint therapy for children who have centrally generated, rhythmic factitial biting and chewing habits is seldom totally satisfactory. Perhaps answers will come with new materials or with a better understanding of the neural mechanisms that drive the involuntary movements that produce oral factitial injuries.

Oral home-care techniques

Stringent preventive measures must be undertaken as soon as the first primary teeth appear in the mouth. Soft baby toothbrushes are readily available, but parents generally will not begin to use them on very young children without reassurance and a demonstration. Parents often do not brush the teeth of very young children for a variety of reasons. A recent study determined that (1) parents were never informed of the need to brush nor shown how to do so, (2) they tried brushing and caused some bleeding, (3) they had no idea of the risk from oral liquid medications and bottle snacking habits, or (4) they were simply delighted that the child wanted to brush and so were able to avoid a daily confrontation.

The authors recommend tooth brushing during normal waking hours. One of the best times is directly before a meal or before oral liquid medication is given. If the plaque bacteria are removed from the teeth before the meal, the fermentable carbohydrate will not be converted to acid. No parent will wake a dozing child to brush the teeth nor will a parent appreciate a confrontation over tooth brushing just before the child is put down for a nap or for the evening. To achieve compliance, oral hygiene practices must be practical and must fit into the normal routine of a child's day.

Children under the age of 5 simply do not have the manual dexterity (although they may have the will) to brush their own teeth adequately, and so this responsibility rests with the parent or caretaker. The brushing of very young children's teeth is best managed when the adult is in a sitting position with the youngster supine on his or her lap. A scrubbing action, strong enough to remove flour and water paste, is required to remove the tenacious plaque. This must be done once every 24 hours, preferably every 12 hours if liquid medication is used or if bottle snacking is necessary. Systemic fluoride should be prescribed by the dentist according to the fluoride levels of the communal water supply and dispensed by the parent. Toddlers should be managed with the child standing in front of the adult, but facing in the same direction as the adult. It is very difficult to brush a child's teeth when facing the child. The child's head should be tipped back against the adult's waist, and the adult should brush the child's teeth by looking into the mouth from above and with the same approach as the adult uses in his or her mouth.

Societal changes have meant that many children are raised by single parents who must leave them with caretakers for significant periods of the day. Parents must be aware of the feeding and oral-hygiene practices of caretakers. Parents who have been away from their children during the day often allow them to stay up later at night than parents did when they were young. This extends the time available for snacking, a habit learned from early demand-feeding practices. Grandparents have fewer grandchildren than one to two generations ago, so they have more time for each grandchild and can supply additional treats, especially if that is their favored means of communication with a developmentally disabled child. Parents must understand such complicated relationships and redirect the attention of grandparents to other means of pleasure for the child.

•   •   •

Pediatric dentistry has much to offer in the evaluation, diagnosis, prevention, and treatment of the developmentally disabled child. Oral care means much more than prevention and treatment of dental caries. Perhaps this extension is a natural outgrowth of a profession that has been overwhelmed by the volume of surgical services required to restore or remove decayed primary teeth. Perhaps as well, the private practice, noninstitutional nature of the specialty has been a factor that has inhibited other health care workers from seeking dental assistance. The increase in multidisciplinary teams that deal with feeding disorders, congenital anomalies, and chronic illnesses will facilitate the intercommunication of professionals and improve access of parents and caregivers to modern dental services as well. It is hoped that the multidisciplinary milieu will encourage more pediatric dentists to become skilled in the management and special needs of developmentally disabled children.

REFERENCES

1. Entwhistle BA, Casamassimo PS: Assessing dental health problems of children with developmental disabilities. *J Dev Behav Pediatr* 1981;2(2):115–121.

2. Kolvin J: Psychoses in childhood: A comparative study, in Rutter M (ed): *Infantile Autism: Concepts, Characteristics and Treatment.* London, Churchill Livingstone, 1971.

3. Kenny DJ, Somaya P: Sugar load of oral liquid medications in chronically ill children. *J Can Dent Assn;* in press.

4. Feigal RJ, Jensen ME, Mensing CA: Dental caries potential of liquid medications. *Pediatrics* 1981;68:416–419.

5. Sochaniwskyj AE, Koheil RM, Bablich K, et al: Oral motor functioning, frequency of swallowing and drooling in normal children and in children with cerebral palsy. *Arch Phys Med Rehabil* 1986;67:866–874.

6. Kleinberg I, Jenkins GN: The pH of dental plaques on the different areas of the mouth before and after meals and their relationship to the pH and rate of flow of resting saliva. *Arch Oral Biol* 1964;9:493–516.

7. Milnes AR, Bowden GH: The microflora associated with developing lesions of nursing caries, abstracted. *J Dent Res* 1988;67(spec):357.

8. Schneyer LH, Pigman W, Hanahan L, et al: Rate of flow of human parotid, sublingual and submaxillary secretions during sleep. *J Dent Res* 1956;35:109–114.

9. Little RM, Girgis SS, Masotti RE: Diphenylhydantoin-induced gingival hyperplasia; its response to changes in drug dosage. *Dev Med Child Neurol* 1975;17:421–424.

10. Levine NL: Injury to the primary dentition, in Levine NL (ed): *Symposium on Dentofacial Trauma.* Toronto, Saunders, 1982, pp 461–480.

11. Kenny DJ, Johnston DH, Bamba S: The composite resin short-post: A review of 625 teeth. *Ontario Dent* 1986;63(5):12–18.

12. Slavkin HC: Distas in developmental craniofacial biology, in Slavkin HC (ed): *Developmental Craniofacial Biology.* Philadelphia, Lea & Febiger, 1979, pp 10–54.

13. Takagi Y, McCalla JL, Bosma JF: Prone feeding of infants with Pierre Robin Syndrome. *Cleft Palate J* 1966;3:232–239.

14. Williams AC, Rothman BN, Seidman IH: Management of a feeding problem in an infant with cleft palate. *J Am Dent Assoc* 1968;77:81–83.

15. Prevention of bacterial endocarditis: A committee report of the American Heart Association. *J Am Dent Assoc* 1985;110:98–100.

16. Payne G, Smith S, MacColl S, et al: Examining the need for clinical prophylactic antibiotic coverage. *Ontario Dent* 1987;64(3):21–26.

17. Harris CS, Baker SP, Smith GA, et al: Childhood asphyxiation by food. A national analysis and overview. *JAMA* 1984;251:2231–2235.

18. Kenny DJ: A review of food asphyxiation mortality and admissions for non-fatal inhalations and accidental swallowing episodes. *INI In-Touch* 1985;3(2):1–3.

19. Mastication, in Dubner R, Sessle BJ, Storey AT (eds): *The Neural Basis of Oral and Facial Function.* New York, Plenum Press, 1978, pp 311–345.

20. McPherson KA: *Clinical evaluation and statistical analysis of ventilation and swallowing in cerebral palsy,* thesis. University of Toronto, Toronto, Canada, 1988.

21. Staff: Summary and recommendations, in *Foods and Choking in Children.* Evanston, Ill, American Academy of Pediatrics, 1983, pp n–q.

22. Blackman JA, Nelson CLA: Reinstituting oral feedings in children fed by gastrostomy tube. *Clin Pediatr* 1985;248):434–438.

23. Geertsma MA, Hyams JS, Pelletier JM, et al: Feeding resistance after parenteral hyperalimentation. *Am J Dis Child* 1985;139:255–256.

24. Dellow PG: The general physiological background of chewing and swallowing, in Sessle BJ, Hannam AJ (eds): *Mastication and Swallowing.* Toronto, University of Toronto Press, 1976, pp 6–21.

25. Rover BC, Morgano SM: Prevention of self-inflicted trauma: Dental intervention to prevent chronic lip chewing by a patient with a diagnosis of progressive bulbar palsy. *Spec Care Dent* 1988;8(1):37–39.

Understanding intraventricular hemorrhage and white-matter injury in premature infants

Yvonne E. Vaucher, MD
Associate Clinical Professor
University of California at San Diego
    School of Medicine
University of California at San Diego
    Medical Center
San Diego, California

PATHOGENESIS

Intraventricular hemorrhage

Intraventricular hemorrhage (IVH) was once thought to be an infrequent, catastrophic, and usually fatal complication of preterm birth. In 1978, based on computerized tomographic (CT) scanning of premature infants at risk, Papile et al[1] reported that IVH was actually quite common, as well as clinically inapparent, except in its most severe form. The availability of head ultrasound examination has further extended knowledge of the natural history of IVH, allowing a description of its time of onset, progression, resolution, and sequelae through serial bedside imaging performed at no risk to the infant.

Subsequent studies have confirmed initial reports that IVH occurs in approximately 40% to 45% of all preterm infants.[2-4] The risk of IVH is highest in the immediate perinatal period, with most bleeds occurring in the first three to four days after birth.[5] Extension of the initial hemorrhage is likewise greatest during this time. Prenatal ultrasound imaging of the fetal brain has confirmed that IVH may be antenatal in onset, occurring in utero days, weeks, or months prior to birth.[6,7] The incidence and severity of IVH are related to the degree of prematurity, with the smallest and most immature infants, especially those weighing less than 1,250 g and born at less than 30 weeks gestation, being at highest risk for IVH and for the most severe degree of bleeding as well.[8]

Hemorrhage is most likely to occur in the germinal matrix layer, which lies in the subependymal region above the roof of the lateral ventricles (Fig 1). In the premature infant, these blood vessels are relatively fragile, with little surrounding support. In addition, autoregulatory mechanisms controlling regional cerebral blood flow are presumed to be immature and inefficient in these infants.[8] As a consequence, too little or too much blood flow in the germinal matrix area may precipitate tissue injury and bleeding. Thus the primary clinical events associated with IVH are those that potentially alter cerebral blood flow substantially, such as shock, hypercarbia, pneumothorax, seizures, or volume expansion.[8]

Although it has been claimed that various pharmacologic agents, including phenobarbital, indomethacin, vitamin E, ethamsylate, and pancuronium bromide decrease the incidence or severity of IVH, evidence remains preliminary.[8] At present, the best preventive measure is to reduce the incidence of prematurity with

Inf Young Children 1988;1(2):31–45

its associated conditions, such as respiratory distress syndrome, which place the infant at high risk for hemorrhage.

Intraventricular hemorrhage continues to be classified largely by the method originally described by Papile et al[1] and depends on the size of the hemorrhage, the amount of blood in the ventricular system, and whether there is intraparenchymal involvement (Figs 1, 2). Grade I hemorrhage involves only small amounts of subependymal bleeding in the germinal matrix area without rupture of blood into the ventricles. A larger Grade II hemorrhage partially fills, but does not distend, the ventricular system with blood. A Grade III hemorrhage results when the ventricles are both filled with and dilated by blood. Grade IV hemorrhage is the most severe form, which results when bleeding extends into the adjacent brain parenchyma. Large amounts of blood within the ventricles form clots that are eventually resorbed very slowly over many weeks.

Fortunately, most premature infants have mild degrees (Grades I and II) of IVH.[9] These infants are usually asymptomatic, with hemorrhage being identified only by routine, cranial ultrasound examination. However, those with more severe Grades III and IV IVH are likely to present with acute deterioration at the time of bleeding, including apnea, bradycardia, shock, hyperglycemia, acidosis, electrolyte imbalance, and seizures. Despite the severity of the presentation, most of these infants will survive if given adequate metabolic, cardiovascular, and respiratory support.

Obstruction to the normal flow of cerebral spinal fluid ([CSF] posthemorrhagic hydrocephalus) may occur as a consequence of blood within the ventricular sys-

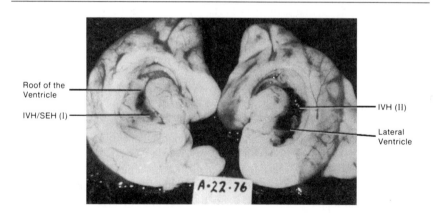

Roof of the Ventricle

IVH/SEH (I)

IVH (II)

Lateral Ventricle

A·22·76

Fig 1. A subependymal (Grade I) intraventricular hemorrhage (IVH/SEH) is present on the left. A Grade II hemorrhage is seen on the right where the blood has ruptured into, but does not fill, the lateral ventricle.

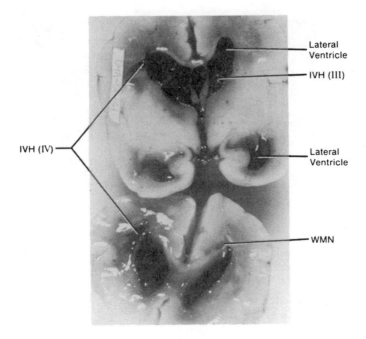

Fig 2. A Grade III hemorrhage has filled and distended the ventricular system with blood in the upper section on the right. An intraparenchymal extension of the hemorrhage (Grade IV) on the left is associated with white-matter necrosis (WMN). Another area of WMN without hemorrhage is present in the bottom section on the right.

tem when clots, protein, and red-blood-cell debris clog either the narrow passages within the ventricular system itself or the small reabsorptive channels over the surface of the brain (Fig 3).[10,11] Obstruction may be partial and subacute, with slow progression of ventricular enlargement and an insidious onset of clinical symptoms, or complete, with acute and rapid distention of the ventricular system associated with marked increases in intraventricular pressure, an inappropriate increase in head circumference, and life-threatening symptoms. Infants may present with apnea and bradycardia, hypertension, lethargy, irritability, and vomiting.

The initial therapy for posthemorrhagic hydrocephalus is palliative, with intermittent drainage of spinal fluid by serial lumbar punctures to temporarily relieve increased intraventricular pressure and alleviate symptoms while awaiting the spontaneous resolution of the obstructive process. Lumbar puncture effectively relieves increased intraventricular pressure if the obstruction is external to the

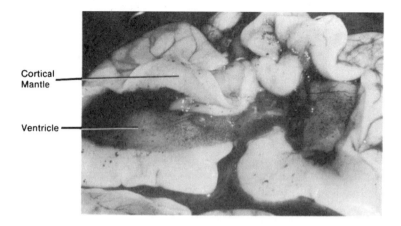

Cortical
Mantle

Ventricle

Fig 3. A severe IVH has resulted in posthemorrhagic hydrocephalus with marked ventricular dilatation and thinning of the overlying cortical mantle. The CSF filling the ventricular system contains residual cellular debris from the resolving hemorrhage.

ventricular system itself, thus allowing decompression of CSF from below. Obstruction to CSF flow within the ventricular system itself necessitates drainage from above with repeated ventricular taps or placement of a temporary drainage tube (ventriculostomy) directly into the ventricles. Over a period of several weeks, blood and protein are gradually cleared from the CSF. If CSF flow is no longer obstructed, ventricular size stabilizes and slowly returns to normal. When the surrounding white matter has been damaged, the ventricles remain enlarged; but without evidence of increased pressure, no further intervention or fluid drainage is necessary (Fig 4).[12]

Some infants with posthemorrhagic hydrocephalus will eventually require an alternative, permanent means of CSF drainage to control intraventricular pressure.[13] Permanent diversion of CSF is accomplished by inserting shunt tubing into the lateral ventricles, the major site of CSF production, with the distal end tunneled beneath the skin to drain into the abdominal cavity where the CSF can be easily reabsorbed. The remaining ventricular system and the areas of resorption over the brain are thus bypassed. Since the presence of a ventriculoperitoneal (VP) shunt seems to irrevocably alter the dynamics of CSF flow, placement is delayed until the permanent need for artificial drainage appears certain. The possibility of VP shunt obstruction and infection remain lifelong problems for the infant. Complete obstruction causes an acute increase in intraventricular and intracranial pressure, which, if unrecognized and not immediately relieved, will result in death. The placement of a foreign body, such as shunt tubing within the central nervous system, substantially increases the risk of bacterial infection within the brain. In-

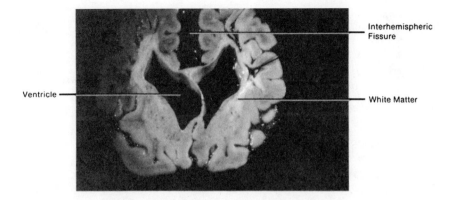

Fig 4. The chronic stage of ventricular dilatation associated with brain atrophy rather than increased pressure is shown here. Markedly enlarged ventricles are surrounded by gliotic scar tissue in the periventricular white matter. Diminished brain volume has resulted in a widened, enlarged interhemispheric fissure.

fection is not only life threatening, but may also have devastating long-term consequences as a result of additional brain damage. The presence of a VP shunt thus requires constant vigilance by family and medical caretakers to detect the earliest and most subtle signs of obstruction or infection.

White-matter necrosis

As the imaging capability of intraventricular ultrasound has improved, additional types of neonatal brain injury to the periventricular white matter, usually too small to be seen on CT scan, have become apparent.[14-16] These areas of white-matter necrosis (WMN) correspond pathologically to periventricular leukomalacia (PVL), literally the loss of white matter surrounding the ventricles. This pathologic abnormality, first described in the brains of preterm infants who died several months after birth, is characterized by necrosis and residual scarring of white matter (Fig 5).[17-19] WMN or PVL can involve frontal, parietal, or occipital areas. The most common site of WMN is at the angle of the lateral ventricles in the region of the corticospinal motor tracts (Fig 6). Damage here is thought to be responsible for spastic diplegia, a form of cerebral palsy seen more often in preterm infants. In contrast, parietal-occipital involvement in the region of the opticothalamic radiations would be expected to result in some type of visual impairment.

As with IVH, serial, bedside, cranial ultrasound examinations have allowed description of the incidence, development, and resolution of WMN in surviving

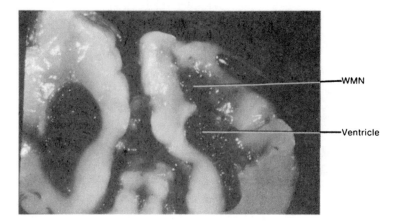

Fig 5. A large area of hemorrhagic WMN is seen communicating with the distended, blood-filled, right lateral ventricle.

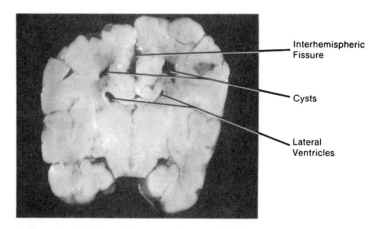

Fig 6. Fluid-filled cysts have replaced the acute white-matter injury at the angle of the lateral ventricles bilaterally. Cysts are surrounded by gliotic scar and do not communicate with the lateral ventricles.

preterm infants.[20] WMN is fairly common, occurring in 15% to 20% of all prematures.[21] In many cases, white-matter injury occurs prior to birth, with the highest antenatal incidence in the smallest and most immature infants.[22,23] WMN can be seen in conjunction with hemorrhage (Fig 5). In fact, the most severe IVH (Grade IV) usually results from secondary hemorrhage into preexisting areas of

WMN, rather than the extension of bleeding into adjacent normal white matter.[24-26]

The ultrasonographic and pathologic evolution of PVL or WMN initially includes an area of echodensity within the white matter, which corresponds to edema, vascular congestion, or tissue necrosis (Fig 7). These echodensities gradually resolve as necrotic white matter is resorbed and removed by scavenger cells (macrophages). Necrotic areas are replaced by fluid-filled cavitations lined by glial scar tissue, which, if large enough, appears on ultrasound as echolucent cysts in the formerly echodense area (Fig 8).[14,23] These cavitations may be small or large, single or multiple, unilateral or bilateral, depending on the extent of the injury (Fig 9). Sometimes very echogenic areas persist for several weeks, but never proceed to definite cavitation. These may represent cystic changes too small to be seen by current ultrasound technology.[23,27] Ultimately, after several months, the cystic changes and echodense areas disappear, and the ultrasound appearance of the brain may return to normal. On direct examination, however, areas of white-matter loss and gliotic scarring remain evident.[19]

Persistent enlargement of the lateral ventricles (ventriculomegaly) occurs if there has been sufficient destruction of surrounding periventricular white matter (Fig 4).[20] Large areas of WMN may communicate with the lateral ventricle, producing an irregular outpouching of the ventricle (porencephalic cyst). Greater degrees of white-matter injury will result in generalized brain atrophy, characterized on ultrasound by an increased width of the subarachnoid space and intrahemisphere fissure, in addition to ventriculomegaly (Fig 10). Destruction or injury of white matter leads to a loss of myelin (the protective sheath surrounding the axons of individual neurons) or a delay in the deposition of myelin by supporting cells in the affected region of the brain. Delay in the rate of white-matter myelination, which is most abnormal in the area of greatest white-matter injury, is best seen by nuclear magnetic resonance (NMR) imaging.[20]

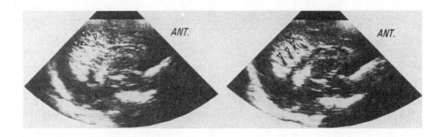

Fig 7. Sagittal sections illustrate the evolution of WMN (arrows), as seen by serial cranial ultrasound with multiple cavitations developing over a one- to two-week period within the echodense area above the roof of the posterior lateral ventricles.

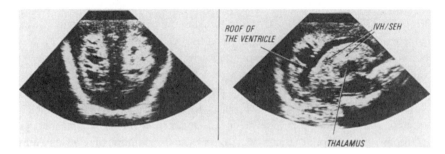

Fig 8. Multiple fluid-filled cysts are seen within an echodense area on a coronal section in the left-hand panel. On the right, multiple cavitations are coalescing to form a large porencephalic cyst in communication with the roof of the lateral ventricle. A Grade I SEH is also present.

WMN or PVL is thought to result from lack of blood and oxygen as a consequence of critically diminished blood flow to susceptible areas in the brain. The periventricular area is particularly sensitive to ischemic injury, probably because the blood vessels in this subcortical region are the most distal branches of the arterial system. Hence, a relatively mild and short-term insult can produce small areas of focal periventricular white-matter injury. A more profound and prolonged decrease in blood flow results in widespread damage, which, if severe enough, leads to destruction of cortical grey matter as well.

Whereas IVH appears to be the most common lesion in extremely preterm infants under 30 weeks gestation, WMN or PVL occurs more frequently than IVH in the infant over 32 weeks gestation. Prenatal factors associated with WMN include evidence of maternal chorioamnionitis and placental vascular anastomosis in twin gestations.[28] Perinatal and postnatal factors associated with WMN include birth asphyxia, placental abruption, hypercarbia, pneumothorax, patent ductus arteriosus, and sepsis. Each of these events may be accompanied by acute changes in cerebral blood flow, which could result in ischemic injury to areas within the brain susceptible to low blood flow.

Infants with WMN are usually asymptomatic in the neonatal period, even when fairly extensive areas are involved, unless there is concomitant hemorrhage and increased intraventricular pressure. Therefore, WMN may not be recognized unless carefully sought on routine ultrasound scan in all preterm infants at risk for the problem. Sometimes even large areas of WMN are identified only incidentally by ultrasound prior to nursery discharge. WMN is relatively insensitive to detection by CT scanning unless cavitations are very large or tissue necrosis is very diffuse.[29] Cavitations are better seen with NMR imaging, although the usefulness of this technique is limited by expense as well as the lack of portability. Abnormal electrical activity emanating from areas of periventricular white-matter damage

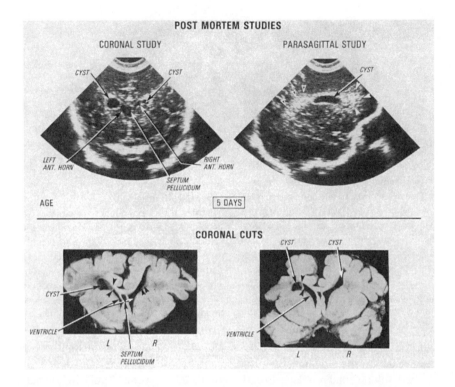

Fig 9. The correspondence between ultrasound and autopsy examination is shown in an infant with well-established, bilateral, cystic WMN. Reprinted with permission from Bejar R, Cohen R, Merritt TA, et al: Focal necrosis of the white matter (periventricular leukomalacia): Sonographic, pathologic, and electroencephalographic features. *J Neurosurg* 1986;7:1077. Copyright by the American Society of Neuroradiology, 1986.

---

may be present on EEG. These discharges, known as positive rolandic or central sharp waves, appear shortly after acute, white-matter injury and subsequently disappear during the chronic phase.[30]

NEURODEVELOPMENTAL OUTCOME

Intraventricular hemorrhage

Approximately 10% to 15% of all very low birth-weight (<1,500 g), preterm infants have significant neuromotor abnormalities (cerebral palsy) in early infancy, with the risk being highest in the smallest, most immature infants.[31-33] A similar incidence of cerebral palsy is seen in infants with mild degrees of hemor-

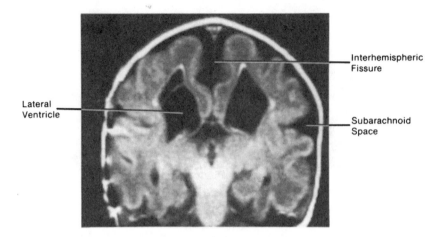

Interhemispheric Fissure

Lateral Ventricle

Subarachnoid Space

Fig 10. Cerebral atrophy is evident on this MRI scan, with an enlarged subarachnoid space surrounding the brain, widened intrahemispheric fissure, and ventricular dilatation. This infant sustained an intraventricular catastrophe in utero following the death of the monozygotic cotwin.

rhage (Grades I-II), as well as in those without IVH. Thus minor amounts of intraventricular bleeding do not seem to be associated with an increased risk of major neurodevelopmental problems in early childhood. The incidence of cerebral palsy and significant developmental delay is clearly higher, however, in those with more severe hemorrhage, such as Grade III (30% to 40%) or Grade IV (75% to 100%), with parenchymal involvement.[34-36] Persistent ventriculomegaly following IVH, even when not associated with increased intraventricular pressure and hydrocephalus, also increases the risk of neurologic abnormality.[3,37,38] Posthemorrhagic hydrocephalus requiring shunt placement is likewise associated with a poor neurodevelopmental prognosis, although even in this group, approximately 20% of infants have normal cognitive and motor development at 2 years of age.[39]

Approximately 15% of infants with IVH experience seizures in the neonatal period.[8] This complication is usually associated with severe hemorrhage (Grades III and IV) and most often occurs in the acute phase of bleeding. The subsequent risk of a seizure disorder requiring anticonvulsant therapy in childhood is unclear. Seizures in the neonatal period, when associated with posthemorrhagic hydrocephalus, are a prognostic sign for neuromotor abnormalities.[35,39]

Mild degrees of hemorrhage are associated with lower, although still normal, developmental scores at 2 years of age.[40] A recent study suggests that selective deficits in expressive-language function do occur even in infants with Grades I and II hemorrhage at 2 years of age.[41]

It is well known that developmental outcome between 2 and 7 years of age in very low birth-weight infants correlates best with parental education and socio-economic status rather than with conditions present at birth.[42] Hence it is not surprising that by 3 years of age, the cognitive outcome for most low birth-weight infants with IVH correlates better with socioeconomic status than with the grade of IVH.[40] On the other hand, children with marked cognitive delay are likely to have had severe hemorrhage and to have been the smallest and most immature at birth.[43]

Although scores from the Bayley Scales of Infant Development at 2 years of age do correlate with results of the Stanford Binet at 5 years, measurements of cognitive function in early infancy are preliminary at best.[44,45] Thus, more extensive psychologic and educational assessment are required at later ages to identify more subtle or isolated defects. Assessment at 5 years of age of infants with a history of IVH substantiates concern that even those with mild degrees of bleeding did sustain some CNS injury that was not evident on earlier testing. Scores of those with a history of IVH were lower on the McCarthy Scales of Children's Abilities when compared with infants of similar birth weight without IVH.[46] Specific deficits were seen in perceptual-motor, verbal, quantitative, and memory scales. Furthermore, according to Williams et al,[46] 76% of infants with a history of hemorrhage, compared with 23% of those without, had educational difficulties, with most requiring special-education intervention.

Thus, neurodevelopmental outcome in early childhood is related to the extent of the IVH. Although small bleeds do not result in major neurologic abnormalities, such as cerebral palsy, more subtle deficits do become apparent in time. Concomitant white-matter damage, such as porencephaly, ventriculomegaly, and atrophy, further increases the risk of poor outcome. Care must be exercised in using a normal neurodevelopmental assessment at 2 years of age to project normal cognitive outcome and academic accomplishment in later childhood. The apparent "normal" outcome of infants with mild degrees of hemorrhage at 2 years of age reflects, in large part, current inability to adequately assess cognitive function, which is itself immature, at this age. Caution is advised when counseling parents about future expectations when early neurodevelopmental evaluation at 2 years of age is without obvious sequelae.

White-matter necrosis

Adverse neuromotor outcome (ie, cerebral palsy) is more frequently associated with cystic WMN or PVL than with IVH.[47–49] Fawer et al[50] described the outcome in preterm survivors with normal neonatal ultrasound scans, IVH alone, or PVL with or without accompanying IVH. Developmental scores, assessed at 18 months of age, were significantly lower in those with PVL in comparison to infants with normal scans or IVH only. No major handicaps were noted in infants with normal scans or isolated IVH, whereas 33% of those with PVL had major handicaps, including cerebral palsy and significant developmental delay. Infants with frontal lesions only had normal neuromotor examinations and developmental quotients. In contrast, those infants with extensive lesions, particularly involving the frontal, lateral, and occipital areas, had significant neuromotor abnormalities, visual impairment, and severe developmental delay.

The author[51] found similar results in a cohort of preterm infants followed from 24 to 36 months of age. All infants with small anterior-frontal lesions had normal neurologic and developmental assessments at 24 months of age. Infants with large parietal lesions had normal cognitive function, significantly lower motor scores, and a higher incidence of motor delay, as well as strabismus compared with control infants or those with small anterior cysts. Infants with large anterior cavitations had severe spastic quadriparesis (Fig 11). Developmental outcome was unrelated to the grade of IVH or to whether the cavitations were prenatal or postnatal in onset.

Calvert et al[52] reported that 93% of infants with cystic periventricular lesions had some motor abnormality in infancy, including 40% with severe spastic quadriparesis and 53% with visual defects. Forty-seven percent had subnormal

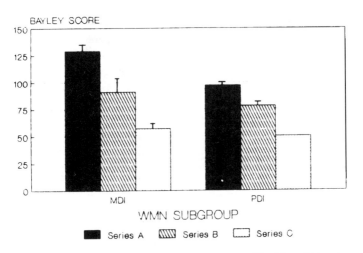

Fig 11. White-matter necrosis developmental outcome. The Mental Development Index (MDI) and Psychomotor Development Index (PDI) (X ± SEM) from the Bayley Scales of Infant Development for 11 infants with cystic WMN is shown. WMN was classified as follows: small frontal cavitations (Series A), large parietoccipital cavitations (Series B), or large anterior cavitations (Series C) (test mean ± SD: 100 ± 16).

intelligence at 5 years of age. Adverse outcome has also been associated with persistent periventricular echodensities,[53-55] with 60% to 75% of these infants having significant motor or cognitive problems at 24 to 60 months of age.

White-matter injury or PVL appears to be the principal brain lesion associated with major neuromotor, visual, and developmental abnormalities in infancy and childhood, with cystic WMN being a highly specific predictor of handicap. Neurodevelopmental outcome is variable, depending on the size and location of the cavitations. The poor outcome previously reported in association with Grade IV hemorrhage may in fact be secondary to the underlying white-matter injury that preceded intraparenchymal bleeding.

INTERVENTION

Because premature infants, especially those less than 1,500 g birth weight, have an increased risk of neurodevelopmental problems, including cerebral palsy, developmental delay, speech and language delay, perceptual-motor abnormalities, behavioral problems, and learning disabilities, much time and effort has been expended on neuromotor screening and early intervention programs. The assumption was that early detection and initiation of therapy would result in an improved prognosis.[56] However attractive this hypothesis, there is little evidence to show a substantial long-term difference in motor function, mental development, or neurologic examination during infancy between children who receive early physical therapy and those who do not.[57-60]

Several factors may relate to the failure of early neuromotor intervention programs to demonstrate improvement in outcome. First, there is no evidence that physical therapy per se changes the natural history of neuromotor development (ie, prevents cerebral palsy). Since only 10% to 15%[31-33] of all high-risk infants will, in fact, develop cerebral palsy and thus require physical therapy, intervention begun for all high-risk infants will treat 85% to 90% of all infants unnecessarily. At best, physical therapy could be expected to improve the outcome of only the small number of infants destined to develop neuromotor problems, although even this assumption has recently been questioned.[59] The most efficient and cost-effective way to provide physical therapy would be to preselect those infants shown to be at highest risk for cerebral palsy, such as those with multicystic WMN or large IVH, thus focusing effort on those infants most likely to benefit from the intervention. Second, many control infants do receive some sort of intervention either because problems develop or because families seek out resources in the community that might help their child. Third, while neonatal factors are the best predictors for outcome in infancy, parental education and socioeconomic status, rather than perinatal or neonatal factors, are the best predictors of outcome in later childhood.[56]

A modest beneficial effect of early "educational" intervention studies was reported in a recent analysis of selected intervention studies in which children were enrolled before 3 years of age.[61] After applying a correction factor that allowed interstudy comparison, the positive effect was identified in programs that provided a structured learning environment and emphasized extensive parental participation. Outcome results did not depend on the specific type or level of disability or on the age at enrollment.

The predominant effect of environment over biologic factors was again emphasized by Slater et al,[62] who compared the outcome at 35 months of age of high-risk, very low birthweight infants participating in a neurodevelopmental follow-up program with those who did not. While no difference was found in the incidence of cerebral palsy or neurologic abnormality, infants enrolled in follow-up had substantially better cognitive scores at 3 years, thought to reflect a better quality of maternal–child interaction as assessed by scales of psychosocial risk, stress, adaptability to change, and attitude toward parenting.

These findings suggest that early educational intervention might benefit more infants than early neuromotor intervention since the long-term positive effects of improved parenting skills and a structured curriculum on cognitive development have been shown at both 2 and 5 years.[60,63] Indeed, the emphasis on constructive parent-child interaction is the common thread that runs through most studies demonstrating any positive effect at all of early intervention. Thus improving the family's perception of and relationship with their individual child may be the critical factor in improving developmental outcome.

•   •   •

Intraventricular hemorrhage and white-matter injury are frequent neurologic sequelae of premature birth. Both are thought to be caused by changes in brain blood flow, which result in injury to either fragile blood vessels or to susceptible periventricular tissue. Most hemorrhages and white-matter injury are clinically silent in the perinatal period. Major neuromotor abnormalities in early childhood are more often associated with cystic WMN than with IVH. Long-term deleterious effects in cognitive function of varying degree appear to be quite common in both IVH and WMN. Infants with either problem identified in the neonatal period require close observation from birth through early school years in order to facilitate appropriate therapy and intervention.

REFERENCES

1. Papile LS, Burstein J, Burstein R, et al: Incidence and evolution of the subependymal intraventricular hemorrhage: A study of infants with weights less than 1,500 grams. *J Pediatr* 1978;92:529–534.

2. Ment LR, Scott DT, Ehrenkranz RA, et al: Neonates of 1,250 grams birth weight. Prospective neurodevelopmental evaluation during the first year post-term. *Pediatrics* 1982;70:292–296.

3. Shankaran S, Slovis TL, Bedard MP, et al: Sonographic classification of intracranial hemorrhage. A prognostic indicator of mortality, morbidity and short-term neurologic outcome. *J Pediatr* 1982;100:469–475.

4. Ahmann PA, Lazzara A, Dykes FD, et al: Intraventricular hemorrhage in the high risk preterm infant: Incidence and outcome. *Ann Neurol* 1980;7:118–124.

5. Perlman JM, Volpe JJ: Cerebral blood flow velocity in relation to intraventricular hemorrhage in the premature newborn infant. *J Pediatr* 1982;100:956–959.

6. Sims ME, Turkel SB, Halterman G, et al: Brain injury and intrauterine death. *Am J Obstet Gynecol* 1985;151:721–723.

7. Pretorius DH, Singh S, Manco-Johnson ML, et al: In utero diagnosis of intracranial hemorrhage resulting in fetal hydrocephalus: A case report. *J Reprod Med* 1986;31:136–138.

8. Ment LR, Duncan CC, Ehrenkranz RA: Intraventricular hemorrhage of the preterm neonate. *Semin Perinatol* 1987;11:132–141.

9. Papile LS, Munsick-Bruno G, Schaefer A: Relationship of cerebral intraventricular hemorrhage and early childhood neurologic handicaps. *J Pediatr* 1983;103:273–277.

10. Ment LR, Duncan CC, Scott DT, et al: Posthemorrhagic hydrocephalus: Low incidence in very low birth weight neonates with intraventricular hemorrhage. *J Neurosurg* 1984;60:343–347.

11. Allan WC, Holt PJ, Sawyer LR, et al: Ventricular dilation after neonatal periventricular-intraventricular hemorrhage. Natural history and therapeutic implications. *AmJ Dis Child* 1982;136:589–593.

12. Levene MI, Starte DR: A longitudinal study of post-haemorrhagic ventricular dilatation in the newborn. *Arch Dis Child* 1981;56:905–910.

13. James HE, Bejar R, Gluck L, et al: Ventriculoperitoneal shunts in high risk newborns weighing under 2,000 grams: A clinical report. *Neurosurgery* 1984;15:198–202.

14. Bejar R, Coen RW, Merritt TA, et al: Focal necrosis of the white matter (periventricular leukomalacia): Sonographic, pathologic, and electroencephalographic features. *J Neurosurg* 1986;7:1073–1080.

15. Sinha SK, Sims DG, Davies JM, et al: Relation between periventricular haemorrhage and ischaemic brain lesions diagnosed by ultrasound in very preterm infants. *Lancet* 1985;2:1154–1156.

16. Chow PP, Horgan JG, Taylor KJW: Neonatal periventricular leukomalacia: Real-time sonographic diagnosis with CT correlation. *J Neurosurg* 1985;145:155–160.

17. Trounce JQ, Fagan D, Levene MI: Intraventricular haemorrhage and periventricular leucomalacia: Ultrasound and autopsy correlation. *Arch Dis Child* 1986;61:1203–1207.

18. Shuman RM, Selednik LJ: Periventricular leukomalacia: A one-year autopsy study. *Arch Neurol* 1980;37:231–235.

19. DeReuckJ, Chattha AS, Richardson EP Jr: Pathogenesis and evolution of periventricular leukomalacia in infancy. *Arch Neurol* 1972;27:229–236.

20. Dubowitz LMS, Bydder GM, Mushin J: Developmental sequence of periventricular leukomalacia. *Arch Dis Child* 1985;60:349–355.

21. Allare M, Bejar R, Wozniak P, et al: White matter necrosis (WMN) in premature infants: Perinatal factors. *Pediatr Res* 1986;20(4):1081.

22. Behar RF, Vaucher YE, Coen RW: Epidemiology of white matter necrosis in preterm infants. *Pediatr Res* 1987;21(4):1308.

23. Fawer C-L, Calame A, Perentes E, et al: Periventricular leukomalacia: A correlation study between realtime ultrasound and autopsy findings. Periventricular leukomalacia in the neonate. *Neuroradiology* 1985;27:292–300.

24. Armstrong DL, Sauls CS, Goddard-Finegold J: Neuropathologic findings in short-term survivors of intraventricular hemorrhage. *Am J Dis Child* 1987;141:617–621.

25. Rushton DI, Preston PR, Durbin GM: Structure and evolution of echo dense lesions in the neonatal brain. A combined ultrasound and necropsy study. *Arch Dis Child* 1985;60:798–808.

26. Hill A, Melson GL, Clark HB, et al: Hemorrhagic periventricular leukomalacia: Diagnosis by real time ultrasound and correlation with autopsy findings. *Pediatrics* 1982;69:282–284.

27. Guzetta F, Shackelford GD, Volpe S, et al: Periventricular intraparenchymal echodensities in the premature newborn: Critical determinant of neurologic outcome. *Pediatrics* 1986;78:995–1006.

28. Bejar R, Wozniak P, Allare M, et al: Antenatal origin of neurologic damage in newborn infants. *Am J Obstet Gynecol*, in press.

29. Schellinger D, Grant EG, Richardson JD: Cystic periventricular leukomalacia: Sonographic and CT findings. *Am J Neurol Res* 1984;5:439–445.

30. Novotny EJ Jr, Tharp BR, Coen RW, et al: Positive rolandic sharp waves in the EEG of the premature infant. *Neurology* 1987;37:1481–1486.

31. Kitchen W, Ford G, Orgill A, et al: Outcome in infants with birth weight 500 to 999 gm: A regional study of 1979 and 1980 births. *J Pediatr* 1984;104:921–927.

32. Kitchen WH, Rickards AL, Ryan MM, et al: Improved outcome to two years of very low-birthweight infants: Fact or artifact? *Dev Med Child Neurol* 1986;28:479–588.

33. Saigal S, Rosenbaum P, Stoskopf B, et al: Outcome in infants 501 to 1,000 gm birth weight delivered to residents of the McMaster Health Region. *J Pediatr* 1984;105:969–976.

34. Papile LA, Munsick-Bruno G, Schaefer A: Relationship of cerebral intraventricular hemorrhage and early childhood neurologic handicaps. *J Pediatr* 1983;103:273–277.

35. Cooke RWI: Early prognosis of low birthweight infants treated for progressive posthaemorrhagic hydrocephalus. *Arch Dis Child* 1983;58:410–414.

36. Ment LR, Scott DT, Ehrenkranz RA, et al: Neurodevelopmental assessment of very low birth weight neonates: Effect of germinal, matrix and intraventricular hemorrhage. *Pediatr Neurol* 1985;1:164–168.

37. Palmer P, Dubowit LM, Levene MI, et al: Developmental and neurological progress of preterm infants with intraventricular haemorrhage and ventricular dilatation. *Arch Dis Child* 1982;57:748–753.

38. Allan WC, Dransfield DA, Tito AM: Ventricular dilation following periventricular-intraventricular hemorrhage: Outcome at age 1 year. *Pediatrics* 1984;73:158–162.

39. Boynton BR, Boynton CA, Merritt TA, et al: Ventriculoperitoneal shunts in low birth weight infants with intracranial hemorrhage: Neurodevelopmental outcome. *Neurosurgery* 1986;18:141.

40. TeKolste KA, Bennett FC, Mack LA: Follow-up of infants receiving cranial ultrasound for intracranial hemorrhage. *Am J Dis Child* 1985;139:299–303.

41. Janowsky JS, Nass R: Early language development in infants with cortical and subcortical perinatal brain injury. *J Dev Behav Pediatr* 1987;8:3–7.

42. Scott DT: Premature infants in later childhood: Some recent follow-up results. *Semin Perinatol* 1987;11(2):191–199.

43. Williamson WD, Desmond MM, Wilson GS, et al: Survival of low-birth weight infants with neonatal intraventricular hemorrhage. *Am J Dis Child* 1983;137:1181–1184.

44. Ware J, Schnell RR: Cognitive assessment, in Taeusch HW, Yogman MW (eds): *Follow-up Management of the High-Risk Infant.* Boston, Little, Brown, 1987, pp 135–148.

45. Sivan AB: Measures of general intellectual development, in Wolraich ML (ed): *The Practical Assessment and Management of Children with Disorders of Development and Learning.* Chicago, Year Book, 1987, pp 85–95.

46. Williams ML, Lewandowski LJ, Coplan J, et al: Neurodevelopmental outcome of preschool children born preterm with and without intracranial hemorrhage. *Dev Med Child Neurol* 1987;29:243–249.

47. DeVries LS, Dubowitz V, Larry S, et al: Predictive value of cranial ultrasound in the newborn baby: A reappraisal. *Lancet* 1985;2:137–140.

48. Graham M, Trounce JQ, Levene MI, et al: Prediction of cerebral palsy in very low birthweight infants: Prospective ultrasound study. *Lancet* 1987;2: 593–596.

49. Low JA, Galbraith RS, Sauerbrei EE, et al: Motor and cognitive development of infants with intraventricular hemorrhage, ventriculomegaly, or periventricular parenchymal lesions. *Am J Obstet Gynecol* 1986;155:750–756.

50. Fawer CL, Diebold P, Calame A: Periventricular leucomalacia and neurodevelopmental outcome in preterm infants. *Arch Dis Child* 1987;62:30–36.

51. Vaucher YE, Bejar RF, Jones BL, et al: Early developmental outcome with cavitary white matter necrosis (WMN). *Pediatr Res* 1987;21:1389.

52. Calvert SA, Hoskins EM, Fong KW, et al: Periventricular leukomalacia: Ultrasonic diagnosis and neurological outcome. *Acta Paediatr Scand* 1986;75:489–496.

53. McMenamin JB, Shackelford GD, Volpe JJ: Outcome of neonatal intraventricular hemorrahge with periventricular echodense lesions. *Ann Neurol* 1984;15:285–290.

54. Guzzetta F, Shackelford GD, Volpe S, et al: Periventricular intraparenchymal echodensities in the premature newborn: Critical determinant of neurologic outcome. *Pediatrics* 1986;78:995–1006.

55. Stewart AL, Reynolds EOR, Hope PL, et al: Probability of neurodevelopmental disorders estimated from ultrasound appearance of brains of very preterm infants. *Dev Med Child Neurol* 1987;29:3–11.

56. Scott DT: Premature Infants in later childhood: Some recent follow-up results. *Semin Perinatol* 1987;11(2):191–199.

57. Goodman M, Rothberg AD, Houston-McMillan JE, et al: Effect of early neurodevelopmental therapy in normal and at-risk survivors of neonatal intensive care. *Lancet* 1985;2:1327–1330.

58. Scherzer AL, Mike V, Ilson J: Physical therapy as a determinant of change in the cerebral palsied infant. *Pediatrics* 1976;58:47–52.

59. Palmer FB, Shapiro BK, Wachtel RC, et al: The effects of physical therapy on cerebral palsy: A controlled trial in infants with spastic diplegia. *N Engl J Med* 1988;318:803–808.

60. Piper MC, Kunos VI, Willis DM, et al: Early physical therapy effects on the high-risk infant: A randomized controlled trial. *Pediatrics* 1986;78:216–224.

61. Shonkoff JP, Hauser-Cram P: Early intervention for disabled infants and their families: A quantitative analysis. *Pediatrics* 1987;80:650–658.

62. Slater MA, Naqvi M, Andrew L, et al: Neurodevelopment of monitored versus nonmonitored very low birth weight infants: The importance of family influences. *J Dev Behav Pediatr* 1987;8:278–285.

63. Resnick MB, Eyler FD, Nelson RM, et al: Developmental Intervention for low birth weight infants: Improved early developmental outcome. *Pediatrics* 1987;80:68–74.

Comprehensive management of the infant with bronchopulmonary dysplasia: A growing challenge

Mary Ellen A. Bozynski, MD, MS
Assistant Professor of Pediatrics
Department of Pediatrics, Section of
 Newborn Services
University of Michigan Medical
 Center
Ann Arbor, Michigan

BRONCHOPULMONARY dysplasia (BPD) was first described by Northway, Rosen, and Porter[1] in 1967 in a group of premature infants recovering from severe hyaline membrane disease or respiratory distress syndrome (RDS). The diagnosis was based on the observation using radiographs of a series of bronchopulmonary changes that appeared in four stages. Stage I (days 2 and 3 of life) was indistinguishable from RDS. Stage II (days 4 through 10 of life) consisted of opacification of the lung fields and was difficult to distinguish from resolving RDS or the presence of a patent ductus arteriosus. In Stage III (days 10 through 20 of life), multiple radiolucencies were seen; and in Stage IV (more than one month of life), radiographs showed areas of incomplete expansion (atelectasis) and hyperinflation.

Since the original description of BPD, however, modern neonatal intensive care has created a growing number of infants with chronic lung disease. Often these infants exhibit neither severe RDS nor the characteristic sequence of changes described above.[2] In particular, many extremely low birth weight infants have an insidious onset of disease, with slowly increasing requirements for oxygen and ventilatory support that appear after an initial period of clinical improvement. Lack of agreement on a new definition of BPD has led to confusion in determining the epidemiology of BPD and in conducting and evaluating related research.[3]

Since detection by radiographs alone appears inadequate and may allow cases to be undetected or misdiagnosed, other clinically based definitions have been proposed.[4] The most widely used of these is that of Bancalari and associates,[5] which includes a requirement for mechanical ventilation in the first three days of life, clinical signs that persist for more than 28 days, a need for supplemental oxygen for more than 28 days to maintain adequate oxygenation, and a chest radiograph consistent with chronic lung disease. Toce and coworkers[6] have suggested the use of a scoring system applied at 21 days of age that combines a history of oxygen or mechanical ventilation with signs of respiratory distress, blood gas measurements, and radiograph confirmation of chronic lung disease.

In addition to the lack of a widely accepted definition of BPD, the incidence and prevalence of the disease have been imprecisely measured because the population at risk has not been well defined. Although the majority of infants with BPD are premature, full-term infants with meconium aspiration, neonatal pneumonia, or other causes of severe respiratory distress may develop BPD. In addition, infants

Inf Young Children 1989;2(1):14–24
© 1989 Aspen Publishers, Inc.

with a family history of reactive airway disease and those with tissue type HLA-A2 are at higher risk.[7–9]

What is clear, however, is that BPD is a significant and growing medical problem with a current estimated annual prevalence of 3,100 cases and a cost of $25 million per year for the initial care of new cases.[3] The cost of care for children with ongoing respiratory or related disorders is currently unknown.

PATHOGENESIS

BPD is a consequence both of lung injury and of repair. Oxygen toxicity and injury from positive pressure ventilation (barotrauma) are both causes; however, other factors, especially prematurity, have also been implicated (see box, "Risk Factors for Bronchopulmonary Dysplasia"). The debate as to whether oxygen or barotrauma is more important in causality continues.[10]

Lung injury is pervasive, affecting all elements of the lung and airways.[11] Oxygen damages the lining cells of the pulmonary capillaries, which then leak fluid into the interstitial spaces.[12,13] Neutrophils, a type of white blood cell, respond to the inflammation and release substances that cause further damage.[14] Injury to the lining cells of the airways results in the production of excessive and abnormal mucous. The loss of cilia, which help to remove mucous, interferes with mucous removal and contributes to blocking the airways. Stimulation of receptors in the airway causes spasm, thickening, and chronic reduction in airway diameter.[15,16]

Type 1 cells, which cover 80% of the surface of the alveoli (air sacs), are also damaged.[17] Hyperplasia of type 2 cells is triggered when type 2 cells attempt to replace damaged type 1 cells. Injury reduces the number of functioning alveoli due to atelectasis or collapse. Hyperinflated (emphysematous) areas occur because of alveolar coalescence following the loss of their cell wall integrity. Other factors may also be important.[18–22]

Risk Factors for Bronchopulmonary Dysplasia

Pulmonary immaturity
Exposure to increased oxygen concentrations
Barotrauma
Intubation
Persistent patent ductus arteriosus
Pulmonary edema
Pulmonary interstitial emphysema or air leak
Family history of reactive airway disease
Tissue type HLA-A2
Vitamin A deficiency

Surfactant, produced by the type 2 cell, plays a role in the protection of the lung by lowering surface tension. This protects the type 2 cell from oxygen injury and plays a part in pulmonary defense mechanisms. With a loss of surfactant production due to type 2 cell injury, alveolar surface tension rises, causing alveolar collapse. The resultant hypoxemia (low blood oxygen level) leads to increased resistance to blood flow to the lung, fluid leakage into the lung, thickening of the interstitium, inflammation, and an accumulation of fluid in the alveoli.[15]

The extent to which the various lung components will heal is unknown. Fibrosis is a dominant feature, and a generally favorable prognosis is largely due to the fact that lung development, especially of the alveoli, continues after birth.[11,23]

DIAGNOSIS

Clinical and laboratory findings

The most common finding in the infant with BPD is an increased respiratory rate (tachypnea). Respiratory distress involving intercostal retractions, nasal flaring, and an increased anteroposterior diameter of the chest (barrel chest) is seen. Auscultation may reveal wheezing, rhonchi, or rales.[5,6]

Infants with severe BPD who require prolonged ventilatory support often have cyanotic (blue) spells during which they are difficult to ventilate. Although these episodes are common, their pathophysiology is not understood.

Blood gas determination typically shows increased Pco_2 and/or decreased Po_2 with resulting acidosis. Noninvasive oxygen saturation monitoring is of great value, especially in the management of oxygen therapy.[24]

Radiographic findings

The chest radiograph of the infant with moderate to severe BPD reveals a flattened diaphragm, areas of atelectasis and hyperinflation, and, in severe cases, an enlarged heart (cardiomegaly). By contrast, radiographic findings in the infant with mild BPD may show only streakiness with mild hyperaeration and atelectasis. Edwards[2] developed a radiographic scoring system for BPD that was used in conjunction with the BPD scoring system suggested by Toce and associates.[6] Edwards[2] has also correlated radiographic staging with pathologic findings at autopsy.

Pulmonary function studies

The common findings on pulmonary function studies include increased resistance to airflow, decreased compliance (increased stiffness) of the lung, and signs of airway obstruction. Increased work of breathing and increased oxygen consumption are also common.

Cardiovascular evaluation

The infant with severe BPD is at risk for pulmonary hypertension and heart failure secondary to lung disease (cor pulmonale).[25] Pulmonary hypertension appears to be the consequence of both constriction of the blood vessels due to low blood oxygen and structural remodelling of the damaged pulmonary bed.[26] Cardiovascular status can be assessed using the electrocardiogram (ECG), noninvasive echocardiography, and cardiac catheterization in some cases. The ECG in severe BPD may show evidence of heart strain or thickening of the walls due to difficulty in pumping blood to the lung because of increased resistance. Echocardiography is used to evaluate pulmonary vascular resistance. In selected cases, cardiac catheterization may be useful to rule out structural heart disease, which can masquerade as BPD or contribute to its severity, and to monitor the response to oxygen therapy and pharmacologic intervention.[27,28]

COMPLICATIONS OF BPD

The infant with BPD may have a number of other medical problems (see box, "Problems Associated with Bronchopulmonary Dysplasia") due to BPD itself or as a complication of its therapy.

Infection

Infants with BPD are at high risk for recurrent lower respiratory infection and sepsis. Those infants with severe disease who receive prolonged mechanical ven-

---

Problems Associated with Bronchopulmonary Dysplasia

Infection
Reactive airway disease
Central airway lesions (eg, tracheomalacia)
Feeding problems
Gastroesophageal reflux
Poor growth
Behavioral disorders
Family stress
Nephrocalcinosis
Osteopenia
Hypertension

tilation and hospitalization are also at risk for fungal infections, especially systemic candidiasis, and for viral infections due to cytomegalovirus or respiratory syncytial virus.[29]

In addition, there is an increased incidence of recurrent otitis media (ear infection) in infants with a history of mechanical ventilation.[30] Oxygen injury to the cells lining the middle ear may contribute to its pathogenesis.[15] Chronic otitis during infancy and early childhood may cause conductive hearing loss and subsequent poor language development. Parents are often unaware of the otitis infection. It is important to examine the ears of the infant with BPD at every opportunity and to verify that infection has been completely resolved. Referral to an ear specialist and placement of tympanotomy tubes may be indicated. If an infant has a speech delay, a thorough evaluation of the ears and hearing is indicated. If the problem is long standing, the infant may benefit from speech therapy. Usually a rapid catch-up is seen.

Nephrocalcinosis

Renal stones have been noted in infants with BPD in association with diuretic therapy, especially furosemide (Lasix).[31] Because increased calcium excretion in the urine may cause stone formation, the concurrent use of a thiazide diuretic is advised. The long-term outcome of nephrocalcinosis is unknown. The lesions are more commonly noted in premature infants and are best diagnosed by ultrasonography.[32]

Osteopenia

Many infants who develop BPD are born extremely prematurely, are unable to tolerate oral feedings, receive prolonged parenteral alimentation, and are given diuretics. Often this results in osteopenia, or fragile, poorly mineralized bones.[33] Other factors may also be operative.[34] Many infants with BPD have osteopenia and sustain fractures of the ribs and long bones. Feedings of formula containing higher calcium and phosphorus content and the use of fortifiers if the infant receives human milk are advised.[35]

Tracheal stenosis, tracheomalacia, or tracheobronchomalacia

The development of tracheal stenosis (narrowing) has been related to the size of the endotracheal tube, to trauma, and to the presence of infection. Tracheomalacia and enlargement of other airways, with collapse on expiration, may also be seen.[2] These lesions may be insidious and result in prolonged intubation because of failed attempts to extubate the infant. In some cases, the diagnosis is made after discharge from the hospital. The infant may have stridor, an abnormal cry, swallowing difficulties, and marked respiratory distress with minor respiratory illnesses.

The optimal time to perform a tracheostomy on an infant with BPD and long-term ventilator dependance is unknown. Since infants with tracheostomies have feeding and speech problems, an occupational therapist or physical therapist, as well as a speech-language pathologist, should join the multidisciplinary team treating the infant. Simon[36] has recently described the role of the speech-language pathologist in caring for the infant with a tracheostomy. This role includes education of parents and other caregivers in proper language stimulation techniques and the use of nonvocal alternative methods of communication.

Gastroesophageal reflux

Infants with BPD have an increased incidence of feeding problems, including gastroesophageal reflux. The reflux may be silent or may present with pneumonia or worsening of the pulmonary status. Diagnosis may be made radiographically and with the use of a pH probe. Treatment therapies include positioning, smaller feedings of thickened foods, and, when delayed gastric emptying complicates the problem, metoclopramide.[15]

Poor growth

The etiology of growth failure in infants with BPD is multifactorial. When correction is made for birth weight, much of the difference between infants with and without BPD disappears.[37] A subgroup of infants with severe BPD, however, has prolonged growth failure due to increased caloric requirements; intolerance to increased fluid volumes or to formulas of increased caloric density; and behavior such as irritability, decreased tolerance to stress, vomiting, and gastroesophageal reflux. The increased caloric requirement in these infants is not solely caused by increased work of breathing and oxygen consumption; other abnormalities (eg, altered substrate utilization, impaired intermediary metabolism) may also contribute to growth failure.[15,38] Later feeding problems include poor tolerance for spoon feeding and for different food textures.

Disturbed family functioning

Prolonged hospitalization, the roller coaster course of the disease, multiple caregivers, physician turnover in the neonatal unit, and the behavior of the infant with BPD result in extreme parental stress that may affect later family functioning.[39–41] Koops et al[30] reported that 33% of families caring for oxygen-dependent infants with BPD underwent major changes in the family unit.

Financial concerns

The hospital costs per infant who survives neonatal intensive care range from $144,616 for infants weighing 501 to 600 g at birth to $50,671 for infants weighing 901 to 1,000 g.[42,43] The majority of infants with BPD fall within this birth weight range; however, costs for infants with BPD are likely to be far above average and are shared by parents, insurance, and hospitals.[44] Many infants are discharged who still require oxygen or other support. Koops[44] has recently documented the financial costs for home care for oxygen-dependent infants with BPD to be $1,450 per month. The list of necessary supplies, medications, and equipment to provide home care is often staggering. The cost of additional hospitalizations associated with BPD are not included in this figure. Infants with BPD are routinely hospitalized for procedures usually performed on an outpatient basis because of anesthetic concerns. Moreover, the cost of follow-up visits, not usually covered by insurance carriers, are not included.

The infant with BPD generally has other problems and may require more visits to a primary physician, a follow-up program, and various consultants. In addition, many infants are on home monitors, the cost of which is usually not fully covered by insurance. A hidden cost arises from loss of work for the parent who takes time off for the child's appointments. Newacheck and McManus[45] found out-of-pocket expenses for chronically ill children to be two to three times higher than for other children.

Other

Because most infants with BPD are premature or have severe respiratory failure following asphyxia, other complications associated with these conditions such as retinopathy of prematurity, intracranial hemorrhage, sensorineural hearing loss, periventricular leukomalacia, and hypoxic-ischemic encephalopathy may also occur.[30,46] The increased incidence of hypertension (high blood pressure) reported in infants with BPD is unclear.[47]

PREVENTION

Since BPD is closely linked to prematurity, prevention of preterm birth and respiratory distress syndrome are the key elements in the primary prevention of BPD. In addition to established strategies such as tocolysis (methods to stop labor) and maternal betamethasone administration to hasten lung maturity, newer approaches may lead to a reduction in the incidence and severity of BPD. These include surfactant therapy and the use of high-frequency ventilation.[48–50] By preventing surfactant deficiency, the exposure to increased oxygen concentrations should be reduced, resulting in less oxidant damage to the lung and at the tissue level. The use of high-frequency ventilation may decrease barotrauma through the use of lower pressures and may also be helpful in the prevention and treatment of air leaks or pneumothorax.

To bolster the defense mechanisms of the lung, a number of antioxidants have been investigated, including vitamins A and E and the antioxidant enzyme superoxide dismutase.[51–53] Recently, vitamin A was shown to decrease the incidence and severity of BPD in a population of susceptible infants.[53] This therapy is especially promising because many infants with BPD are vitamin A deficient, and many of the pathologic findings in BPD have been seen in vitamin A deficiency.

On the other hand, vitamin E does not appear to be efficacious, and the research on superoxide dismutase has produced conflicting results. Blocking destructive proteolytic enzymes using inhibitors and suppressing the influx of protease-releasing neutrophils by administering steroids is also being explored.[54–56] Steroids also stabilize cells and membranes, increase surfactant synthesis, and stimulate antioxidant enzyme activity.[56]

Als and associates[57] recently researched a novel approach to prevention—the impact of an individualized multidisciplinary care plan on the incidence and outcome of infants at high risk for BPD. They found not only a decreased incidence of BPD, but also less intracranial hemorrhage, better weight gain, earlier discharge, and better short-term developmental outcome in treated infants.

MANAGEMENT

Management goals include the prevention of further pulmonary damage, the diagnosis and treatment of complications of BPD and its therapy, and the promotion of optimal growth and development. A full discussion of inpatient and outpatient care, including the management of the infant requiring home ventilation, is beyond the scope of this article but is available in a number of excellent references.[24,30,37,58]

To prevent further pulmonary damage, the infant must be weaned from the ventilator and high oxygen concentrations. This must be balanced, however, with the risk of inadequate oxygenation leading to pulmonary hypertension and poor growth. The use of bronchodilating agents to ameliorate airway spasm and diuretics to remove fluid may be useful both during weaning and on a continuing basis after discharge.[59] The bronchodilating agents most often used include theophylline and betaadrenergic agonists, usually administered by aerosol.[60] Theophylline may also be used with premature infants to treat apnea of prematurity or to improve diaphragmatic performance.

Diuretics are commonly used in the treatment of BPD and have been shown to be effective.[30,61] To avoid increased calcium loss in the urine, a thiazide diuretic (usually chlorothiazide) and spironolactone are used, rather than furosemide. Electrolyte supplements, including sodium and potassium, are often necessary; electrolyte levels must be monitored.

Steroids may also be useful in weaning the infant from the ventilator.[54,62] The exact mechanism is unknown at this time, and potential adverse effects require that further studies be completed to define which infants may benefit from steroid therapy. A new area of investigation is the link between BPD and arachidonic acid metabolites (eg, leukotrienes), which may be related to problems seen in infants with BPD such as reactive airway disease and pulmonary hypertension. Both steroids and cromolyn are useful for treatment if such metabolites are important.

Many infants are discharged on low-flow oxygen delivered by nasal cannula. Preliminary data indicate better weight gain in these infants.[30,63] After discharge, oxygen and other therapy should be slowly withdrawn only after the infant has demonstrated good growth—perhaps the most sensitive indicator of adequate oxygenation. Monitoring oxygen saturation on an outpatient basis may be useful, but since the infant's saturation is often lowest during sleep and feeding, caution must be used in weaning solely on the basis of outpatient saturation monitoring.[24,30]

Discharge planning is a complex process that must be begun early and includes a number of important steps.[30,64] Good communication with the infant's parents and primary care physician is essential for a successful transition to the home and is crucial if hospitalization is to become less common.[65,66]

A developmental program that begins during hospitalization and continues after discharge is essential. Since the infant with BPD is often fragile, the caregivers and therapists must be well acquainted with signs of stress or overstimulation in the infant, such as hiccups, gagging, color change, and spitting up.[67] Awareness of and response to environmental and parental concerns are particularly important in optimizing the outcome for these infants.[67,68]

EARLY OUTCOME

Mortality

The reported mortality due to BPD is 20% to 40%; the wide range is not unexpected due to varying definitions of BPD. Although mortality due to BPD cannot be precisely measured, the duration of ventilatory support and oxygen therapy and length of hospitalization are probably good predictors of late neonatal death.[69]

Diagnosis of pulmonary hypertension confers an added risk for both morbidity and mortality.[27] Recently Campbell and associates[70] reported a syndrome of progressive neurological deterioration and death in a subgroup of infants with BPD. These infants presented with intractable seizures, deterioration, and eventual death. The etiology and incidence of this syndrome remain unclear.

Growth

Although many studies have demonstrated poor growth in infants with BPD, there is evidence that unless BPD is severe, the primary reason for this finding is birth weight.[37,71–73] On the other hand, infants with severe BPD may sustain growth failure affecting not only weight, but head growth as well.[74] Head growth during hospitalization and in the first year of life is a strong predictor of later cognitive outcome.[75] Studies assessing the various perinatal variables affecting CNS development will clarify the role of BPD. In any event, careful attention must be paid to nutritional factors, and a dietitian must be part of the team. Kurzner and associates[38] recently found evidence for a relative state of protein-calorie malnutrition in infants with BPD and growth failure.

Health status

Infants with BPD are hospitalized more often in the first year of life for pneumonia, viral illnesses (eg, respiratory syncytial virus), and reactive airway disease.[65,66] It is unclear whether they are at increased risk for apnea; however, due to their fragile condition, even minor illnesses can place them at risk for respiratory failure.[76]

EARLY DEVELOPMENT

Motor

Infants with BPD are generally extremely premature and have other confounding problems such as intracranial hemorrhage. It is therefore difficult to assess the contribution of BPD to delayed motor development. Although some short-term follow-up studies[71,72] indicate a poor outcome in infants surviving BPD, confounding variables such as birth weight and intracranial hemorrhage were not controlled for. To control for these confounding factors, a study of extremely low birth weight infants was performed and analyzed using multivariable techniques.[77] The impact of mechanical ventilation for more than three weeks (a marker for BPD) and intracranial hemorrhage on developmental progress were assessed longitudinally through the first 18 months using the Bayley Scales of Infant Development.[77] Birth weight, gestational age, and socioeconomic status were controlled using analysis of covariance. The variable of prolonged mechanical ventilation was associated with poorer developmental progress, both motor and cognitive, through 18 months of age.

Future studies will clarify the prognosis for infants with BPD if they control for confounding variables such as birth weight, gestational age, and severity of BPD. Koops and Lam[78] have suggested a standard definition of neurological handicap and a handicap score that are clear and address the functional abilities of the child with BPD.

Behavior

Sell and Vaucher[37] found evidence for poorer behavioral organization and regulation during the neonatal period and at discharge in infants with BPD. Als and associates[57] found improvement in behavioral regulation in infants at risk for BPD who received individualized behavioral and environmental intervention. The work of Als and associates suggests that behavioral and environmental issues in the neonatal unit are important factors in outcome. If confirmed by other studies, this work could have a major impact on how care is organized for these infants both in the hospital and at home.

Cognitive and socioemotional development

In early studies, few developmental sequelae attributable to BPD were identified.[79,80] However, a study comparing 17 infants with BPD and 20 with RDS found that BPD contributed significantly to differences in group cognitive outcomes.[81] Results from cognitive, sensorimotor, and language measures demonstrated that in the second year of life, infants with BPD performed significantly less well than those with RDS. Moreover, regression analyses showed that the type of respiratory illness (ie, RDS or BPD) explained more of the variance in cognitive outcomes than such neonatal factors as birth weight or gestational age.

In this sample, however, no reliable differences were found between RDS and BPD infants on indicators of socioemotional development and psychosocial adaptation.[81] When RDS and BPD infants were compared to healthy preterm infants free of respiratory illness, differences emerged on attachment, affect expression, and capacity to become involved in tasks and to be responsive to the examiner.[82-84] At 36 months of age, similar relationships were found with no significant differences between infants having RDS and those having BPD, but significant differences were found between these infants as a group and low-risk, healthy preterm infants. Among the parameters studied at 36 months were stranger sociability and socioemotional adaptation.[85,86] These studies indicate that BPD has its greatest effect on early cognitive development, and its effects on psychosocial development are indistinguishable from those of other significant respiratory diseases during early infancy.

Pulmonary function

Long-term follow up of children with a history of chronic lung disease has shown a persistence of airway obstruction.[87,88] Since similar findings have been noted in survivors of RDS without BPD, Boynton[3] has suggested that these abnormalities reflect residua from early lung injury that then alter subsequent growth and development.

LATE OUTCOME

Few studies have been done of school age children who survive BPD. Northway[89] found a 34% incidence of severe handicap at age three. On the other hand, Sauve and Singhal[74] followed 141 infants with BPD and 66 control infants, some to 8 years of age. There were no differences between the groups on developmental testing; however, abnormal speech and language assessments were found in 22% of children with a history of BPD.

In general, the pulmonary status of survivors improves yearly, with few children manifesting obvious sequelae by school age. It is hoped that ongoing studies will provide a clearer, more comprehensive answer to the question of long-term developmental sequelae in children who have survived modern neonatal intensive care for respiratory disease.

•   •   •

This is an exciting era for research in bronchopulmonary dysplasia. Current studies may provide new information on the prevention and management of BPD, as well as the definition of specific risk for sequelae. With this information, specific treatment and intervention strategies to ameliorate the impact of BPD can be developed and tested. The potential for benefit to the child, the family, and the larger society is enormous.

REFERENCES

1. Northway WH Jr, Rosen RC, Porter DY: Pulmonary disease following respirator therapy of hyaline membrane disease: Bronchopulmonary dysplasia. *N Engl J Med* 1967;276:357–368.

2. Edwards DK: The radiology of bronchopulmonary dysplasia and its complications, in Merritt TA, Northway WH Jr, Boynton BR (eds): *Bronchopulmonary Dysplasia*. Boston, Blackwell Scientific, 1988.

3. Boynton BR: Epidemiology of BPD, in Merritt TA, Northway WH Jr, Boynton BR (eds): *Bronchopulmonary Dysplasia*. Boston, Blackwell Scientific, 1988.

4. Tooley WH: Epidemiology of bronchopulmonary dysplasia. *J Pediatr* 1979;95:851–858.

5. Bancalari E, Adenenour GE, Feller R, et al: Bronchopulmonary dysplasia: Clinical presentation. *J Pediatr* 1979;95:819–823.

6. Toce SS, Farrell PM, Leavitt LA, et al: Clinical and roentgenographic scoring systems for assessing bronchopulmonary dysplasia. *Am J Dis Child* 1984; 138:581–585.

7. Nickerson BG, Taussig LM: Family history of asthma in infants with bronchopulmonary dysplasia. *Pediatrics* 1980;65:1140–1144.

8. Fineberg M, Stabile MW, Lew CD, et al: Bronchial hyperactivity in parents of infants with bronchopulmonary dysplasia. *Am Rev Respir Dis* 1985;131:A265.

9. Clark DA, Pincus LG, Oliphant M, et al: HLA-A2 and chronic lung disease in neonates. *JAMA* 1982; 248:1868–1869.

10. Goetzman BW: Understanding bronchopulmonary dysplasia. *Am J Dis Child* 1986;140:332–334.

11. Bonikos DS, Bensch KG, Northway WH Jr, et al: Bronchopulmonary dysplasia: The pulmonary pathologic sequelae of necrotizing bronchiolitis and pulmonary fibrosis. *Hum Pathol* 1976;7:643–666.

12. Bonikos DS, Bensch KG, Ludwin SK, et al: Oxygen toxicity in the newborn. The effect of prolonged 100 percent O_2 exposure on the lungs of newborn mice. *Lab Invest* 1975;32:619–635.

13. Kistler GS, Calswell PRB, Weibel ER: Development of fine structural damage to alveolar and capillary lining cells in oxygen-poisoned rat lungs. *J Cell Biol* 1967;32:605–628.

14. Fantone JC, Ward PA: Polymorphonuclear leukocyte-mediated cell and tissue injury: Oxygen metabolites and their relations to human disease. *Hum Pathol* 1985;16:973–979.

15. Platzker ACG: Chronic lung disease of infancy, in Ballard RA (ed): *Pediatric Care of the ICN Graduate*. Philadelphia, W.B. Saunders, 1988.

16. Johnson DE, Lock JE, Elde RP, et al: Pulmonary neuroendocrine cells in hyaline membrane disease and bronchopulmonary dysplasia. *Pediatr Res* 1982;16:446–454.

17. Evans MJ, Cabral LJ, Stephens RJ, et al: Transformation of alveolar type 2 cells to type 1 cells following exposure to NO_2. *Exp Mol Pathol* 1975;22:142–150.

18. Stahlman MT, Cheatham W, Gray ME: The role of air dissection in bronchopulmonary dysplasia. *J Pediatr* 1979;95:878–882.

19. Bonikos DS, Bensch KG: Pathogenesis of bronchopulmonary dysplasia, in Merritt TA, Northway WH Jr, Boynton BR (eds): *Bronchopulmonary Dysplasia*. Boston, Blackwell Scientific, 1988.

20. Janoff A: Proteases and lung injury: A state of the art minireview. *Chest* 1983;83(suppl):54–58

21. Gadek JE, Fella GA, Zimmerman RL, et al: Antielastases of the human alveolar structures: Implications for the protease-antiprotease theory of emphysema. *J Clin Invest* 1981;68:889–898.

22. Bruce MC, Wedig KE, Jentoft N, et al: Altered urinary excretion of elastin cross-links in premature infants who develop bronchopulmonary dysplasia. *Am Rev Respir Dis* 1985;131:568–572.

23. Avery ME, Fletcher BD, Williams RG: *The Lung and its Disorders in the Newborn Infant*, ed 4. Philadelphia, W.B. Saunders, 1981.

24. Bernbaum J, D'Agostino J: The NICU graduate: Managing the major complications. *Contemp Pediatr* 1986;3:69–82.

25. Fouron JC, LeGuenner JC, Villemant, et al: The outcome of bronchopulmonary dysplasia of the newborn. *Pediatrics* 1980;65:529–535.

26. Tomashefski JF Jr, Opperman HC, Vawter GF, et al: Bronchopulmonary dysplasia: A morphometric study with emphasis on the pulmonary vasculature. *Pediatr Pathol* 1984;2:469–487.
27. Sherman FS: Cor pulmonale, in Ballard RA (ed): *Bronchopulmonary Dysplasia.* Boston, Blackwell Scientific, 1988.
28. Brownlee JR, Beekman RH, Rosenthal A: Acute hemodynamic effects of nifedipine in infants with bronchopulmonary dysplasia and pulmonary hypertension. *Pediatr Res* 1988;24:186–190.
29. Myers MG, McGuinness GA, Lachenbruch PA, et al: Respiratory illnesses in survivors of infant respiratory distress syndrome. *Am Rev Respir Dis* 1986;133: 1010–1011.
30. Koops BL, Abman SH, Accurso FJ: Outpatient management and follow-up of bronchopulmonary dysplasia. *Clin Perinatol* 1984;11(1):101–122.
31. Hufnagle KG, Khan SN, Penn D, et al: Renal calcifications: A complication of long-term furosemide therapy in preterm infants. *Pediatrics* 1982; 70:360–363.
32. Gilsanz V, Fernal W, Reid BS, et al: Nephrolithiasis in premature infants. *Radiology* 1985;154:107–110.
33. Steichen JJ, Gratton TL, Tsang RC: Osteopenia of prematurity: The cause and possible treatment. *J Pediatr* 1980;96:528–534.
34. Klein GL, Targoff GM, Ament ME, et al: Bone disease associated with total parenteral nutrition. *Lancet* 1980;2:1041–1044.
35. Greer FR, Tsang RC: Calcium, phosphorus, magnesium, and vitamin D requirements for the preterm infant, in Tsang, RC (ed): *Vitamin and Mineral Requirements in Preterm Infants.* New York, Marcel Deckek, 1985.
36. Simon BM: Speech and language development in the high risk infant, in Ahmann E (ed): *Home Care for the High Risk Infant.* Rockville, Aspen Publishers, 1986.
37. Sell EJ, Vaucher Y: Growth and neurodevelopmental outcome of infants who had bronchopulmonary dysplasia, in Merritt TA, Northway WH Jr, Boynton BR (eds): *Bronchopulmonary Dysplasia.* Boston, Blackwell Scientific, 1988.
38. Kurzner SI, Garg M, Bautista DB, et al: Growth failure in infants with bronchopulmonary dysplasia: Nutrition and elevated resting metabolic expenditure. *Pediatrics* 1988;81:379–384.
39. Minde KK: Parenting the premature infant: Problems and opportunities, in Taeusch HWO, Yogman MW (eds): *Follow-Up Management of the High-Risk Infant.* Boston, Little, Brown, 1987.
40. Beckwith L: Adverse reactions, in Taeusch HWO, Yogman MW (eds): *Follow-Up Management of the High-Risk Infant.* Boston, Little, Brown, 1987.
41. McCauley BB, McCauley JE: Continuing care: Parent's retrospective, in Taeusch HWO, Yogman MW (eds): *Follow-Up Management of the High-Risk Infant.* Boston, Little, Brown, 1987.
42. Hernandez JA, Offutt DPA, Butterfield JA: The cost of care of the less-than-1000-gram infant. *Clin Perinatol* 1986;13:461–476.
43. Shankaran S, Cohen SN, Linver M, et al: Medical care costs of high-risk infants after neonatal intensive care: A controlled study. *Pediatrics* 1988;81:372–378.
44. Koops BL: Commitment to long-term support: Clinical, economic, and ethical issues, in Bancalari E, Stocker JT (eds): *Bronchopulmonary Dysplasia.* Washington, DC, Hemisphere, 1988.
45. Newacheck PW, McManus MA: Financing health care for disabled children. *Pediatrics* 1988;81:385–394.
46. Saigal S, O Brodovich H: Long-term outcome of preterm infants with respiratory disease. *Clin Perinatol* 1987;14:635–650.

47. Sheftel DN, Hustead V, Friedman A: Hypertension screening in the follow-up of premature infants. *Pediatrics* 1983;71:763–766.

48. Notter RH, Shapiro DL: Lung surfactants for replacement therapy: Biochemical, biophysical, and clinical aspects. *Clin Perinatol* 1987;14:433–480.

49. Bancalari E, Goldberg RN: High-frequency ventilation in the neonate. *Clin Perinatol* 1987;14:581–598.

50. Donn SM, Nicks JJ, Bandy KP, et al: Proximal high frequency jet ventilation of the newborn. *Pediatr Pulmon* 1985;1:267–271.

51. Rosenfeld W, Evans H, Concepcion L, et al: Prevention of bronchopulmonary dysplasia by administration of bovine superoxide dismutase in preterm infants with respiratory distress syndrome. *J Pediatr* 1984;105:781–785.

52. Enrenkranz RA, Ablow RA, WarsnawJB: Prevention of bronchopulmonary dysplasia with vitamin E administration during the acute stages of respiratory distress syndrome. *J Pediatr* 1979;95:873–878.

53. Shenai JP, Stahlman MT, Chytil F, et al: Clinical trial of vitamin A supplementation in infants susceptible to bronchopulmonary dysplasia. *J Pediatr* 1987;111:269–277.

54. Bruce MC, Wedig E, Jentoft N, et al: Altered urinary excretion of elastin cross-links in premature infants who develop bronchopulmonary dysplasia. *Am Rev Respir Dis* 1985;131:568–572.

55. Rosenfeld W, Concepcion K, Evans H, et al: Serial trypsin inhibitory capacity and ceruloplasmin levels in prematures at risk for bronchopulmonary dysplasia. *Am Rev Respir Dis* 1986;134:1229–1232.

56. Ariagno RL: Use of steroids, in Merritt TA, Northway WH Jr, Boynton BR (eds): *Bronchopulmonary Dysplasia*. Boston, Blackwell Scientific, 1988.

57. Als H, Lawhorn G, Brown E, et al: Individualized behavioral and environmental care for the very low birth weight preterm infant at high risk for bronchopulmonary dysplasia: Neonatal intensive care unit and developmental outcome. *Pediatrics* 1986;78:1123–1132.

58. Ballard RA (ed): *Pediatric Care of the ICN Graduate*. Philadelphia, W.B. Saunders, 1988.

59. Monin P, Vert P: The management of bronchopulmonary dysplasia. *Clin Perinatol* 1987;14:531–549.

60. Kao LC, Warburton D, Platzker ACG, et al: Effect of isoproterenol inhalation on airway resistance in chronic bronchopulmonary dysplasia. *Pediatrics* 1984; 73:509–514.

61. Patel H, Yeh TF, Jain R, et al: Pulmonary and renal response to furosemide in infants with stage III-IV bronchopulmonary dysplasia. *Am J Dis Child* 1985; 139:917–920.

62. Mammel MC, Green TP, Johnson DE, et al: Controlled trial of dexamethasone in respirator-dependent infants with bronchopulmonary dysplasia. *Lancet* 1983;1:1356–1358.

63. Groothuis JR, Rosenberg AA, Zerbe GO: Home oxygen promotes weight gain infants with bronchopulmonary dysplasia. *Pediatr Res* 1986;20:227A.

64. Colangelo AL, Vento TB, Taeusch HW: Discharge planning, in Taeusch HWO, Yogman MW (eds): *Follow-Up Management of the High-Risk Infant*. Boston, Little, Brown, 1987.

65. McCormick MC, Shapiro S, Starfield BH: Rehospitalization in the first year of life for high-risk survivors. *Pediatrics* 1980;66:991–999.

66. Hack M, De Monterice D, Merkatz IR, et al: Rehospitalization of the very-low-birth-weight infant: A continuum of perinatal and environmental morbidity. *Am J Dis Child* 1981;135:263–266.

67. Boynton BR, Jones B: Nursing care of the infant with bronchopulmonary dysplasia, in Ballard RA (ed): *Bronchopulmonary Dysplasia*. Boston, Blackwell Scientific, 1988.

68. Ramey CT, Bryant DM: Environmental interventions, in Taeusch HWO, Yogman MW (eds): *Follow-Up Management of the High-Risk Infant.* Boston, Little, Brown, 1987.

69. Shankaran S, Szego E, Eizert D, et al: Severe bronchopulmonary dysplasia: Predictors of survival and outcome. *Chest* 1984;86:607–610.

70. Campbell LR, McAllister W, Volpe JJ: Neurologic aspects of bronchopulmonary dysplasia. *Clin Pediatr* 1988;27:7–13.

71. Yu VYH, Orgill AA, Lim SB, et al: Growth and development of very low birth weight infants recovering from bronchopulmonary dysplasia. *Arch Dis Child* 1983;58:791–794.

72. Vohr BR, Bell EF, Oh W: Infants with bronchopulmonary dysplasia: Growth pattern and neurologic and developmental outcome. *Am J Dis Child* 1982; 136:443–447.

73. Meisels SJ, Plunkett JW, Roloff DW, et al: Growth and development of preterm infants with respiratory distress syndrome and bronchopulmonary dysplasia. *Pediatrics* 1986,77:345–352.

74. Sauve RS, Singhal N: Long-term morbidity of infants with bronchopulmonary dysplasia. *Pediatrics* 1985; 76:725–733.

75. Hack M, Breslau N: Very low birth weight infants: Effects of brain growth during infancy on intelligence quotient at 3 years of age. *Pediatrics* 1986;77:196–202.

76. Werthammer J, Brown E, Neff RK, et al: Sudden infant death syndrome in infants with bronchopulmonary dysplasia. *Pediatrics* 1982;69:301–304.

77. Bozynski ME, Nelson MN, Matalon TAS, et al: Prolonged mechanical ventilation and intracranial hemorrhage: Impact on developmental progress through 18 months in infants weighing 1,200 grams or less at birth. *Pediatrics* 1987;79:670–676.

78. Koops BL, Lam C: Outcome in bronchopulmonary dysplasia: Mortality risks and prognosis for growth, neurological integrity, and developmental performance, in Bancalari E, Stocker JT (eds): *Bronchopulmonary Dysplasia.* Washington, DC, Hemisphere, 1988.

79. Taussig LM: Bronchopulmonary dysplasia, in Sell EJ (ed): *Followup of the High-Risk Newborn— A Practical Approach.* Springfield, Ill, Charles C Thomas, 1980.

80. Markestad T, Fitzhardinge PM: Growth and development in children recovering from bronchopulmonary dysplasia. *J Pediatr* 1981;98:597–602.

81. Meisels SJ, Plunkett JW, Roloff DW, et al: Growth and development of preterm infants with respiratory distress syndrome and bronchopulmonary dysplasia. *Pediatrics* 1986;77:345–352.

82. Plunkett JW, Meisels SJ, Stiefel GS, et al: Patterns of attachment among preterm infants of varying biological risk. *J Amer Acad Child Psychol* 1986;25:794–800.

83. Stiefel GS, Plunkett JW, Meisels SJ: Affective expression among preterm infants of varying roles of biological risk. *Infant Behav Dev* 1987;10:151–164.

84. Meisels SJ, Plunkett JW, Cross DR: Use of the Bayley Infant Behavior record with preterm and full term infants. *Dev Psychol* 1987;23:475–482.

85. Plunkett JW, Klein T, Meisels SJ: The relationship of preterm infant-mother attachment to stranger sociability at 3 years. *Infant Behav Dev* 1986;11:83–96.

86. Plunkett JW, Meisels SJ: Socio-emotional adaptation of preterm infants at three years. *J Infant Mental Health,* to be published.

87. Smyth JA, Tabachnik E, Duncan WJ, et al: Pulmonary function and bronchial hyperactivity in longterm survivors of bronchopulmonary dysplasia. *Pediatrics* 1981;68:336–340.

88. Heldt GP: Pulmonary status of infants and children with bronchopulmonary dysplasia, in Merritt TA Northway WH Jr, Boynton BR: *Bronchopulmonary Dysplasia.* Boston, Blackwell Scientific, 1988.

89. Northway WH Jr: Observations on bronchopulmonary dysplasia. *J Pediatr* 1979;95:815–818.

A genetics primer for early service providers

Elizabeth J. Thomson, RN, MS
Coordinator, Genetic Counseling
  Services
Division of Medical Genetics
Department of Pediatrics
University of Iowa Hospitals and
  Clinics
Iowa City, Iowa

EARLY SERVICE providers come into frequent contact with children who are born with birth defects, genetic disorders, or other disabling conditions. Many of these problems have a specific genetic or environmental etiology that can be identified; the children affected with such disorders may benefit from a genetic consultation.

It is important to be aware of how frequently these problems occur. One in 30 babies is born with a birth defect. Of those, 20% to 30% of defects are due to genetic influences (a chromosome abnormality, a single gene disorder, or multiple genes working together), and approximately 10% are due to prenatal environmental influences. In 60% to 70% of children born with such problems, the cause remains virtually unknown. Nevertheless, for those 30% to 40% of children born with problems in which the cause can be delineated, understanding the underlying genetic or environmental contribution to the problem may assist the professional providing early services in better understanding the pathogenicity and natural history of the disorder and anticipate future needs for the affected children and their families. This article reviews the basic principles of human genetics so that early care providers can begin to apply the information in the setting in which they provide services.

PRINCIPLES OF HUMAN GENETICS

Genes are the basic unit of inheritance and are composed of deoxyribonucleic acid (DNA). DNA is a double-stranded molecule that is presented in the nucleus of the cell and is shaped like a coiled ladder. DNA has several functions including replication during cell division, coding for the production of structural proteins and enzymes, and regulating the rate of synthesis of these proteins and enzymes. Genes are arranged linearly along the chromosomes with each gene having a particular location (locus). A gene locus on one chromosome has a matching gene locus on its paired chromosome, so that genes, like chromosomes, come in pairs with one member of each pair inherited from each parent. It is estimated that there are between 30,000 and 50,000 gene pairs that make up the human genome. Of that number, only approximately 2,300 have been identified to be present at a specific gene locus. In another 2,200, the location of the gene has been suggested but not proven. To date, some 500 disorders have been identified in which a spe-

Inf Young Children 1989;2(1):37–48
© 1989 Aspen Publishers, Inc.

cific genetic change (mutation) has been mapped to a specific gene location. These numbers continue to grow at a rapid rate.

In humans there are 46 chromosomes, or 23 chromosome pairs. Twenty-two pairs of chromosomes are identical in males and females and are referred to as the autosomes. The 23rd pair determines the sex of an individual and thus are called the sex chromosomes. Females have two X chromosomes and males have one X chromosome and one Y chromosome (Fig 1).

Cell division

In humans there are two types of cell division— mitosis and meiosis. Mitosis almost always occurs in the body cells. The body grows and damaged or dead cells are replaced via this type of cell division. In mitosis the 46 chromosomes duplicate within the parent cell. The duplicate strands align themselves along the equator of the cell. These duplicate strands then separate and migrate (pulled by spindle fibers) to opposite poles of the cell. As the duplicate strands complete their migration to the poles, the material surrounding the DNA, the cytoplasm, divides and two separate daughter cells, identical to the original parent cell, are formed (Fig 2).

Meiosis is a specialized type of cell division that occurs during gametogenesis (egg and sperm cell formation). Meiosis in women takes place in the ovaries and

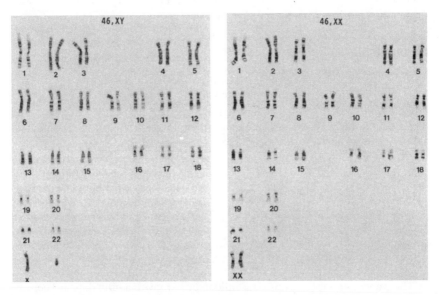

Fig 1. Normal chromosome complements—male (A) and female (B).

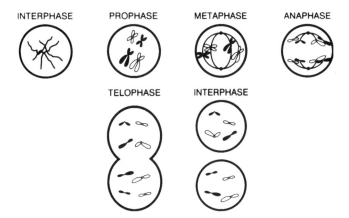

Fig 2. Mitosis.

results in the production of ova (egg) cells. In men, meiosis occurs in the testes and results in the production of sperm cells. Like mitosis, meiosis begins with the duplication of the genetic material contained in the chromosomes. This duplication, however, is followed not by one, but by two successive divisions of the chromosome strands. Thus, meiosis results in the formation of four daughter cells, each with only half (one member of each pair) of the chromosomes that were present in the original parent cell (Fig 3).

Fertilization

Since sperm cells and egg cells have only a half set of chromosomes (ie, 23), it is necessary for a sperm cell to unite with an egg cell to regain a full chromosome complement. During fertilization, an egg and a sperm cell unite to form a zygote. The single fertilized egg cell then begins to undergo mitotic cell division, which initiates embryonic and subsequently fetal development.

Although all of the cells in a human body have the same genetic material present (barring new mutations), these cells have different genes active at any given time. The result during embryogenesis is cell differentiation, in which some cells become nerves, some become muscles, some become bones, and so forth, even though the genetic material in each of these cells is identical.

GENETIC CAUSES OF BIRTH DEFECTS

There are numerous reasons for a child to be born with a birth defect. There are genetic factors, including chromosome abnormalities and gene disorders. There

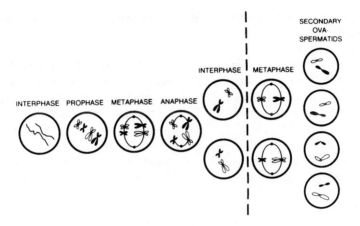

Fig 3. Meiosis I (left) and II (right).

are environmental factors, and there are combinations of genetic and environmental factors, which are known as multifactorial problems.

Chromosome abnormalities

Chromosomes can be considered packages of genetic material. These packages can be examined under the microscope through a process called chromosome analysis, or karyotyping. The actual number of chromosomes in humans became known only in 1956.[1] Although initially described much earlier, Down syndrome was the first birth defect problem that was associated with a specific chromosome abnormality. This chromosome abnormality was identified in 1959.[2]

In the early years, when a chromosome analysis was carried out, chromosomes were simply dark staining bodies that were grouped together by size and location of the constricted area (the centromere). At that time only the actual number of chromosomes present could be well identified. Although large structural chromosome abnormalities were occasionally identified, it was not possible to identify small structural changes or rearrangements by the early techniques.

Since the early 1970s, a variety of chromosome staining techniques have been developed. These techniques have allowed for evaluation of the finer structure of the chromosome complement. Each chromosome has now been identified to have a specific banding pattern, so that it is now possible to differentiate among all of the individual chromosome pairs. By 1986, there had been approximately 1,000 distinct bands identified in the human chromosome complement with high resolution banding.[3] Thus it has become increasingly possible to evaluate finer structural abnormalities of the chromosomes. Despite these recent advances, however, it is important to realize that each individual chromosome band still represents a small number to several hundred gene loci. Thus the presence of a normal chromosome complement does not in any way rule out all forms of genetic abnormalities.

Chromosome abnormalities may occur as a result of an abnormal number or an abnormal structure of the chromosomes. Aneuploidy, or problems of chromosome number, include monosomies, trisomies, and mosaicisms. Structural chromosome abnormalities include deletions, additions, inversions, and translocations. Chromosome abnormalities are further defined as being autosomal in nature (involving one of the first 22 pairs of chromosomes) or sex chromosomal (involving the X or the Y chromosomes). In any of these abnormalities, the child has received an abnormal amount of genetic material (either too much or too little). The presence of this abnormal number of genes usually results in alterations in growth and development.

Chromosome abnormalities arise from an error that has occurred in cell division either in the formation of the egg or sperm cell contributing to the formation of the individual or in one of the individual's ancestors. Whereas chromosome abnormalities can be inherited from one parent or the other, the vast majority of chromosome abnormalities occur sporadically during gametogenesis. Sporadic chromosome abnormalities are most often due to nondisjunction (lack of separation) of the paired chromosomes during meiosis. When nondisjunction occurs, both members of a chromosome pair go to an individual egg or sperm cell. The result is a gamete that has an extra chromosome or is missing one of the chromosomes. When fertilization occurs, the zygote will have either a trisomy (47) or a monosomy (45) of the chromosomes. Occasionally, nondisjunction occurs after fertilization during mitotic cell division. The result of such a chromosome accident is a mosaicism. In mosaicism, the individual ends up having two or more cell lines. Although it is possible that the individual may have two abnormal cell lines, usually some cells of the individual are normal, while other cells have an extra chromosome or are missing a chromosome.

Structural chromosome abnormalities involve the gain, loss, or rearrangement of some of the genetic material. When a chromosome acquires extra genetic material, it is usually called a "duplication" or "addition" and is also sometimes referred to as a "partial trisomy." The loss of genetic material is called a "deletion" and is usually referred to as a "partial monosomy." Additions and deletions result when a portion of one chromosome breaks off and is lost or becomes attached to another chromosome. An inversion occurs when there are two breaks in a single chromosome followed by a reattachment, with the section of the chromosome material between the breaks having been inverted.

The exchange of chromosome material between two chromosomes is referred to as a translocation. Such structural rearrangements usually occur during the meiotic cell division of gametogenesis. These structural rearrangements may be present in a balanced or unbalanced form. Only if present in an unbalanced form does it lead to a problem in an individual. If an individual has a balanced chromosome rearrangement, that individual is usually entirely normal, but may pass an abnormal amount of genetic material to his or her children, thus potentially causing problems in the children. The specific risk is dependent on many factors, including what specific chromosomes are involved and how large an area of chromosome material is rearranged.

It has been estimated that 40% to 60% of conceptions begin with a chromosome abnormality; however, the vast majority of these conceptions results in a pregnancy not compatible with life, and a spontaneous abortion or miscarriage occurs. It is known, however, that approximately 1 in 200 children born alive has a chromosome abnormality present.

Examples of chromosome abnormalities

The most frequently observed numerical autosomal chromosome abnormality is Down syndrome, or trisomy 21. Down syndrome occurs in approximately one in 800 live births.[4] Of children born with Down syndrome, 95% to 96% have nondisjunction trisomy 21. In nondisjunction trisomy 21, there is an extra separate copy of the 21st chromosome (Fig 4). It results when during meiosis, the 21st pair of chromosomes does not separate during gametogenesis (in either egg or sperm cell formation). Nondisjunction trisomy 21 is usually not considered to be "inher-

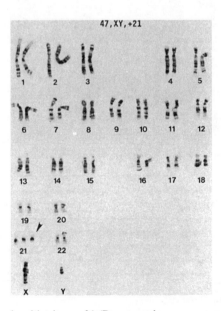

Fig 4. Karotype of male with trisomy 21 (Down syndrome, see arrowhead).

ited," in spite of the fact that it involves the genetic material. Nondisjunction trisomy 21 usually occurs sporadically in a family; however, once a couple has had one child with trisomy 21, their risk of having a second affected child is somewhat higher than the general population risk (1/2% to 1% above their age-specific risk).

Approximately 4% of children born with Down syndrome have a translocation type of Down syndrome. In this disorder, the extra 21st chromosome is attached to another chromosome (usually the 14th) (Fig 5a). In approximately half of the children born with translocation Down syndrome, the chromosome rearrangement is inherited from one parent or the other (Fig 5b). If such a translocation is present in the family, individuals will be at a significantly increased risk of having similarly affected children (5% to 15% depending on which parent is the carrier).

The third form of Down syndrome is Down syndrome mosaicism, which results when nondisjunction occurs some time after conception, usually within the first few mitotic cell divisions. In Down syndrome mosaicism, the child will have some cells that have the normal number of chromosomes (46), and some cells with an extra number 21 chromosome present. Down syndrome mosaicism may result in a somewhat less severe degree of altered growth and development. However, in

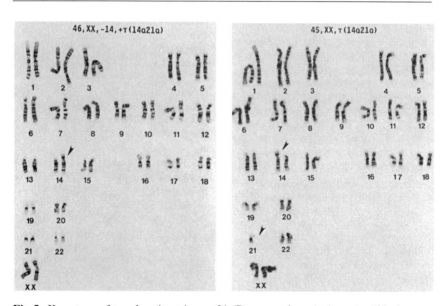

Fig 5. Karyotype of translocation trisomy 21 (Down syndrome). An extra #21 chromosome is attached to the #14 (arrowhead) chromosome (A). Karyotype of normal female with balanced translocation. One of the #21 (arrowhead) chromosomes is attached to the #14 (arrowhead) chromosome (B).

any individual child with this disorder, it is impossible to predict how well or how poorly the child may do in the long term, since the actual percentage and distribution of the abnormal cells cannot be ascertained by chromosome analysis on blood or skin.

Other numerical autosomal chromosome abnormalities that occur with relatively high frequency are trisomies 18 and 13. Children with these disorders have a much poorer outcome than children born with Down syndrome. These children will have multiple malformations involving many organ systems at birth. Fewer than 20% of children born with either of these disorders survive beyond the first year of life. Those children who do survive display a serious failure to thrive and have severe mental deficiency.

The most frequent numerical sex chromosome abnormality that occurs is Klinefelter syndrome, or 47,XXY. This disorder occurs in approximately one in 1,000 newborn boys.[5] Klinefelter syndrome results when there is nondisjunction in gametogenesis resulting in the presence of two X chromosomes and a Y chromosome at the time of conception. Studies have suggested that in approximately 60% of the boys born with Klinefelter syndrome, the extra X chromosome is maternal in origin. In the remaining 40% the extra chromosome is paternally derived. Approximately 15% of males with Klinefelter syndrome have mosaicism.[4] Klinefelter syndrome usually leads to tall stature, an increased risk for learning and behavior problems, and infertility. Additionally, at puberty, many will begin to show feminization of their physical features rather than masculinization.

A second common numerical sex chromosome abnormality is Turner syndrome, or 45,X. This disorder occurs in approximately 1 in 2,500 newborn girls.[6] Girls with Turner syndrome receive only a single X chromosome from their parents. That means that either the egg or the sperm cell lost the sex chromosome during gametogenesis. Approximately 40% of girls with clinical features of Turner syndrome have either a structural alteration of the X chromosome or a sex chromosome mosaicism.

Girls with Turner syndrome often show puffiness of their hands and feet at birth. They may have a low posterior hairline and extra skin in the neck region (sometimes neck webbing). They may have a heart murmur due to some cardiovascular anomaly. As they grow, their stature is shorter than average, with full adult height usually less than five feet. They have a somewhat increased risk for learning disabilities, although intelligence is usually normal. Without hormonal treatment, girls with Turner syndrome will not go through puberty and feminize normally. Even with treatment, infertility usually occurs.

Numerous other numerical sex chromosome abnormalities have been reported. Girls have been born with three, four, and five X chromosomes. There have also been boys identified as having XYY, XXYY, XXXY, and XXXXY. Such sex chromosome abnormalities result in varying degrees of defects. The general rule is that the higher number of extra sex chromosomes present, the poorer the outcome for the affected individuals.

One of the most commonly recognized structural chromosome abnormalities is cri du chat or 5p— syndrome. It is referred to as 5p— because there is a deletion (—) of one portion of the short arm (p) of chromosome number 5. (The long arm of chromosomes are referred to as the q arm.) Cri du chat syndrome occurs in approximately one in 50,000 live births.[7] The severity of this disorder is dependent on the amount of chromosome material that has been deleted. Most children born with cri du chat syndrome have the disorder as a result of a sporadic loss of chromosome material. However, 10% to 15% of children born with cri du chat syndrome inherit this deletion from one parent or the other, who is later identified to be a balanced translocation carrier.[4]

Children with cri du chat syndrome are usually smaller than average at birth. The name of the syndrome comes from their cry, which has been described as sounding like that of a mewing cat. They have atypical physical appearance including microcephaly, wide-spaced down slanting eyes, epicanthal folds, low-set, poorly formed ears, and facial asymmetry. They grow and develop poorly after birth with severe mental retardation.

There are many other possible structural chromosome rearrangements. Cases have been reported of children with deletions or additions involving essentially all of the 23 pairs of chromosomes. The outcome for the children born with structural chromosome abnormalities is dependent on which chromosome is involved and the amount of genetic material that is added or deleted.

Single gene abnormalities

Single gene disorders are caused by an alteration (mutation) in the chemical makeup of a single gene or a single gene pair. There are four types of single gene patterns of inheritance: autosomal dominant, autosomal recessive, X-linked dominant, and X-linked recessive. While individually single gene disorders may not be common in the population, in the aggregate, these disorders are common, having been diagnosed in approximately 2% to 3% of the population by 1 year of age.

Autosomal dominant disorders are caused by a single altered gene along one of the autosomes. The disorder may be present in several generations, having been passed from parent to child, or it may be due to a new mutation. An individual affected with an autosomal dominant disorder has a 50% risk of passing the gene to each of his or her offspring. Males and females are equally likely to be affected, since the altered gene is along one of the autosomes. Individuals who do not have the gene have essentially no risk of passing the disorder to their offspring (barring a new mutation). There are presently 1,443 known autosomal dominant disorders. Another 1,114 disorders are suspected to be dominant in origin.[8] Fig 6 demonstrates autosomal dominant inheritance and shows examples of somewhat more frequent autosomal dominant disorders.

Autosomal recessive disorders result when both members of an autosomal gene pair are altered. It is estimated that every human carries approximately four to

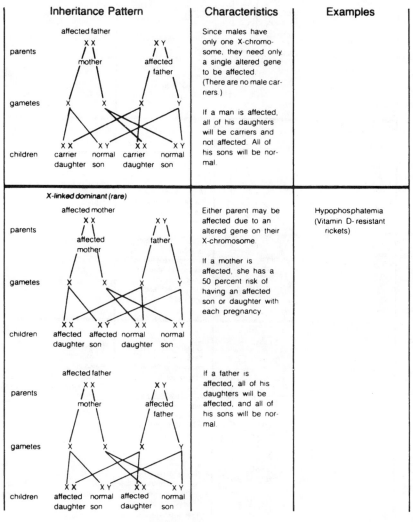

continues

Fig 6. Types of single-gene disorders.

Inheritance Pattern	Characteristics	Examples

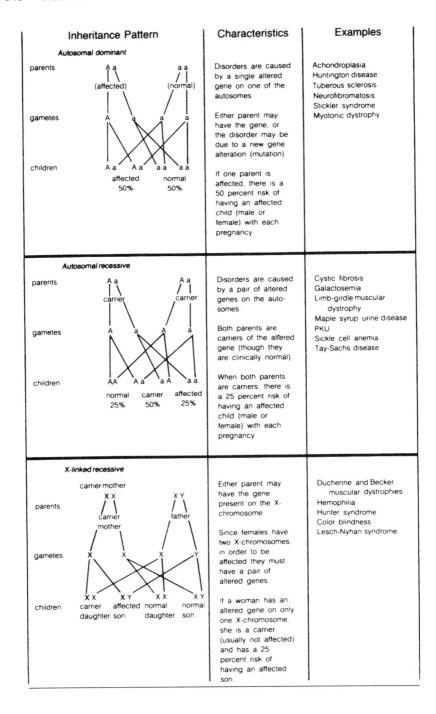

Autosomal dominant

Characteristics:

Disorders are caused by a single altered gene on one of the autosomes.

Either parent may have the gene, or the disorder may be due to a new gene alteration (mutation)

If one parent is affected, there is a 50 percent risk of having an affected child (male or female) with each pregnancy

Examples:

Achondroplasia
Huntington disease
Tuberous sclerosis
Neurofibromatosis
Stickler syndrome
Myotonic dystrophy

Autosomal recessive

Characteristics:

Disorders are caused by a pair of altered genes on the autosomes.

Both parents are carriers of the altered gene (though they are clinically normal)

When both parents are carriers, there is a 25 percent risk of having an affected child (male or female) with each pregnancy

Examples:

Cystic fibrosis
Galactosemia
Limb-girdle muscular dystrophy
Maple syrup urine disease
PKU
Sickle cell anemia
Tay-Sachs disease

X-linked recessive

Characteristics:

Either parent may have the gene present on the X-chromosome

Since females have two X-chromosomes, in order to be affected they must have a pair of altered genes

If a woman has an altered gene on only one X-chromosome, she is a carrier (usually not affected) and has a 25 percent risk of having an affected son.

Examples:

Duchenne and Becker muscular dystrophies
Hemophilia
Hunter syndrome
Color blindness
Lesch-Nyhan syndrome

eight recessive altered genes. These genes, when present in a single dose, usually do not cause any significant health problems. The problem arises, however, when two individuals carrying the same recessive altered gene by chance pass the altered gene to their offspring. When both members of a couple are carriers of an autosomal recessive disorder, they have a 25% risk of passing the disorder to each offspring. Thus, in a family with an autosomal recessive disorder, affected individuals will usually only be observed in one generation in one immediate family. Males and females are again equally likely to be affected, since the altered genes are present along the autosomes. There are 626 known autosomal recessive genetic disorders at the present time. Another 851 disorders are suspected to be autosomal recessive in origin.[8]

There are 139 known X-linked single gene disorders. An additional 171 are suspected to be inherited in this fashion.[8] Both X-linked dominant and X-linked recessive disorders have been described; however, X-linked dominant disorders are extremely rare. In an affected family, an X-linked dominant disorder will occur twice as often in females as in males, since females have two X chromosomes and males have just one. X-linked dominant disorders will be passed from an affected male to all of his daughters (to which he contributes his X chromosome) and to none of his sons (to which he contributes his Y chromosome). Females with an X-linked dominant disorder will pass the disorder to half of her offspring, either sons or daughters, making the inheritance pattern difficult to distinguish from an autosomal dominant disorder in a family.

X-linked recessive disorders are much more common than X-linked dominant disorders. They occur much more frequently in males than in females. Since males have just one X chromosome, if they have the gene in a single dose, they display the disorder. Females have two X chromosomes; therefore, they must have the gene present in a double dose in order to be affected with the disorder. A female who is a carrier of an X-linked recessive disorder has a 25% risk of having an affected son. A male who is affected with an X-linked recessive disorder will most likely have no affected children. However, all of his daughters (since they receive his X chromosome) will be carriers of the disorder, while none of his sons will be affected with the disorder (since they receive his Y chromosome).

Multifactorial birth defects

Birth defects that are multifactorial in origin occur as a result of an interaction of many genetic and environmental influences working together. By far the most frequent birth defects are multifactorial in origin. Many theories have been proposed regarding the mechanisms of multifactorial inheritance. None of the theories, however, have been readily accepted by all scientists and clinicians. Multifactorial disorders tend to cluster in families; that is, they occur more frequently than one would expect by chance, and yet not frequently enough to be attributed to a single gene inheritance pattern.

Examples of multifactorial birth defects include neural tube defects, clefts of the lip and palate, many forms of congenital heart defects, pyloric stenosis, congenital dislocation of the hip, situs inversus, and club foot. Later onset disorders that are common and are often multifactorial in origin are many forms of cancer, diabetes, adult onset heart disease, epilepsy, and familial mental retardation.

GENETIC EVALUATION AND COUNSELING

Genetic evaluation and counseling should be offered to the parents of any child who is born with a birth defect or who is known or suspected to have a genetic disorder. Some families may be referred for genetic evaluation in order to attempt to establish a specific underlying cause for the child's problems. In other instances, the diagnosis may already be established and the family may be referred for genetic evaluation and counseling so that they may receive further information and support regarding the specific diagnosis established for their child. The genetic evaluation and counseling process includes four components: diagnosis, information, support, and follow-up counseling.

Diagnosis

The first component of the genetic counseling process is to attempt to establish a specific diagnosis; a specific diagnosis may be extremely difficult and many times is not possible. The diagnostic evaluation entails a review of family history, history of the pregnancy, age, ethnic background, medical records, school records, psychological testing, and any other information that may contribute to the diagnosis. An examination of the affected child is carried out. Specific diagnostic evaluations such as chromosomal analysis, molecular or biochemical genetic testing, specific consultative evaluations, and radiographs may be carried out. If a specific diagnosis cannot be established, it is extremely difficult to provide the family with accurate information about what they can expect for their child in the future or what their specific risk of recurrence is.

Informative counseling

The second component of the genetic evaluation and counseling process is informative counseling. Information about the disorder and its prognosis, medical management, and available treatment programs is provided. This information is provided to the immediate family and also to extended family members, local health care professionals, and other individuals who may be involved with the family should they so desire. Whenever possible, the family is given not only verbal but also written information to take home to review. If the family is considering future pregnancies, information is provided to the family regarding reproductive options.

Supportive counseling

Supportive counseling is the third component of the genetic evaluation and counseling process. It is provided in order to help the family deal with the grief process that they may encounter because of their child's birth defect or genetic disorder. Families may need to be reassured that their child's problems are not due to anything they did or did not do. It is also important for families to understand that the resolution of their grief may not be easy and may continue as long as their child is alive and continues to exhibit these problems. Referrals to parent support groups, a member of the clergy, or a psychological or psychiatric counselor may be offered, and the parents are encouraged to identify their own support people and to call on them as they need support.

Support must also be provided to families during their reproductive decision-making process. There are many factors that may be weighed in making reproductive decisions. These factors include how strong the couple's desire is for more children, their interpretation of their risk of recurrence, their past experience with the disorder, their own financial situation, and certainly their ethical, moral, and religious values. It is vitally important for a couple to have support during this decision-making process so that they can reach a decision with which they will be happy.

Follow-up counseling

The fourth component of the genetic evaluation and counseling process, follow-up counseling, provides the counselors with the opportunity to have further discussions with the family, to provide additional information, and to correct any possible misconceptions the family may have about the previously received information. Follow-up counseling also allows for an assessment of the family's reaction to the presence of a child with a birth defect or genetic disorder and to determine how the family has integrated the child and the information they received into their lives.

The genetic evaluation and counseling process has evolved over time. It began as a service that primarily provided reproductive information and options. Most genetic counseling services today provide diagnostic consultation and confirmatory testing and use a case management approach for providing information, support, and follow-up to individuals affected with birth defects and genetic disorders and their families.

• • •

Early service providers deal with children with genetic factors that contribute to their problems. When suspected, the early service provider should refer the child and family for genetic evaluation and counseling. The information the early service provider knows about the child and family may contribute significantly to the genetics team's ability to identify a specific diagnosis. Early service providers should be able to briefly explain what the family may expect from this evaluation. They should also understand enough about human genetic principles to reinforce information received at a genetics visit. With parental permission, the early service provider may wish to participate in the genetic evaluation and counseling session to receive first-hand information about what the family was told at the visit and allow for further exchange of information and ideas. Additionally, early service providers are in a unique position to provide ongoing support to a family in which there is a child with a birth defect or genetic disorder. Working together with the genetic health care team, early service providers have an opportunity to maximize the child's potential and better promote the integration of the child into the family.

REFERENCES

1. Tjio HJ, Levan A: The chromosome numbers of man. *Hereditas* 1956;42:1–6.

2. Lejeune J, Gautier M, Turpin MR: Étude des chromosomes somatiques de neus enfants mongoliens, *CR ACAD SCI (Paris)* 1959;248:1721–1722.

3. Francke U: Elusive chromosome anomalies. *Hosp Pract* 1986;21(5):175–178,182,191–193.

4. Thompson JS, Thompson MW: *Genetics in Medicine*, ed 2. Philadelphia, W.B. Saunders, 1986.

5. de la Chapelle A: Sex chromosome abnormalities, in Emery AE, Rimoin DL (eds): *Principles and Practice in Medical Genetics*. Edinburgh, Churchill Livingstone, 1983.

6. Smith DW: *Recognizable Patterns of Human Malformations*, ed 4. Philadelphia, W.B. Saunders, 1988.

7. deGrouchy J, Turlean C: Autosomal disorders, in Emery AE, Rimoin DL (eds): *Principles and Practice in Medical Genetics*. Edinburgh, Churchill Livingstone, 1983.

8. McKusick V: *Mendelian Inheritance in Man*, ed 8. Baltimore, Johns Hopkins University Press, 1988.

Brain injury in premature infants: Patterns on cranial ultrasound, their relationship to outcome, and the role of developmental intervention in the NICU

John F. Mantovani, MD
Director of Child Neurology
St. John's Mercy Medical Center
Instructor in Clinical Pediatrics and
    Neurology
Washington University School of
    Medicine
St. Louis, Missouri

JoAnn Powers, OTR
Clinical Coordinator of Neonatal
    Services
St. John's Mercy Child Development
    Center
St. Louis, Missouri

NEURODEVELOPMENTAL abnormalities in surviving premature infants of less than 1,500-g birth weight (very low birth rate [VLBW]) are all too familiar to those of us caring for them in the neonatal intensive care unit (NICU) and later. Although a variety of disabilities affect these infants, only spastic motor dysfunction (cerebral palsy) and associated mental retardation are felt to be due to perinatal brain injury per se.[1,2] These major deficits are reported in 10% to 15% of surviving VLBW infants and appear to result largely from the effects of two neuropathologically defined lesions: intraventricular hemorrhage (IVH) and periventricular leucomalacia (PVL).

Frequent evaluation by computed tomography (CT) scanning and cranial ultrasonography has greatly expanded our understanding of the clinical and prognostic features of IVH and periventricular pathology in living infants.[3,4] Cranial ultrasound is now the mainstay of brain imaging in the NICU although magnetic resonance imaging (MRI)[5] and investigative applications of cerebral blood flow studies,[6] positron emission tomography (PET) scanning,[7,8] and continuous electroencephalogram (EEG) monitoring[9] are continuing to provide insights and hope for expanded applications.

The opportunity to visualize infant brain injury patterns in the NICU has also led to an increased demand for prognostic statements—"telling the future," as described by Levene[10]—and is frequently a major reason for neurologic consultation. A large body of literature correlating ultrasound patterns and outcome has therefore developed and will provide the basis for much of this article. It is most important to emphasize at the outset, however, that such correlations are not perfect and that we should not mistake the statistical relationships between imaging studies and outcomes for certainty when dealing with individual patients.[10–12]

The authors thank Janice Figueroa and Lonnie Gatlin for expert technical assistance and the pediatric, neonatology, and nursing staffs of St. John's Mercy Medical Center for involving us in the care of their patients.

Inf Young Children 1991;4(2):20–32
© 1991 Aspen Publishers, Inc.

153

The first section of this article will review several patterns of brain injury as identified by cranial ultrasound in VLBW infants (diagnosis) and discuss their anticipated outcomes (prognosis). The second section will deal with an approach to early intervention used for infants with these lesions in our NICU (treatment). The coupling of these perspectives is intended to emphasize the interrelationships of diagnostic, therapeutic, and prognostic approaches in these smallest of patients.

We believe that recognition of brain injury patterns will improve our understanding of the infants' neurologic and developmental conditions in the NICU, permit informed discussion with parents and caretakers, and encourage the early institution of appropriate measures to maximize the infants' outcomes.

INTRAVENTRICULAR HEMORRHAGE

IVH is a frequent neurologic lesion in VLBW infants but is rarely found in infants more than 34 weeks of gestational age at birth. Despite a decreasing incidence within the last decade, IVH still occurs in 20 to 30 percent of VLBW infants.[13] The hemorrhage begins in the germinal matrix region beneath the lateral ventricle and can remain there (called a germinal matrix hemorrhage [GMH]), can break through the ependymal wall into the ventricle (called IVH), or can extend into the brain parenchyma itself (called intraparenchymal hemorrhage [IPH]). These lesions comprise the IVH complex hereafter simply termed IVH. The pathophysiology of IVH relates to a variety of anatomic, metabolic, and vascular factors that are well described elsewhere.[14,15] Figure 1 shows a brain demonstrating the typical pattern of IVH as seen at autopsy.

Although clinical signs suggesting IVH have been described,[16,17] many hemorrhages are recognized only by screening ultrasound, which has shown an accurate correlation with autopsy and CT scan diagnosis in more than 90 percent of cases.[18] Figure 2 shows an IVH as it appears on cranial ultrasound. IVH is most often classified according to the system initially developed by Papile et al[3] for CT scan grading: grade I (GMH only), grade II (IVH without ventricular dilatation), grade III (IVH with ventricular dilatation), and grade IV (IVH with intraparenchymal extension). Although infants with IVH have higher neonatal mortality rates, much of the clinician's interest in this lesion relates to its effects on prognosis. Studies have shown a bimodal distribution of outcome. Grades I and II hemorrhages precede major deficits in approximately 20% of cases (similar to VLBW infants without IVH), while grades III and IV IVH are associated with major deficits in 50% to 90% of survivors.[19,20] Spastic hemiparesis, quadriparesis, and mental retardation are the major sequelae of large IVH.[21]

Although ventricular enlargement (ventriculomegaly) occurs by definition in grade III IVH, progressive or persistent ventriculomegaly is often seen after both grades III and IV IVH. An ultrasound of a patient with posthemorrhagic

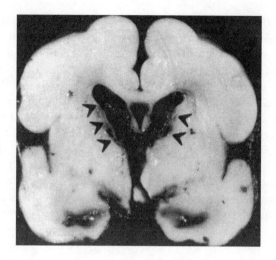

Fig 1. An autopsy specimen showing the brain of a premature infant in coronal section (frontal view). The arrows show the margins of the lateral ventricles with a large IVH filling the entire ventricular system.

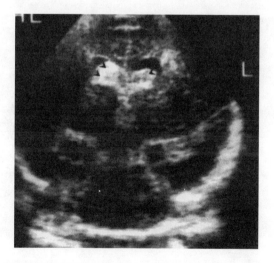

Fig 2. Coronal view of a cranial ultrasound of a 3-day-old premature infant showing a large IVH with blood (in white) filling most of the lateral ventricles.

ventriculomegaly (PHV) is shown in Fig 3. This entity has attracted considerable attention with respect to its impact on outcome. The central question is whether PHV is the cause or the result of brain injury leading to poor outcome. PHV has been treated with a variety of approaches including osmotic drugs, diuretics, and serial lumbar punctures, without demonstrated long-term benefit.[21,22] Ventriculoperitoneal shunts have often been recommended in hopes of reducing further brain injury.[23] Current views suggest, however, that the majority of such patients have reversible or static ventriculomegaly, do not deteriorate clinically, and do not require shunt procedures.[24] A second, smaller group develops symptomatic hydrocephalus with rapid progression of symptoms, including increased intracranial pressure and rapid head growth (exceeding 2 cm per week). These infants may require external drainage or ventriculoperitoneal shunting procedures.[23,24] Interestingly, the outcomes of the two groups appear to be quite similar, indicating that the need for a shunt is not a distinguishing prognostic feature.[24,25]

The prognostic importance of PHV is clouded by its frequent association with the larger grades of hemorrhage. Most studies and our own experience suggest that the prognosis for infants with PHV correlates best with the grade of associated IVH. The worst outcomes occur in infants with intraparenchymal echodensity (IPE) in addition to ventriculomegaly; these infants have major deficits in 60 to 90 percent of cases.[25,26]

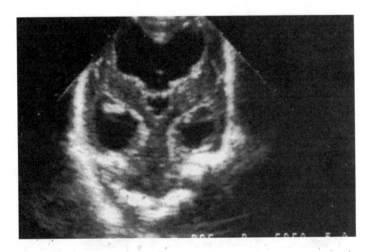

Fig 3. Coronal view of a cranial ultrasound in a 32-day-old infant showing posthemorrhagic ventriculomegaly. Note the enlargement of both lateral ventricles without echodensities as compared to Fig 2.

Several other subgroups of infants with ventriculomegaly have also been identified. They include those with asymmetrical ventricular enlargement following large IVH and those with isolated ventriculomegaly but no preceding IVH, both of which groups have had major deficits in more than 50 percent of cases.[27,28]

The second prognostically important ultrasonographic feature of patients with IVH is intraparenchymal hemorrhage, also termed IPE, in which abnormal echodensities involve the brain substance itself.[29,30] Such echodensity within the brain substance is the defining feature of grade IV IVH. The echodensities are typically asymmetrical, tend to develop 1 to 2 days after the IVH, and occupy the areas lateral to the angle of the ventricles, as shown in Fig 4. These lesions can vary considerably in size, which leads to a distinction between extensive IPE, which fills most of the affected hemisphere, and localized IPE, which appears in only a single anatomic region.[30] Although the pathophysiology of these lesions is controversial, most authors now agree that hemorrhagic venous infarction is the most frequent cause.[1,31] Despite the fact that IPE is often due to venous infarction and is pathophysiologically distinct from PVL (which results from arterial insufficiency), these two lesions may be very difficult to distinguish by ultrasound alone.

Virtually all investigators have found patterns of IPE to be highly associated with mortality and major deficits.[11,29,30] Infants with localized IPE appear to have a

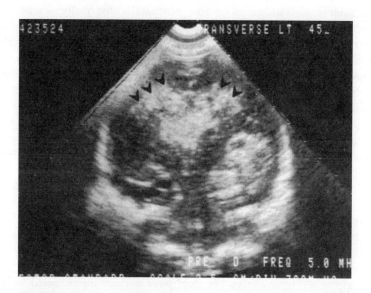

Fig 4. Coronal view of a cranial ultrasound in a 5-day-old infant with IVH and large bilateral areas of intraparenchymal echodensity (indicated by arrows).

lower mortality and a good cognitive outcome in up to one-third of cases. Nonetheless, they frequently develop porencephalic cysts and almost invariably suffer from cerebral palsy.[11,30] Unilateral lesions are often followed by spastic hemiparesis and bilateral lesions by spastic quadriparesis.

In summary, IVH is the classic hemorrhagic lesion of the premature newborn and is reliably diagnosed by cranial ultrasound. Lower grades of hemorrhage (grades I and II) are not associated with an increased incidence of major deficits. PHV leads to such deficits in 30% to 90% of affected patients, depending on the degree of preceding IVH, and IVH with intraparenchymal extension leads to major disabilities in 75% to 90% of survivors.

PERIVENTRICULAR ECHODENSITY

The other commonly recognized pattern of brain injury diagnosed by ultrasound of VLBW infants in the NICU is bilateral periventricular echodensity (PVE).[1,2,10] There are no early clinical manifestations of such lesions, although infants subject to cerebral ischemia from a variety of causes appear to be at increased risk. Like IVH, these abnormalities are usually identified on screening ultrasound and occur in 25 to 50 percent of VLBW infants in several series.[30,32] The abnormal echoes are often visualized during the first week of life but can appear later and continue to evolve postnatally for many weeks. These echodensities have usually been attributed to PVL, a pathologic term used to describe cerebral white matter infarction occurring in a characteristic periventricular location.[33] PVL is felt to result from circulatory insufficiency (ischemia) based on regional anatomic and metabolic vulnerabilities.[34] Figure 5 shows an autopsy specimen from an infant with this lesion. Studies are mixed with respect to the accuracy of the ultrasound diagnosis of PVL as compared with autopsy study, ranging from 28 percent to greater than 70 percent correlation.[18,35] More extensive lesions termed subcortical leucomalacia have also been described and may coexist or occur independently of classic PVL.[36] These data suggest that PVL may be difficult to diagnose by ultrasound alone, and we therefore prefer the term PVE when describing abnormalities on ultrasound. The timing of the ultrasound and the duration and evolution of echodensities over time are critically important in determining their correlation with PVL and prognostic significance.[37,38] Figure 6 shows an ultrasound of an infant with bilateral PVEs proven at autopsy to be due to PVL.

Infants with PVE lesions have varied outcomes. Early periventricular echoes that disappear during the second or third week and are unassociated with later ventriculomegaly or cystic changes are not likely to correlate with major disabili-

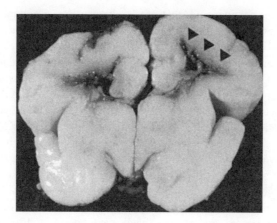

Fig 5. An autopsy specimen showing the brain of a premature infant in coronal section with bilateral and severe PVL (indicated by the arrows above the lesion on the right).

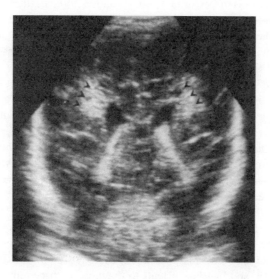

Fig 6. Coronal view of a cranial ultrasound of an 18-day-old premature infant with bilateral PVE. Note also the anechoic, darker cystic areas medial to the middle arrow on the left and the top arrow on the right.

ties.[39,40] Similar echodensities that persist, however, and one pattern with more extensive periventricular involvement, called "prolonged flare," are associated with PVL and cerebral palsy in more than 50% of cases.[32,37,38]

Cystic degeneration of echogenic areas (which typically occurs 2 to 3 weeks after the initial lesion) has, however, shown a strong correlation with later cerebral palsy and cognitive deficits.[41,42] Cysts are anechoic areas within PVE that are due to dissolution of brain tissue secondary to infarction.[35,41] They develop from 2 to 6 weeks postnatally and continue to evolve for weeks[41,43] (see Fig 6).

Despite the overall frequency of later deficits in patients with cystic lesions, cerebral palsy is not invariable.[11,12] The anatomic location of the PVE and the size of the cysts are prognostically important. Small cysts in frontal regions may have a better prognosis, leading to major deficits in 25% to 40% of such patients.[11,12] Infants with large (>3 mm in diameter) bilateral cystic lesions located in the parietal or occipital areas, on the other hand, have been found to develop cerebral palsy in more than 90% of cases.[44,45] Even when these larger cystic lesions are transient and develop a solid appearance on ultrasound within several weeks, the outcome remains the same. This resolution of ultrasonographic findings appears to be due to gliosis (brain "scarring").[18,44]

Because of the importance of the evolution of PVE with respect to prognosis, serial studies are often performed. Some studies indicate that ultrasound performed later in the hospital course or at term age may correlate better with outcome than earlier studies. Cystic PVE or ventriculomegaly on later ultrasounds has been followed by cerebral palsy in 50 percent to 100 percent of affected patients.[43,46]

MRI has also shown promise in improving our ability to predict severe sequelae in infants with PVE.[47] The MRI findings prior to discharge in a number of our patients have been remarkable (Fig 7) and appear to be particularly helpful in those with equivocal ultrasound findings. MRIs performed in infants more than 8 months of age have also been shown to be quite reliable in documenting anatomic abnormalities in patients with later cerebral palsy.[48,49] Whether MRI prior to discharge will prove to be cost-effective and more predictive than serial ultrasounds remains to be seen.

In summary, PVEs are a common finding in VLBW infants. The duration and pattern of abnormality on serial scanning are critically important in determining their prognostic significance. PVL is a histopathologic term that represents the classic ischemic lesion in this population, bears a definite relationship to long-term disabilities, and can be difficult to diagnose with certainty by ultrasound alone. Developing a consistent terminology for PVE, continuing investigations with neuropathologic correlations and MRI, PET scan, and other techniques may be helpful in clarifying the pathophysiology of these abnormalities and improving our ability to anticipate their outcomes.

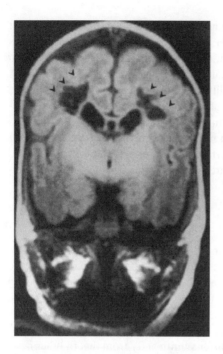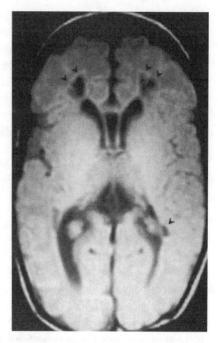

Fig 7. (a) Coronal view of a magnetic resonance imaging (MRI) scan of a 42-day-old infant with extensive cystic periventricular leucomalacia (PVL) indicated by the arrows. (b) A horizontal view of the same MRI showing cystic PVL in both the frontal and the left parietal regions.

INTERVENTION IN THE NICU

There is continuing controversy regarding the potential benefits and hazards of stimulation therapies for neonates.[50–52] Nonetheless, NICU staff members frequently request consultations by therapists to obtain a developmental perspective and to consider appropriate interventions. Among VLBW infants, those with demonstrated cranial ultrasound abnormalities comprise an interesting subgroup but also may prove particularly vulnerable to the negative aspects of such approaches.[51]

The primary focus of any intervention, therefore, must begin with a sensitivity toward the timing of involvement and full awareness of the therapists' responsibility—"First, do no harm." Therapists working with brain-injured newborns also benefit from a realistic attitude toward what can be accomplished by intervention and must acknowledge that present therapies are not able to undo or repair structural neurologic injuries of the types discussed in the first section of this article. It may be reasonable, however, to expect that appropriate stimulation activities might "assist to some extent in the resumption of a process that may have been abruptly interrupted by the infant's premature birth,"[52(p174)] or even by brain injury. The goal, therefore, becomes one of facilitating development to the extent that it is biologically possible. An additional benefit is the gaining of information regarding the child's maturational age (ie, the infant's functional level), which may differ from the postconceptional age. Such information may impact nursing care or feeding approaches. Perhaps most important, interventional approaches can also form the basis of enlightened parental care taking and enhance the parents' understanding of their infant's developmental functioning.

Assessment

Referral for intervention tends to occur somewhat earlier in infants with known brain injury. In our NICU, such referrals are made for infants with an average age of 32 to 34 weeks. Discussions with neonatology and nursing staff members and the pediatric neurologist and the review of pertinent brain imaging studies may be helpful for the consulting therapist and may provide a realistic view of the infant's neurologic condition. Despite some unique features, however, the actual assessment of brain-injured infants does not differ significantly from that of other newborns.[53,54] An occupational therapist performs most of the evaluation. The assessment process begins with an evaluation of the infant's maturational age regarding sensorimotor and behavioral responsivity as well as feeding behaviors.

SENSORIMOTOR AND BEHAVIORAL EVALUATION

Evaluation of the preterm infant's sensorimotor development can usually begin around 32 to 33 weeks' postconceptional age and uses an observational approach. The exact timing depends on the infant's general status, overall maintenance of homeostasis, observed rest-activity cycle, and the presence of any obvious deviant motor behaviors as noted in consultation with NICU staff. The observation of movements in premature infants has been well described and provides a basis for assessing the duration and character of movement with respect to fluency and variability.[53,54] Neurologically abnormal infants typically produce disorganized movement patterns and other atypical movements, which have been described.[54]

The Assessment of Preterm Infant Behaviors (APIB) instrument, as well as its adaptation, The Naturalistic Observational Assessment (NOA) instrument, can be used for such observations.[55,56] The APIB requires extensive training to administer and has been used to identify subsystems of behavioral functions, which include autonomic, motor, state organizational, attentional, interactional, and self-regulatory systems, and provides an excellent model for evaluation.[56] A variety of dysfunctions in these areas, and particularly inconsistency in state organization during the neonatal period, may be associated with later developmental disabilities.[57] The NOA provides an instrument for the observation of sleep and arousal states before the infant is fed and of self-regulatory behaviors following feeding.

Following the sensorimotor and behavioral assessment, an evaluation of feeding may be performed. Efficient and nonefficient feeders can be distinguished by empirical means as well as by experienced clinical judgment.[58,59] A neonatal oral motor assessment has been developed to quantify normal and deviant oral motor patterns in neonates.[60] Poor feeders are distinguished by abnormalities in sucking rhythm and rate, fatigability, long pauses between sucks, and inability to establish a rhythmic pattern.[61]

Through this three-part evaluation, the therapist gains an understanding of the infant's developmental status with respect to sensory responses and motor patterns, sleep-wake activity, and feeding ability. This information provides the basis for individualized handling and intervention strategies, and the results are shared with the NICU staff and the infant's parents. Recommendations for handling and care-taking activities are made at this time and are aimed at minimizing stress on the infant.

INDIVIDUALIZED TREATMENT PROGRAM

Treatment of deficient sensorimotor, behavioral, and feeding patterns is usually begun as soon as the infant's responsivity, coping ability, and overall status permit.[52,62] Treatment strategies for infants who exhibit motor dysfunction or are at risk for motor problems should begin with a synactive model of intervention.[56,63] This model uses the infant's approach behaviors such as coordination of hand-to-mouth behavior to balance avoidance movements such as grimace, startle, truncal arch, and finger splay.[55]

A number of intervention programs have been described to ameliorate behavioral disorganization and dysfunction.[52,62,64] These models include modulation techniques, handling, positioning, and treatment of oral and feeding problems. Field[64] has shown that treated infants averaged greater weight gain per day, had better organization of state development, and had more mature habituation, orientation, and motor activity than control infants. Resnick et al[65] reported a significantly lower incidence of developmental delay in low birth weight infants enrolled in a multidisciplinary family-centered treatment program compared to controls when treatment began in the NICU and continued for 2 years.

Abnormalities such as persistent or obligate postures, reduced range of joint mobility, and even associated contractures are treated by the physical therapist in the NICU. Supportive positioning techniques are used and are intended to stimulate normal flexion of the trunk and limb, activate head rotation, and facilitate a balance between flexion and extension postures.[66] Symmetrical postures are encouraged, since they enhance midline orientation and facilitate smooth antigravity limb movement. Persistent retraction and elevation of the shoulders or froglike postures of the legs are reduced by gentle position changes. Splinting is indicated in rare infants to prevent progressive deformity when postural approaches are insufficient.[67]

Intervention for feeding is based on a consideration of the maturational factors rather than the child's postconceptional age alone and is coordinated by the occupational therapist. Although many neonatal poor feeders are "disorganized" and require therapeutic measures to help coordinate breathing, sucking, and swallowing, brain-injured infants are more often in the "dysfunctional" group. In this group, the feeding difficulties often relate to abnormalities of arousal mechanisms and muscle tone. For such infants, nurses and parents are instructed to prepare the infants for feeding by gradually increasing stimulation contingent on the infant's responses, that is, following the infant's cues.[68] Additionally, the timing of the feeding should be based on the individual infant's historical pattern, rather than "by the clock." Specific approaches to gentle stimulation and arousal of the infant, followed by appropriate feeding techniques, may be videotaped and then shared with the parents and other caretakers.[64] These approaches have also been shown to improve parent-infant interactions.[69] An example of an evaluation and interventional approach used for a single patient is shown in Table 1.

Parental involvement

Parents are included in their child's intervention program. The goal is not to train parents to become therapists, but rather to educate the parents and to enhance their sense of confidence in caring for their infant. This participation also provides an opportunity for parents to work through their feelings and to discuss a wide range of concerns with staff members.

Involvement of parents in the intervention program begins with helping them understand their infant's behavior and suggesting methods of response to their baby's individual cues. Parents are taught approaches that follow a sensory sequence of tactile, proprioceptive, vestibular, and finally, visual interaction.[52,68] These activities can be easily incorporated into the parents' caregiving role as their child progresses from the NICU to discharge; they also permit better adaptation by the infant, which facilitates parent–child interaction.[69]

Intervention guidelines and summary

To develop an appropriate plan of intervention, certain guidelines may be helpful.

Table 1. Sample evaluation and intervention in a 36-week-old infant*

Behavioral observations	36-week expected neonatal behavior	Responses from this infant	Intervention
Rest	Defined and regular cycles of rest and activity	Short rest periods; more frequent stretching and movements	Modify environment (reduce light, noise, traffic); position appropriately
Spontaneous movement	Alternating flexion and extension; variable and fluent movements	Tremors, restricted monotonous movements	Position for support of weak muscles in cervical alignment; relaxation of restricted movements
Level of arousal	High threshold of stimulation; inhibition of startle and muscle contraction; brief eye closure or fixation on light	Grimaces, startles, and tenses muscles with handling and position change; avoidance of light by head-turning	Schedule manipulations in clusters according to infant responses; handle with limb flexed toward midline; slow and gentle handling
Self-regulatory controls	Good self-quieting; gradual state changes; focuses attention on examiner's face; quiets to voice	Hyperexcitable, irritable, and panicky with stimulation; worried, dull facial expression.	Reduce intensity of stimuli; modulate voice and touch according to infant's facial expression
Feeding patterns	Mature sucking with regular bursts, pauses, rests, and breaths	Jaw clenching, breath holding; tongue retracted and pulled back into pharynx	Stimulate rooting response for jaw opening and to facilitate tongue protrusion; provide appropriate nipple and rest periods

*The infant's magnetic resonance image is shown in Fig 7.

- Infants with known brain injury often have maturational rates that deviate from their post-conceptional age. The child's maturational age should be used as an overall guide for any intervention program.
- Evaluation methods should be short and nonintrusive and should rely on direct observation, including videotaping. Quantitative as well as qualitative measurements should be used when possible.
- The responsiveness of the infant to the environment can be evaluated by observation during routine caregiving. Additional evaluation techniques can then be used for more detailed and quantitative measurement, as the infant can tolerate.

- Sensorimotor interventions may facilitate functional responses in motor, behavioral, and feeding development if the approach is based on an individual evaluation.
- Any therapeutic program should be designed to foster parental interaction with the infant and to enhance feelings of parental competence.

In summary, this approach to assessment and treatment recognizes the special needs of the brain-injured neonate. It begins with observational approaches that cause minimal stress for the infant and proceeds to an individualized assessment and intervention approach. Goals are to facilitate and enhance the infant's development while recognizing the reality of biologic limits and involving the parents in an educational approach to foster their own sense of competency.

The importance of qualitative and quantitative aspects of the interventions, the specific populations of infants and families most likely to benefit, and the question of whether such interventions significantly alter outcomes across a range of functions remain fertile areas for thoughtful and controlled studies. The risks, as well as the benefits, of such interventions also require additional analysis. For the present, continued involvement by therapists in the NICU is likely to remain a controversial but often-requested service. It is necessary for those of us involved in the care of these infants to temper our enthusiasm for early intervention with continued evaluation of these approaches and their effects.

REFERENCES

1. Volpe JJ. Brain injury and the premature infant: Is it preventable? *Pediatr Res.* 1990;27 :28–33.
2. Allan WC. The IVH complex of lesions: Cerebrovascular injury in the preterm infant. *Neurol Clin.* 1990;8:529–552.
3. Papile L, Burstein J, Burstein R, Koffer H. Incidence and evolution of subependymal hemorrhage: A study of infants with birth weight less than 1500 grams. *J Pediatr.* 1978;92:529–534.
4. Volpe JJ. Evolution of neonatal periventricular-intraventricular hemorrhage: A major advance. *Am J Dis Child.* 1980;134:1023–1025.
5. Dubowitz LMS, Bydder GM. MRI of the brain in neonates. *Semin Perinatol.* 1990;14:212–223.
6. Griesen G, Trojaberg W. Cerebral blood flow, $PaCO_2$ changes, and VER in mechanically ventilated preterm infants. *Acta Pediatr Scand.* 1987;76: 394–400.
7. Altman DI, Powers WJ, Perlman JM, Herscovitch P, Volpe S, Volpe JJ. Cerebral blood flow requirements for brain viability in newborn infants is lower than in adults. *Ann Neurol.* 1988;24:218–226.
8. Volpe JJ, Herscovitch PI, Perlman JM, Raichle ME. Positron emission tomography in the newborn: Extensive impairment of regional cerebral blood flow with intraventricular hemorrhage and hemorrhagic intracerebral involvement. *Pediatrics.* 1983; 72:589–601.
9. Connell J, Oozeer R, Regev R, DeVries LS, Dubowitz LMS, Dubowitz V. Continuous four channel EEG monitoring in evaluation of echodense ultrasound lesions and cystic leucomalacia. *Arch Dis Child.* 1987;62:1019–1024.

10. Levene MI. Cerebral ultrasound and neurological impairment: Telling the future. *Arch Dis Child.* 1990;65:469–471.

11. Blackman JA, McGuiness GA, Bale JF, Smith WL. Large postnatally acquired porencephalic cysts: Unexpected outcomes. *J Child Neurol.* 1991;6:58–64.

12. Bennett FC, Silver G, Leung EJ, Mack LA. Periventricular echodensities detected by cranial US: Usefulness in predicting neurodevelopmental outcome in low birth weight, preterm infants. *Pediatrics.* 1990;85:400–404.

13. Philip AGS, Allan WC, Tito AM, Wheeler LR. IVH in preterm infants: Declining incidence in the 1980's. *Pediatrics.* 1989 ;84 :797–801.

14. Volpe JJ. IVH and brain injury in the premature infant: Neuropathology and pathogenesis. *Clin Perinatol.* 1989;16:361–386.

15. Ment LR, Duncan CC, Ehrenkranz RA. IVH of the preterm neonate. *Semin Perinatol.* 1987; 11:132–141.

16. Lazzara A, Ahmann PA, Dykes F, Brann AW, Schwartz J. Clinical predictability of intraventricular hemorrhage. *Pediatrics.* 1980;65:30–34.

17. Dubowitz LMS, Levene MI, Marante A. Neurologic signs in neonatal intraventricular hemorrhage: A correlation with real time ultrasound. *J Pediatr.* 1981;99:127–133.

18. Hope PL, Gould SJ, Hovard S, Hamilton PA, Costello AM, Reynolds EO. Precision of ultrasound diagnosis of pathologically verified lesions in the brains of very preterm infants. *Dev Med Child Neurol.* 1988;30:457—471.

19. Papile LA, Munsick-Bruno G, Schaeffer A. Relationship of cerebral intraventricular hemorrhage and early childhood neurologic handicaps. *J Pediatr.* 1983;103:273–277.

20. Shankaran S, Slovis TL, Bedard MP, Poland RL. Sonographic classification of intracranial hemorrhage: A prognostic indicator of mortality, morbidity, and short term neurologic outcome. *J Pediatr.* 1982;100:469–475.

21. Volpe JJ. *Neurology of the Newborn.* Philadelphia: W.B. Saunders, 1987.

22. Mantovani JF, Pasternak JF, Matthew O, et al. Failure of daily lumbar punctures to prevent development of hydrocephalus following intraventricular hemorrhage. *J Pediatr.* 1980;97:278–281.

23. Boynton BR, Boynton CA, Merritt A, Vaucher YE, James HE, Bejar RF. VP shunts in low birth weight infants with intracranial hemorrhage: Neurodevelopmental outcome. *Neurosurgery.* 1986;18:141–145.

24. Allan WC, Dransfield DA, Tito AM. Ventricular dilation following periventricular-intraventricular hemorrhage: Outcome at age 1 year. *Pediatrics.* 1984;73:158–162.

25. Shankaran S, Koepke T, Woldt E, et al. Outcome after post hemorrhagic ventriculomegaly in comparison with mild hemorrhage without ventriculomegaly. *J Pediatr.* 1989;114:109–114.

26. Dykes FD, Dunbar D, Lazarra A, Ahmann P. Post hemorrhagic hydrocephalus in high risk preterm infants: Natural history, management and long term outcome. *J Pediatr.* 1989;114:611–618.

27. Graziani LJ, Parto M, Stanley C, et al. Neonatal sonographic correlates of cerebral palsy in preterm infants. *Pediatrics.* 1986;78:88–95.

28. Garfinkel E, Tejani N, Boxes HS, et al. Infancy and early childhood follow-up of neonates with periventricular or intraventricular hemorrhage or isolated ventricular dilation: A case controlled study. *Am J Perinatol.* 1988;5: 214–219 .

29. McMenamin JB, Shackleford GD, Volpe JJ. Outcome of neonatal intraventricular hemorrhage with periventricular echodense lesions. *Ann Neurol.* 1984;15:285–290.

30. Guzetta F, Shackleford GD, Volpe S, Perlman JM, Volpe JJ. Periventricular intraparenchymal

echodensity in premature newborns: Critical determinant of neurologic outcome. *Pediatrics.* 1986;78:995–1006.

31. Gould SJ, Howard S, Hope PL, Reynolds EOR. Periventricular intraparenchymal cerebral hemorrhage in preterm infants: The role of venous infarction. *J Pathol.* 1987;151:197–202.

32. Graham M, Leven MI, Trounce JQ, Rutter N. Prediction of cerebral palsy in VLBW infants: Prospective ultrasound study. *Lancet.* 1987;2:593–596.

33. Banker BQ, Larroche JC. Periventricular leucomalacia of infancy. *Arch Neurol.* 1962;7:32–50.

34. DeReuck JL. Cerebral angioarchitecture and perinatal brain lesions in premature and full-term infants. *Acta Neurol Scand.* 1984;70:391–399.

35. Nwasei CG, Pape KE, Martin DJ, Becker LE, Fitz CR. Periventricular infarction diagnosed by cranial ultrasound: A postmortem correlation. *J Pediatr.* 1984;105:106–110.

36. Paneth N, Rudelli R, Monte W, et al. White matter necrosis in VLBW infants: Neuropathologic and ultrasonographic findings in infants surviving six days or longer. *J Pediatr.* 1990;116:775–784.

37. Rushton DI, Preston PR, Dunkin GM. Structure and evolution of echodense lesions in the neonatal brain. *Arch Dis Child.* 1985;60:798–808.

38. Cooke RWI. Early and late cranial ultrasonographic appearance and outcome in VLBW infants. *Arch Dis Child.* 1987;62:931–937.

39. Laub MC, Ingrisch H. Increased periventricular echogenicity (periventricular halos) in neonatal brain: A sonographic study. *Neuropediatrics.* 1986;17:39–43.

40. Devries LS, Dubowitz LMS, Dubowitz V, et al. Predictive value of cranial ultrasound: A reappraisal. *Lancet.* 1985;2:137–140.

41. Weindling AM, Rocheport MJ, Calvert SA, Fok TF, Wilkinson A. Development of cerebral palsy after ultrasonographic detection of periventricular cysts in the newborn. *Dev Med Child Neurol.* 1985;27:800–806.

42. Calvert SA, Hoskins EM, Fong KW, Forsyth SC. Periventricular leucomalacia: Ultrasonic diagnosis and neurological outcome. *Acta Pediatr Scand.* 1986; 75:489–496.

43. Bozynski MEA, Nelson MN, Genaze D, Rosati-Skevitch C, Matalan TA, Vasan U. Cranial ultrasonography and the prediction of cerebral palsy in infants weighing less than 1200 grams at birth. *Dev Med Child Neurol.* 1988;30:342–348.

44. Pidcock FS, Graziani LJ, Stanley C, Mitchell DG, Merton D. Neurosonographic features of periventricular echodensities associated with cerebral palsy in preterm infants. *J Pediatr.* 1990;116:417–422.

45. Hansen NB, Kopechek J, Miller RR, Menke JA, Cordero L. Prognostic significance of cystic intracranial lesions in neonates. *J Dev Behav Pediatr.* 1989;10:129–133.

46. Nwasei CG, Allen AC, Vincer MJ, et al. Effect of timing of cerebral ultrasonography on the prediction of later neurodevelopmental outcome in high risk preterm infants. *J Pediatr.* 1988;112:970–975.

47. Devries LS, Connell JA, Dubowitz LMS, Oozer RC, Dubowitz V. Neurological, electrophysiological and magnetic resonance imaging abnormalities in infants with extensive cystic leukomalacia. *Neuropediatrics.* 1987;18:61–66.

48. Feldman HM, Sher MS, Kemp SS. Neurodevelopmental outcome of children with evidence of periventricular leucomalacia on late MRI. *Pediatr Neurol.* 1990;6:296–302.

49. Byrne P, Welch R, Johnson MA, Dauah J, Pipe M. Serial MRI in neonatal hypoxic-ischemic encephalopathy. *J Pediatr.* 1990;117:694–700.

50. Strauss MS, Brownell CA. A commentary on infant stimulation and intervention. *J Child Contemp Soc.* 1985;17:133–139.

51. Sweeney JK. The physiologic adaptations of neonates to neurological assessment. In: Sweeney JK, ed. *The High Risk Neonate: Developmental Therapy Perspectives.* New York: Haworth Press, 1986.

52. Korner AF. Infant stimulation issues of theory and research. *Clin Perinatol.* 1990;17:173–183.

53. Prechtl HFR. Qualitative changes of spontaneous movement in fetus and preterm infant are a marker of neurological dysfunction. *Early Hum Dev.* 1990; 23:151–157.

54. Ferrari F, Cioniand G, Prechtl HFR. Qualitative changes of general movements in preterm infants with brain lesions. *Early Hum Dev.* 1990;23:193–231.

55. Als H, Lester BM, Tronick E, Brazelton TB. Towards a research instrument for the assessment of preterm infants' behavior (APIB). In: Fitzgerald HE, et al, eds. *Theory and Research in Behavioral Pediatrics.* New York: Plenum, 1982.

56. Als H. A synactive model of neonatal behavioral organization: Framework for the assessment of neurobehavioral development in the preterm infant and for support of infants and parents in the neonatal intensive care environment. In: Sweeney JK, ed. *The High Risk Neonate: Developmental Therapy Perspectives.* New York: Haworth Press, 1986.

57. Thoman EB, Denenberg VH, Sievel J, Zeidner LP, Becker P. State organization in neonates: Developmental inconsistency indicates risk for developmental dysfunction. *Neuropediatrics.* 1981;12:10–18.

58. Dubignon J, Cooper D. Good and poor feeding behavior in the neonatal period. *Inf Behav Dev.* 1980;3:395–408.

59. Rybski D, Gisel E. Optimal and sub-optimal feeding behavior of neonates. *Phys Occup Ther Pediatr.* 1984;4:37–46.

60. Braun MA, Palmer MA. A pilot study of oral motor dysfunction in "at risk" infants. *Phys Occup Ther Pediatr.* 1985;5:13–25.

61. Case-Smith J, Cooper P, Scala V. Feeding efficacy of premature neonates. *Am J Occup Ther.* 1989;43:245–250.

62. Anderson J. Sensory intervention with the preterm infant in the neonatal intensive care unit. *Am J Occup Ther.* 1986;40:19–26.

63. Fetters L. Sensorimotor management of the high risk neonate. In: Sweeney JK, ed. *The High Risk Neonate: Developmental Therapy Perspectives.* New York: Haworth Press, 1986.

64. Field T. Interventions for premature infants. *J Pediatr.* 1986;109:183–190.

65. Resnick MB, Eyler FD, Nelson RM, Eitzman OV, Buciarelli RL. Developmental intervention for low birth weight infants: Improved early developmental outcome. *Pediatrics.* 1987;80:68–74.

66. Updike C, Schmidt RE, Macke C, Caheen J, Miller M. Positional support for premature infants. *Am J Occup Ther.* 1986;40:712–715.

67. Anderson LJ, Anderson JM. Hand splinting for infants in the intensive care and special care nurseries. *Am J Occup Ther.* 1988;42:222–226.

68. Blackburn S. Fostering behavioral development of high-risk infants. *J Gynecol Nurs.* 1983;(May/June)(Suppl):76–86.

69. Rauh VA, Nurcombe B, Achenbach J, Howell C. The mother-infant transaction program. *Clin Perinatol.* 1990;17:31–45.

Congenital infections: Clinical outcome and educational implications

W. Daniel Williamson, MD
Assistant Professor
Section of Developmental Pediatrics
Department of Pediatrics
Baylor College of Medicine
Meyer Center for Developmental
  Pediatrics
Texas Children's Hospital
Houston, Texas

Gail J. Demmler, MD
Assistant Professor
Section of Infectious Diseases
Department of Pediatrics
Department of Microbiology and
  Immunology
Baylor College of Medicine
Houston, Texas

CONGENITAL infections affect at least 40,000 newborn infants each year in the United States. This number includes those infants with infections classically referred to as the TORCH infections, caused by *Toxoplasma gondii* (toxoplasmosis), rubella virus, cytomegalovirus (CMV), herpes simplex virus (HSV), and *Treponema pallidum* (syphilis). Although there are many similarities among the early manifestations as well as the long-term sequelae of this group of intrauterine infections, various differences warrant an individual review of each infection.

This review describes the method of transmission of these prenatal infections, their initial symptomatology and long-term effects, and the appropriate ongoing management required by infected infants. The fact that each of these infections results in significant neurodevelopmental damage to affected infants underscores the educational impact of these diseases.

CONGENITAL TOXOPLASMOSIS

Toxoplasma gondii, a parasite with worldwide distribution, has been known to cause significant prenatal infections since the 1920s.[1] The frequency of congenital toxoplasmosis is estimated to be approximately 2.3 per 1,000 live births in the United States, with a much higher frequency in Europe and South America.[2]

Epidemiology

Toxoplasma organisms are acquired by ingesting the parasites in raw or poorly cooked infected meat or by exposure to infected cat feces. Initial (primary) infections are usually subclinical but occasionally present with a mild febrile illness similar to infectious mononucleosis. The prevalence of *Toxoplasma* infections ranges from 5% to 95% of the young adults throughout the world.[3] In the United States the prevalence of positive antibodies for *Toxoplasma* organisms by the second decade of life ranges from 3% to 20%.[1]

170

Inf Young Children 1992;4(4):1–10
© 1992 Aspen Publishers, Inc.

Intrauterine transmission of *Toxoplasma* organisms occurs only during a primary maternal infection, when the parasite goes from the mother's blood to infect the placenta and the fetus. The overall transmission rate from mother to fetus is approximately 39%, with a lower rate during the first trimester (20%) than during the second or third trimester (25% to 65%).[2] When the fetus is infected during the first trimester, however, the severity of the infection is likely to be greater.[3] In the third trimester, more than 90% of the infections are subclinical in the infant. It is estimated that nearly three fourths of the infants born with congenital toxoplasmosis lack symptoms at birth.[3]

Neonatal and long-term outcome

The classic features of congenital toxoplasmosis—inflammation of the retina (retinochoroiditis), hydrocephalus or microcephaly, and intracranial calcification—occur in only a small proportion of cases. Occasionally, enlargement of the spleen and liver (hepatosplenomegaly) and jaundice accompany the initial clinical picture. However, abnormalities of the eye occur in nearly three fourths of infants with neonatal symptoms and in more than 80% of infants who have subclinical disease.[4,5]

The most frequent ocular lesion is retinochoroiditis, usually with bilateral involvement.[4] Visual impairment will depend on the size and the location of the lesion. In either subclinical or symptomatic neonatal disease, reactivation of old retinochoroiditis or late onset of new lesions can occur months to years after birth, causing significant visual impairment.[6] Abnormally small eyes (microphthalmus) occur in 20% of infants with eye abnormalities.[7] Other abnormalities may include cataracts, strabismus, nystagmus, swelling and inflammation of the optic nerve (papilledema), and optic atrophy.

Neurodevelopmental outcome of infants with congenital toxoplasmosis is directly associated with the degree of symptomatology at birth. Nearly 90% of the neonates with classic features of eye and brain abnormalities will exhibit later mental retardation; almost as many will have seizures or cerebral palsy.[8] Some 20% of the infants who have serologic evidence of congenital toxoplasmosis but who lack symptoms at birth will have later neurodevelopmental abnormalities, and most will have retinochoroiditis of at least a mild degree.[5]

Treatment and prevention

Congenital toxoplasmosis can be prevented by eliminating primary maternal *Toxoplasma* infections during pregnancy. Prevention can be achieved by eating only well-cooked meats and washed fruits and vegetables and by avoiding direct contact with or inhalation of material containing infected cat feces (eg, cat litter, garden soil, and open sandboxes). Because there are no widely available screening programs for *T gondii*, one must either request serologic studies or attempt to practice the above mentioned preventive measures. Such preventive measures are important because between 85% and 95% of women in many areas of the United States have never had a primary *Toxoplasma* infection.[1]

If a maternal *Toxoplasma* infection is confirmed, specific antiparasitic drug treatment and counseling are recommended.[9] Treatment appears to reduce the transmission of the maternal infection to the fetus and may reduce the sequelae experienced by the infected fetus.[9] It is recommended that the congenitally infected infant, whether symptomatic or not, receive treatment with pyramethiamine and sulfadiazine or with spiramycin.[9] Such early treatment may reduce the incidence of sequelae caused by the intrauterine infection. In addition, routine ophthalmologic follow-up is necessary because late-onset retinochoroiditis may occur and require medical intervention. Certainly, infants with congenital toxoplasmosis who have obvious ophthalmologic or neurodevelopmental sequelae should receive ongoing educational intervention. Enrollment of these infants in early childhood intervention programs does not present health risks to the education staff because there is no postnatal human-to-human transmission of *Toxoplasma* organisms.

CONGENITAL RUBELLA SYNDROME

It has been 50 years since the relationship between maternal rubella (German measles) during pregnancy and congenital cataracts of the neonate was first described.[10] This discovery during the Australian epidemic of 1939–1941 was followed by the documentation of hearing loss in infants exposed to rubella during fetal life.[11,12] The rubella epidemic of 1964–1965 in the United States resulted in more than 20,000 neonates born with congenital rubella syndrome. Because of the numerous developmental and physical problems, the cost of this epidemic was estimated to be more than $2.2 billion.[13] Although the development of the rubella vaccine has significantly reduced the occurrence of congenital rubella syndrome, 17 confirmed or compatible cases and an additional 5 possible cases of congenital rubella infection for 1990 were reported to the Centers for Disease Control.[14] This is an increase over previous years and mirrors the rise in cases of postnatal rubella in 1990, representing the largest number since 1982.

Epidemiology

Rubella virus has a worldwide distribution. In studies done before the widespread use of the rubella vaccine begun in the late 1960s, some 70% to 80% of adults were seroimmune.[15] The incidence of congenital rubella syndrome during periods of epidemics is estimated to be 4 to 30 cases per 1,000 live births.[3] During interepidemic periods, however, the incidence decreases to 0.2 to 0.5 per 1,000 live births.

Acquisition of postnatal rubella usually begins with a 2- to 3-week incubation period between the time of contact with the virus and onset of the rash. Virus can be recovered from the nasopharynx as early as 1 week before the onset of the rash and for up to 2 weeks after the rash disappears. The virus can also be recovered from the blood for up to 1 week before the rash appears but then becomes unobtainable. This period of maternal viremia is the critical phase for transmission of the virus to the fetus via maternal blood and the placenta.[15] During the first 12 to 14 weeks of pregnancy, the risk of transmission varies from 67% to 80%. The risk of transmission drops at the end of the second trimester to 25% but increases to more than 90% in the last trimester.

The timing of the transmission of the rubella virus from mother to fetus is important to the ultimate postnatal outcome. Fetal infections occurring during the first 16 weeks of gestation are likely to produce major physical, neurologic, and developmental problems. The risk for the fetus to be affected decreases with each month of gestation, and after 4 months damage to the fetus is uncommon.[16]

Neonatal and long-term outcome

The neonate with congenital rubella syndrome is likely to have multiple organ involvement and to be born at term but to exhibit intrauterine growth retardation.[17] More than half the congenitally infected infants will have an enlarged liver and spleen (hepatosplenomegaly), decreased number of platelets (thrombocytopenia), anemia, hepatitis, and jaundice. At least 40% of the congenitally infected infants will exhibit abnormalities of the eye, including cataracts, pigmentary retinopathy, retinal degeneration, glaucoma, microphthalmus, strabismus, or nystagmus. Nearly half those infected will have early and significant sensorineural hearing loss, and a similar proportion will have congenital heart defects such as pulmonary arterial lesions and persistent ductus arteriosus. Early neurologic abnormalities may include generalized encephalitis (lethargy, hypotonia, and irritability) and seizures.[18]

The neonate with congenital rubella syndrome requires lifelong follow-up for potential complications from the intrauterine infection. In a longitudinal study of adolescents with congenital rubella syndrome, it was found that the most frequently occurring chronic problem was sensorineural hearing loss, which occurred in more than 90% of the youths by age 16 to 18 years.[19] The majority with hearing loss had experienced deterioration in hearing; by adolescence, 70% had severe to profound bilateral hearing loss. Manual communication was used by more than half the group with hearing loss. Significant visual impairment occurred in 56% of the group; 19% had both visual and hearing impairment. Other chronic neurologic problems included cerebral palsy (19%), epilepsy (8%), and behavioral disorders (32%). Although congenital heart disease was diagnosed in 68% of those followed, only one adolescent had functional heart disease. Diabetes mellitus had developed in one subject by adolescence.

Nearly half the adolescents in the prospective study had average or above average intellectual functioning; 28% functioned within the mentally retarded range, and the remaining one fourth functioned as slower learners. Some type of special education services, however, was required by three fourths of the entire group; one fourth of the group was being served through state residential schools for students with sensory impairments.

Treatment and prevention

The development of the rubella vaccine has resulted in a significant decrease in the incidence of congenital rubella syndrome. The disease is not eradicated, however, in part because not all children are adequately immunized.[20] There is no specific antiviral treatment available for rubella virus infection. An infant with congenital rubella syndrome requires lifelong medical follow-up to monitor general health, to anticipate the development of late-onset disease such as diabetes mellitus, and to manage persistent problems such as seizure disorders, cerebral palsy, cardiac defects, and behavioral problems. In addition, repeated ophthalmologic examinations are necessary to observe for progressive eye disease, and routine audiologic reassessment must continue through adulthood because of the potential for progressive hearing loss. Enrollment in an early intervention program usually is a necessity. Although the infected infant may excrete the virus in the nasopharynx and urine for months, the condition is considered noncontagious after the first 3 to 6 months because the concentration of virus decreases dramatically.

CONGENITAL CYTOMEGALOVIRUS INFECTION

CMV, a member of the herpes virus family, is the most frequent cause of congenital infections in humans, affecting from 0.5% to 2.5% of all live births in the United States.[21] Although human CMV was not isolated in the laboratory until 1956, the pathologic changes in tissue infected with CMV were described in the late 1800s and early 1900s.[21] The prefix *cytomegalo-* has long been used to describe the abnormal microscopic changes of infected tissue.[22,23]

Epidemiology

CMV is a frequently occurring viral infection in humans. The prevalence of CMV infections in children worldwide has varied from 30% to 90%.[21] By adulthood 35% to 77% of pregnant women in the United States have positive serology, indicating previous exposure to CMV.[24]

CMV is transmitted to children and adults through various routes, and postnatal transmission of CMV may occur at any age. In children there appear to be peak times of acquisition in infancy and early childhood and again in puberty.[21] Transmission at the earliest ages is probably related to several factors, including breast feeding and group child care settings. Another factor related to earlier transmission is hygiene; studies indicate CMV transmission in settings such as hospitals and day care centers may be related to certain hygienic practices.[25,26] Acquisition of CMV at a later date may be related to sexual activity, and CMV transmission at any age may occur through blood transfusions as well as solid organ and bone marrow transplantation. In most instances a postnatal CMV infection causes no symptoms, or it may cause mild symptoms such as a flu-like illness or infectious mononucleosis type illness. Postnatal infections with CMV usually cause no long-term effects unless the infected person has an immune deficiency.

The maternal CMV infection transplacentally transmitted to the fetus in a congenital infection may be either primary (first-time infection) or recurrent (reactivation of a previous infection). Currently, available data suggest that primary maternal CMV infections usually are acquired from other family members, particularly children, who are unknowingly excreting CMV.[27,28] Transmission of the virus from mother to fetus in a primary infection occurs in approximately 40% of the cases.[24] A recurrent infection means that the pregnant woman has had a CMV infection before pregnancy that reactivates during pregnancy. When that reactivation occurs, CMV may be transmitted from mother to fetus in approximately 0.5% to 1.4% of cases.[24] Neonates who are symptomatic at birth probably are born to mothers who experienced primary CMV infections during pregnancy.[24] Data are accumulating, however, that suggest that infants without symptoms at birth but who have long-term sequelae such as hearing loss may be born to mothers with either primary or recurrent CMV infections during pregnancy.[29]

Neonatal and long-term outcome

Although congenital CMV infection is the most frequently occurring congenital infection, only 10% of the infected neonates are identified at birth.[21] These infants have symptoms classically associated with congenital infections such as petechiae, hepatosplenomegaly, jaundice, thrombocytopenia, microcephaly, intracranial calcifications, retinochoroiditis, and intrauterine growth retardation. With supportive management, most of these infants survive. The remaining 90% of infected infants are asymptomatic at birth and look no different than any other infant in a full-term nursery unit.[21] These infants usually are identified only when born in hospitals having CMV screening programs.

Long-term outcome for infants with symptomatic congenital CMV infections has been well documented in the literature. Virtually all symptomatic infants have some neurologic, audiologic, or developmental sequelae.[30,31] Sensorineural hearing loss and mental retardation are the most frequent sequelae, occurring in half the symptomatic infants. Although the hearing loss is usually congenital, late-onset sensorineural hearing loss also has been documented, and deterioration in hearing over time may occur.[31] Other long-term problems include cerebral palsy and visual impairment secondary to retinochoroiditis or optic atrophy. Initially symptomatic infants who have normal hearing are at risk for language disorders caused by problems such as developmental verbal dyspraxia; those with normal intelligence are at risk for specific learning disabilities.[31]

The long-term outcome for asymptomatic, congenitally infected neonates is less well documented. Studies suggest that 15% of the initially asymptomatic neonates have sensorineural hearing loss; again, the hearing loss is usually congenital but may be of later onset, and progressive deterioration in hearing loss may occur.[32-34] Another 5% have other significant neurologic and developmental abnormalities, such as mental retardation and cerebral palsy accompanying hearing loss. Conflicting data are available about the school performance of the asymptomatic group who escape neurologic, audiologic, and intellectual deficits.[35,36] Until further comprehensive studies can be completed, it must be assumed that the asymptomatic group also is at risk for language disorders and learning disabilities.

Treatment and prevention

Currently, there are no routine treatments available for infants with congenital CMV infections other than supportive measures. Nevertheless, restricted experimental therapies with antiviral medications such as ganciclovir are in progress for infants who are symptomatic at birth. At this time there is no CMV vaccine available for widespread use to prevent congenital CMV infections, although clinical trials are in progress. Therefore, measures to prevent primary CMV infection during pregnancy are limited at this time.

CMV-seronegative women who are pregnant should avoid intimate contact such as kissing or sharing food or drink with persons actively shedding CMV or who are likely to be shedding CMV, such as young children who attend group day care. Also, diapering should be avoided, and hand washing after casual contact should be practiced. These practices should be used by seronegative pregnant women who work with young children, such as day care workers, teachers, and therapists, and should be applied to all children in the group setting rather than only to the child known to be excreting CMV.

NEONATAL HERPES SIMPLEX VIRUS INFECTION

Neonatal HSV infection has been recognized as a significant cause of neonatal illness and long-term neurologic sequelae since the 1930s.[37] The infection is usually caused by HSV-2, the type most often causing herpetic genital infections. HSV-1 ("oral" herpes), however, also may cause both genital herpes and neonatal HSV infections. It is estimated that congenital HSV infections occur in 1 in 7,500 live births in the United States.

Epidemiology

Both HSV-1 and HSV-2 infections are frequent. HSV-1 infections are usually acquired in childhood; by adulthood some 50% to 75% of individuals have had HSV-1 infections.[38] HSV-2 is usually transmitted by sexual contact and thus is usually acquired after puberty. Serologic studies indicate that from 10% to 60% of individuals have positive serology.[39]

Transmission of HSV requires close contact with someone actively shedding the virus. Transmission can occur not only from contact with herpetic lesions but also from asymptomatic viral shedding from the genitourinary tract.[3] HSV infections with viral shedding may be due to a primary infection, reactivation of a latent infection, or reinfection with a new strain of the virus.

In contrast to the other congenital infections, which have the transplacental route as the primary route of transmission to the fetus, neonatal HSV infection is thought to occur primarily by an ascending infection via ruptured amnionic membranes or by direct exposure to the virus during delivery. The risk for neonatal HSV infection is approximately 10% when an infant is born to a mother with proven HSV infection present after gestation week 32 but increases to 40% to 50% if the virus is present at delivery, unless the infant is delivered by Cesarean section within 4 hours of rupture of the amnionic membranes.[40]

Neonatal and long-term outcome

When a neonate has actually acquired an HSV infection prenatally, he or she is probably born with microcephaly, hydranencephaly, microphthalmus, intracranial calcification, retinal dysplasia, and herpetic skin lesions or scars. Such exposure usually results in severe cognitive, motor, and visual deficits or death.[37,41]

Neonates who acquire their HSV infections nearer the time of delivery usually develop symptoms during the first 2 weeks of life but may go as long as 1 month before symptoms appear.[3] It is unusual for an infant with a congenital/intrapartum HSV infection to remain asymptomatic. Most develop either localized or disseminated disease. In localized disease, the infection may be limited to the skin, the eye, or the mucous membranes. If treated, survival without sequelae is likely. In contrast, disseminated disease may include both meningoencephalitis and liver and adrenal failure as well as fever, vomiting, respiratory distress, and bleeding.[37] If untreated, the mortality rate is 70% to 80% with virtual certainty of long-term neurodevelopmental deficits in survivors.[42] If treated, the mortality rate decreases to 15% to 20%, but at least half the survivors are left with significant neurologic and developmental impairments.[42]

Treatment and prevention

Reduction of the risk for congenital HSV infection appears to be possible in instances where the mother has overt HSV genital lesions and delivery by Cesarean section can be performed within 4 hours of membrane rupture.[40] If delivery is delayed for 6 hours or more after the membranes rupture, however, the chance for reducing fetal acquisition of HSV is poor. Once HSV infection is identified, institution of antiviral therapy with either acyclovir or vidarabine is indicated.[42]

Most infants with neonatal HSV infections will require special education services from birth. In general, they present no major risks to providers of such services. Nevertheless, specific precautions should be taken to cover active herpetic lesions when possible. Good hygienic techniques, including washing of hands and toys, is recommended.

CONGENITAL SYPHILIS

Syphilis, which is caused by the organism *Treponema pallidum*, was described at least as early as the 13th century, and congenital syphilis was first described in 1858.[43] Congenital syphilis, which follows the trend of adult acquired sexually transmitted diseases, is on the rise in the United States.[44] In the United States, the incidence of syphilis rose from 13.7 cases per 100,000 persons in 1981 to 18.4 cases per 100,000 persons in 1989. This incidence was the highest since 1949. From 1985 to 1989, the number of reported cases of congenital syphilis rose from 266 to 859. Although historically the oldest and one of the most easily preventable of the group of congenital diseases described in this review, congenital syphilis is an increasingly frequent disease encountered in infants in neonatal units and subsequently in early childhood intervention programs.

Epidemiology

The transmission of *Treponema pallidum* through sexual contact is the means by which the pregnant woman first acquires syphilis. In many instances, syphilis, at the time of acquisition, is a silent infection. During the primary stage of syphilis a single lesion (chancre) develops at the site of penetration of the bacteria, usually on the external genitalia. If untreated, the primary lesion heals, and after 6 to 8 weeks the secondary stage of the disease is heralded by a generalized maculopapular skin rash, often with lesions on the palms and soles. Accompanying the rash may be generalized symptoms including enlarged lymph nodes (lymphadenopathy), fever, weight loss, and joint pain (arthralgia). The signs and symptoms of secondary syphilis disappear over 4 to 6 weeks even without treatment.

The latent phase of syphilis, during which the disease remains quiescent, may follow the secondary stage. Neurosyphilis develops in 8% to 9% of untreated patients.[45] If left untreated, this stage may be characterized by various neurologic abnormalities, including meningitis, degeneration of the spinal cord, and dementia.

If the pregnant infected woman goes untreated, she may transmit the infection to her unborn child through the transplacental route at any time during pregnancy and in any stage of the disease.[46] Of the fetuses with congenital syphilis, 30% to 40% are stillborn.[47]

Neonatal and long-term outcome

Neonates with congenital syphilis will have laboratory evidence of the congenital infection, but two thirds may have no clinical signs.[47] In other instances infected neonates may have nonspecific findings common to any congenital infection, including intrauterine growth retardation, hepatosplenomegaly, anemia, thromocytopenia, and jaundice. The young infant may develop a bloody rhinitis (snuffles), which may be followed by a diffuse, maculopapular, red rash. Additional early manifestations may include skin lesions (condylomata lata) and bone abnormalities (osteochondritis), which may cause pain and inhibition of limb movement. If left untreated, an acute or subacute syphilitic meningitis can develop after several months.

Even when an infant with congenital syphilis receives treatment after birth, late abnormalities secondary to inflammatory and hypersensitivity reactions may occur. These include dental abnormalities (irregularly shaped upper central incisors and lower first molars), inflammation and clouding of the cornea (interstitial keratitis, which may result in visual impairment if untreated), and neural deafness (which may be progressive).

Treatment and prevention

Congenital syphilis is a preventable congenital infection. The first stage in prevention is to prevent maternal infections. The second stage is to test for maternal syphilis during the initial trimester of pregnancy and at delivery and to institute antibiotic treatment to the mother whenever prenatal maternal syphilis is documented.[48] Finally, the neonate with congenital syphilis should receive appropriate antibiotics after confirmation of the congenital infection and should also have ongoing serologic studies as well as ophthalmologic, audiologic, and neurodevelopmental assessments. Once treated with appropriate antibiotics, and after the initial skin lesions and nasopharyngeal discharge disappear, the infant is noninfectious and warrants no unusual hygiene procedures in an infant intervention program.

•   •   •

Congenital infections caused by *Toxoplasma gondii*, rubella virus, CMV, HSV, and *Treponema pallidum* are often associated with significant long-term developmental, neurologic, and sensory impairments. Infected infants frequently require early intervention programs to provide both general developmental support and motor and speech therapies. Additional services may be needed from specialists skilled in serving infants with sensory impairments. Case management and social services are usually necessary to ensure that the Individualized Family Services Plan is adequately developed and followed. Careful medical follow-up for congenitally infected infants is required to address ongoing as well as newly developing problems. If the guidelines provided in this review are followed, affected infants can be safely served in early intervention programs. However, close, ongoing coordination among medical and educational service providers is necessary to ensure that programs are effective, appropriate, and safe. Furthermore, long-term sequelae from congenital infections require that these infants receive careful educational, audiologic, ophthalmologic, and motor assessments through school age. These later services are necessary to maximize the benefits received from early intervention.

REFERENCES

1. Feldman HA. Toxoplasmosis. *N Engl J Med.* 1968; 279: 1275–1370.

2. Desmonts G, Couvreur J. Toxoplasmosis: Epidemiologic and serologic aspects of perinatal infection. In: Krugman S, Gershon AA, eds. *Infections of the Fetus and the Newborn Infant.* New York, NY: Liss, 1975;3.

3. Alford CA, Pass RF. Epidemiology of chronic congenital and perinatal infections in man. In: Plotkin SA, Starr SE, eds. *Clinics in Perinatology: Symposium on Perinatal Infections.* Philadelphia, Pa: Saunders; 1981;8.

4. Couvreur J, Desmonts G. Congenital and maternal toxoplasmosis: Review of 300 congenital cases. *Dev Med Child Neurol.* 1962;4:519–530.

5. Wilson CB, Remington JS, Stagno S, et al. Development of adverse sequelae in children born with subclinical congenital toxoplasma infection. *Pediatrics.* 1980;66:767–774.

6. Shaffer DB. Eye findings in intrauterine infections. In: Plotkin SA, Starr SE, eds. *Clinics in Perinatology: Symposium on Perinatal Infections.* Philadelphia, Pa: Saunders; 1981;8.

7. Remington JS, Desmonts G. Toxoplasmosis. In: Remington JS, Klein JO, eds. *Infectious Diseases of the Fetus and Newborn Infant.* Philadelphia, Pa: Saunders; 1976.

8. Eichenwald H. A study of congenital toxoplasmosis. In: Sirim JC, ed. *Human Toxoplasmosis.* Copenhagen, Denmark: Munksgaard; 1960.

9. Daffos F, Forestier F, Capella-Pavlovsky M, et al. Prenatal management of 746 pregnancies at risk for toxoplasmosis. *N Engl J Med.* 1988;318:271–275.

10. Gregg NM. Congenital cataract following German measles in the mother. *Trans Ophthalmol Soc Aust.* 1941;3:34–45.

11. Gregg NM. Further observations on congenital defects in infants following maternal rubella. *Trans Ophthalmol Soc Aust.* 1944;4:119–131.

12. Swan C, Tostevin AL, Moore B, Mayo H, Black GHB. Congenital defects in infants following infectious diseases during pregnancy. *Med J Aust.* 1943; 2:201–210.

13. Cooper LZ, Ziring PR, Ockerese AB, Fedun BA, Kiely B, Krugman S. Rubella: Clinical manifestations and management. *Am J Dis Child.* 1969;118: 18–29.

14. Cases of selected notable diseases, United States, weeks ending May 25, 1991, and May 26, 1990. *MMWR.* 1991;40:348.

15. Hanshaw JB, Dudgeon JA, Marshall WC. *Viral Diseases of the Fetus and Newborn.* 2nd ed. Philadelphia, Pa: Saunders, 1985.

16. Miller E, Craddock-Watson JE, Pollock TH. Consequences of confirmed maternal rubella at successive stages of pregnancy. *Lancet.* 1982;2:781–784.

17. Desmond MM, Wilson GS, Verniaud WM, Melnick JL, Rawls WE. The early growth and development of infants with congenital rubella. In: *Advances in Teratology.* New York, NY: Academic Press; 1970;4.

18. Desmond MM, Wilson GS, Melnick JL, et al. Congenital rubella encephalitis: Course and early sequelae. *J Pediatr.* 1967;71:311–331.

19. Desmond MM, Wilson GS, Vordeman AL, et al. The health and educational status of adolescents with congenital rubella syndrome. *Dev Med Child Neurol.* 1985;27:721–729.

20. Kaplan KM, Cochi SL, Edmonds LD, Zell ER, Preblud SR. A profile of mothers giving birth to infants with congenital rubella syndrome: An assessment of risk factors. *Am J Dis Child.* 1990;144:118–123.

21. Hanshaw JB, Dudgeon JA, Marshall WC. *Viral Diseases of the Fetus and Newborn.* 2nd ed. New York, NY: Saunders; 1985.

22. Goodpasture E, Talbot FB. Concerning the nature "protozoan-like" cells in certain lesions of infancy. *Am J Dis Child.* 1921;21:415–425.

23. Weller TH, Hanshaw JB, Scott DE. Serological differentiation of viruses responsible for cytomegalic inclusion disease. *Virology.* 1960;12:130–132.

24. Stagno S, Pass RF, Cloud G, et al. Primary cytomegalovirus infection in pregnancy: Incidence, transmission to fetus and clinical outcome. *JAMA.* 1986;256: 1904–1908.

25. Balcarek KB, Bagley RN, Cloud GA, Pass RF. Cytomegalovirus infection among employees of a children's hospital: No evidence of increased risk associated with patient care. *JAMA.* 1990;263:840–844.

26. Murph JR, Baron JC, Brown CK, Ebelhack CL, Bale JF. The occupational risk of cytomegalovirus infection among day care providers. *JAMA.* 1991;265:603–608.

27. Yeager A. Transmission of cytomegalovirus to mothers by infected infants: Another reason to prevent transfusion-acquired infections. *Pediatr Infect Dis J.* 1983;2:295–297.

28. Taber LH, Frank AL, Yow MD. Acquisition of cytomegalovirus infections in families with young children: A serological study. *J Infect Dis.* 1985;151:948–952.

29. Williamson WD, Demmler G, Percy AK, Catlin F. Asymptomatic congenital CMV infection: Association of congenital and progressive sensorineural hearing loss (SNHL) with recurrent as well as primary maternal CMV infection. *Pediatr Res.* 1991;29:167A. Abstract.

30. Pass RF, Stagno A, Myers JJ, Alford CA. Outcome of symptomatic congenital cytomegalovirus infection: Results of long-term longitudinal follow up. *Pediatrics.* 1980;66:758–762.

31. Williamson WD, Desmond MM, LaFevers N, Taber L, Catlin FI, Weaver TG. Symptomatic congenital cytomegalovirus: Disorders of language, learning and hearing. *Am J Dis Child.* 1982;136:902–905.

32. Williamson WD, Percy AK, Yow MD, et al. Asymptomatic congenital cytomegalovirus infection: Audiologic, neuroradiologic and neurodevelopmental abnormalities during the first year. *Am J Dis Child.* 1990;144:1365–1368.

33. Saigal S, Lunyk O, Larke RPB, Chernesky MA. The outcome of children with congenital cytomegalovirus infection: A longitudinal follow-up study. *Am J Dis Child.* 1982;136:896–901.

34. Pearl KN, Preece PM, Ades A, Peckham CS. Neurodevelopmental assessment after congenital cytomegalovirus infection. *Arch Dis Child.* 1986;61:323–326.

35. Hanshaw JB, Scheiner AP, Mosley A, Gaw L, Abel V, Scheiner B. CNS effects of "silent" cytomegalovirus infection. *N Engl J Med.* 1976;295:468–470.

36. Conboy TJ, Pass RF, Stagno S, et al. Intellectual development in school-aged children with asymptomatic congenital cytomegalovirus infection. *Pediatrics.* 1986;77:801–806.

37. Hanshaw JB, Dudgeon JA, Marshall WC. *Viral Diseases of the Fetus and Newborn.* 2nd ed. Philadelphia, Pa: Saunders; 1985.

38. Nahmias AJ, Visintine AM. Perinatal herpes simplex virus infection. In: Remington JS, Klein JO, eds. *Congenital and Perinatal Infection.* Philadelphia, Pa: Saunders; 1974.

39. Nahmias AJ, Roizman B. Infection with simple viruses 1 and 2. *N Engl J Med.* 1973;289:667–674, 719–725, 781–789.

40. Nahmias AJ, Josey WE, Naib ZM, Freeman MG, Fernandez RJ, Wheeler JH. Perinatal risk associated with maternal genital herpes simplex virus infection. *Am J Obstet Gynecol.* 1971;110:835–837.

41. Hutto C, Arvin A, Jacobs R, et al. Intrauterine herpes simplex virus infections. *J Pediatr.* 1987;110:97–101.

42. Whitley R, Arvin A, Prober C, et al. A controlled trial comparing vidarabine with acyclovir in neonatal herpes simplex virus infection. *N Engl J Med.* 1991;324:444–449.

43. Bell WE, McCormick WF. *Neurologic Infections in Children.* 2nd ed. Philadelphia, Pa: Saunders; 1981.

44. Rolfs RT, Nakashima AK. Epidemiology of primary and secondary syphilis in the United States, 1981 through 1989. *JAMA.* 1990;264:1432–1437.

45. Termini BA, Music SI. The national history of syphilis: A review. *South Med J.* 1972;65:241–245.

46. Harter CA, Benirschke K. Fetal syphilis in the first trimester. *Am J Obstet Gynecol.* 1976;7:705–711.

47. Centers for Disease Control. Guidelines for the prevention and control of congenital syphilis. *MMWR.* 1988;37(suppl 1):1–13.

48. Ikeda MK, Jenson HB. Evaluation and treatment of congenital syphilis. *J Pediatr.* 1990;117:843–852.

Disorders of brain development

Robert E. Nickel, MD
Associate Professor
Department of Pediatrics
Oregon Health Sciences University
Portland, Oregon

Clinical Director
Regional Service Center
Child Development and Rehabilitation
   Center
Eugene, Oregon

CURRENT NEUROLOGIC imaging techniques have markedly improved the ability to identify disorders of brain development in early childhood. Many of the children in early intervention (EI) services have an identifiable disorder of brain development either as an isolated problem or as part of a multiple congenital anomaly syndrome. These children manifest a variety of clinical and developmental problems including mental retardation and seizure disorders. EI professionals should have an understanding of each child's medical diagnosis and potential medical and developmental problems in order to develop appropriate intervention plans.

This article reviews the major events in normal brain development and presents examples of the most common brain disorders specific to each process. Where available, it provides information on the developmental significance of each disorder and the implications for EI service providers. Readers can find further information about the specific syndromes mentioned in this article elsewhere.[1,2]

DEVELOPMENT OF THE CENTRAL NERVOUS SYSTEM

The development of the central nervous system (CNS) can be separated into six major events that generally occur in a temporal sequence (Table 1).[3] These events, which are discussed separately in the sections that follow, are dorsal induction, ventral induction, neuronal proliferation, neuronal migration, organization, and myelination.

Dorsal induction

Induction refers to the influence of one tissue on another so that the second tissue differentiates into a completely different tissue than the first. In the developing embryo, cells segregate to form three germ layers: the endoderm, the ectoderm, and the mesoderm. The nervous system begins to develop from the ectodermal tissue on the back of the embryo. The underlying mesoderm induces the ectoderm to differentiate into the neural plate at approximately 18 days of gestation.[4] This process is referred to as dorsal induction. The neural plate invaginates to form neural folds and then closes dorsally to form the neural tube. Closure of the neural tube is complete by 26 days of gestation.[3] Meningomyelocele and anencephaly are disorders of neural tube closure. The clinical aspects of

Inf Young Children 1992;5(1):1–11
© 1992 Aspen Publishers, Inc.

Table 1. The major events in brain development

Major event	Timing	Example of disordered development
Dorsal induction	18–26 d	Meningomyelocele, anencephaly
Ventral induction	4–10 wk	Holoprosencephaly, Dandy-Walker syndrome
Neuronal proliferation	2–4 mo	Primary microcephaly
Neuronal migration	2–5 mo	Lissencephaly, schizencephaly, polymicrogyria, heterotopias, agenesis of the corpus callosum
Organization	6 mo of gestation to postnatal	?
Myelination	6 mo of gestation to adulthood	?

A portion of this table is adapted with permission from Volpe JJ. *Neurology of the Newborn.* Philadelphia, Pa: WB Saunders; 1987:3.

meningomyelocele have been reviewed previously and are not discussed further in this article.[5,6]

Ventral induction

Ventral induction refers to the inductive events involving mesoderm at the rostral (head) end of the embryo and the developing neural tube that result in the formation of the face and brain.[7] The neural tube undergoes a series of cleavages to form paired cerebral hemispheres and basal ganglia, to separate the hypothalamus and thalamus, and to separate the paired optic (vision) and olfactory (smell) structures.[3,7,8] Holoprosencephaly, an example of a ventral induction disorder, is a disorder of cleavage of the embryonic forebrain that occurs by the fourth week of gestation.[8] In holoprosencephaly, the brain fails to make the normal cleavages and retains a large single ventricle (Fig 1). Warkan et al[9] theorize that deficient rostral mesoderm results in lack of stimulation of the primitive forebrain.

Holoprosencephaly is classified as alobar, semilobar, and lobar in order of descending severity. In alobar holoprosencephaly, severe facial deformities may accompany the brain anomalies. The eyes may be fused or nearly fused and nasal structures are absent. More commonly, the nose is small and flat, the eyes are close together (hypotelorism), and there is a midline cleft of the lip. In milder forms of this disorder, facial findings are less dramatic. However, alobar holoprosencephaly has been associated with normal facial findings.[10] Fig 1 presents the computed tomography (CT) scan of a child with alobar holoprosencephaly. There is a single ventricle and a dorsal midline cyst. In lobar holo-

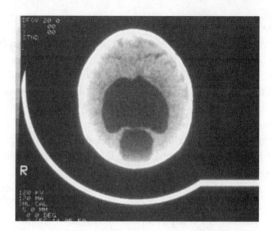

Fig 1. CT scan of a male infant with alobar holoprosencephaly showing large single ventricle and dorsal midline cyst.

prosencephaly, there is partial separation of the lateral ventricles. The anterior part of the ventricles continues to be fused, and the structure that normally separates them—the septum pellucidum—is absent.[6] Infants usually have microcephaly, or less commonly, accompanying hydrocephalus. The prevalence of holoprosencephaly in newborns is approximately 1.26 per 10,000.[2] The majority of cases are sporadic with no identifiable cause. Nevertheless, holoprosencephaly can be part of chromosomal (trisomy 13) and nonchromosomal syndromes, caused by single gene defects (both autosomal recessive and dominant inheritance) or by environmental factors (1% to 2% incidence in infants of diabetic mothers).[2] In addition, there are a number of suspected teratogens (agents that cause physical defects in the embryo) including fetal dilantin exposure.[2]

Infants with alobar holoprosencephaly have a bleak medical and developmental prognosis. They experience recurrent apnea, seizures, poor temperature regulation, and failure to thrive. They demonstrate little environmental interaction and usually die during infancy.[2,8,11] EI services for these infants should focus on family support and basic care services such as specialized feeding programs. Open communication among health care professionals, families, and EI staff members is essential. Infants with semilobar holoprosencephaly also are severely to profoundly impaired, and most infants with lobar holoprosencephaly are severely mentally retarded. A few infants with lobar holoprosencephaly may be only mildly to moderately retarded and may remain seizure free. The EI staff should expect that infants with lobar holoprosencephaly will make consistent develop-

mental progress and incorporate realistic goals for infant behavior change into the
EI program.

The syndrome of septo-optic dysplasia may be confused with lobar
holoprosencephaly. These children lack the septum pellucidum (the wall between
the anterior part of the ventricles), which is associated with deficiencies of pitu-
itary hormones, and have small optic nerves with variable visual impairment.[2]
Children lacking the septum pellucidum clearly need to be evaluated for this disorder.

Some authors[7] include malformations of the cerebellum as ventral induction
disorders. These authors argue that ventral inductive events are important both for
forebrain and hindbrain development. The Dandy-Walker syndrome is a developmental anomaly of the cerebellum and related structures that occurs at 7 to 10
weeks of gestation.[7] The cerebellar hemispheres are widely separated by a cyst
that is continuous with the fourth ventricle, and the vermis (middle lobe of the
cerebellum) is partially or completely absent (Fig 2).[12,13] The diagnosis of Dandy-
Walker syndrome also requires the presence of hydrocephalus, which may not
develop during the first weeks of life.[13] Dandy-Walker syndrome, which is estimated to be involved in about 4% of cases of hydrocephalus,[12] is often associated
with other CNS anomalies (eg, agenesis of the corpus callosum). It can occur as
part of chromosomal and nonchromosomal syndromes (Cornelia de Lange) and
single-gene disorders (Meckel-Gruber syndrome and Joubert syndrome).[1,2] In addition, it can be caused by teratogens (fetal anticoagulant exposure) and can occur
as an isolated anomaly.[12]

Studies of individuals with Dandy-Walker syndrome generally report a poor
intellectual prognosis. In one study, 75% of the patients had intellectual quotients
of less than 70,[12] and in another study only 33% had normal intelligence.[13] Mental
retardation is due to the presence of other brain anomalies. By contrast, a number
of asymptomatic adults with Dandy-Walker syndrome have been reported.[12]
Maria et al[14] noted that 12 of 14 children with Dandy-Walker syndrome and no
other brain anomaly were developing normally. Thus, Dandy-Walker syndrome
can be associated with normal development or a prognosis that is similar to other
individuals with treated hydrocephalus. EI staff members who serve children with
Dandy-Walker syndrome should request medical information concerning the
presence of additional CNS anomalies and should be knowledgeable about the
treatment of hydrocephalus.[15]

Neuronal proliferation

As the neural tube forms, primitive neuroepithelial cells occupy the zone that
surrounds the central canal or the future ventricular system.[16] This ventricular

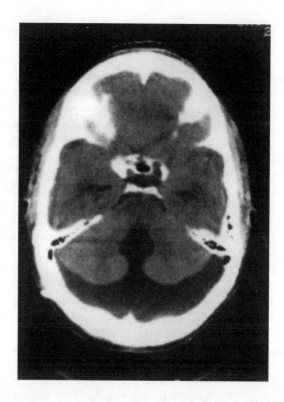

Fig 2. CT scan of an 11-year-old boy with Dandy-Walker syndrome and hydrocephalus. The fourth ventricle is large, and the cerebellar hemispheres are separated by an apparent cyst. The vermis is absent.

zone is the site of proliferation of neuroblasts (cells that will form neurons in the mature brain) and glioblasts (cells that will form basic support structures in the mature brain). The time of most rapid neuronal proliferation is 2 to 4 months of gestation, and the time of most rapid glial proliferation is 5 to 12 months or more postnatally.[3] A surplus of neurons is produced; the excess is estimated to be 40% to 50% more than present in the mature brain.[17,18]

True or primary microcephaly is classified by Volpe[3] as a disorder of proliferation. Microcephaly refers to a head size that is more than two or three standard deviations below the mean for age and sex. More than 200 syndromes that involve microcephaly have been reported.[1,19,20] Many of these syndromes are due to chromosomal abnormalities, while many are related to single-gene mutations including autosomal dominant, autosomal recessive, and X-linked dominant or recessive inheritance. Many of these children have other malformations such as cleft lip and palate.

Isolated or nonsyndromic primary microcephaly has been reported to have autosomal dominant and autosomal recessive inheritance.[20] Individuals in some families with autosomal dominant microcephaly have normal intelligence, while individuals in other families have mild to moderate mental retardation. Motor development is normal, and seizures may occur. Children with autosomal recessive microcephaly have been reported to have mild to moderate mental retardation and no spasticity or seizures, or severe spastic quadriplegia, seizures, and severe mental retardation. The neuropathology of one severely affected child showed a thin cortex with a paucity of cells in each layer.[20]

Teratogens, including fetal alcohol exposure, fetal dilantin exposure, and high blood phenylalanine levels due to maternal phenylketonuria, can also cause microcephaly.[1] In these situations microcephaly is presumed to be the result of interference with neuroblast proliferation at 2 to 4 months of gestation.[3] Sarnat[21] notes that neuronal proliferation ends with induction of the ependymal cells, which replicate and line the ventricles. He speculates that teratogens may act as natural inducers with early induction of the ependyma and thus early cessation of the cell proliferation phase.

Neuronal migration

Beginning at 6 to 8 weeks of gestation, neurons begin to migrate away from the proliferation zone.[17] In the cerebral cortex those cells that migrate first usually migrate to the deepest layers of the cortex; neurons produced later migrate the greater distances to the superficial layers.[17,18] The first cortical layer is present at 8 weeks. By 8 months of gestation all six layers of the cerebral cortex are clear and have the same appearance as that found in older children.[18] The process of cell migration is not well understood, but it appears to involve both cellular and extracellular cues. The migration of cells to the cerebral cortex is along a system of radial glial fibers that extends from the ventricular surface to the cortical surface.[3,17,18,22,23] Extracellular matrix proteins known as substrate adhesion molecules and neural cell adhesion molecules also play a significant role.[18,23]

Abnormal neuronal migration results in abnormal brain gyral patterns (convolutions) and heterotopias (collections of neurons in abnormal locations). These are generally rare disorders. Lissencephaly, or smooth brain, is the most severe manifestation of a neuronal migration disorder (NMD) (Fig 3). The lack of gyri may not be complete[24-26]; in such cases the remainder of the brain usually has pachygyria or a few thick gyri, and the cerebral cortex is thick and possesses four layers rather than the normal six.[25] Lissencephaly represents a disruption to neuronal migration at 11 to 13 weeks of gestation.[27-29] It can result from a chromosomal microdeletion syndrome (Miller-Dieker syndrome), occur as part of an autosomal recessive disorder (Walker-Warburg syndrome), result from an in utero infection with cytomegalovirus, or occur as an isolated anomaly.[25,30,31]

Children who completely lack gyri experience apnea, poor feeding ability, seizures, and profound mental deficiency.[25-29] All are microcephalic, and most die during infancy, although survival to the age of 10 years has been reported.[26] The focus of EI services for many of these infants and families will be similar to that described for infants with alobar holoprosencephaly: family support and basic care services. Children with predominant pachygyria are also severely mentally retarded but may be able to crawl and develop limited speech. Children with Walker-Warburg syndrome also have hydrocephalus, congenital muscular dystrophy, and visual impairment due to ocular disorders.[25]

Schizencephaly refers to bilateral clefts of the cerebral hemispheres that result when a portion of the cerebral wall fails to develop[32-34] (Fig 4). Some investigators[23,35] feel that schizencephaly results from very early disruption of a normally developing brain with secondary neuronal migration problems. The timing of this

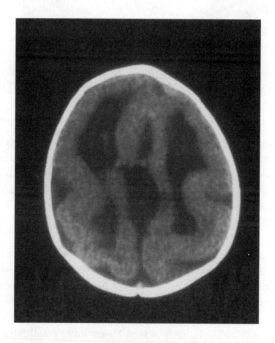

Fig 3. CT scan of female infant with lissencephaly. Note the smooth cerebral surface and figure of eight shape due to agyria or pachygyria.

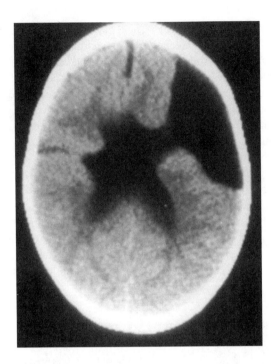

Fig 4. CT scan of a 15-month-old girl with a left hemiplegia and bilateral asymmetric schizencephaly. Note that the lips of the cleft are widely separated on one side and fused on the other.

disorder is no later than the 8th week of gestation.[3,35] The lips of the clefts are fused or separated, and the walls of the clefts show other evidence of migration problems such as polymicrogyria and heterotopias. The septum pellucidum is absent in 75% to 100% of the cases.[35] Magnetic resonance imaging (MRI) has significantly increased the identification of schizencephaly and has improved understanding of its variability. The spectrum includes individuals with single fused clefts with normal intelligence[35] to individuals with severe bilateral clefts and severe spastic quadriplegia and mental retardation.[36,37] The child whose CT scan is shown in Fig 4 has normal intelligence and a left-sided spastic hemiplegia. Most, if not all, individuals with schizencephaly have seizures. Schizencephaly has not been associated with multiple congenital anomaly syndromes, chromosomal or genetic disorders, or teratogens.[23] Schizencephaly and septo-optic dysplasia can co-exist.[35]

Polymicrogyria (PMG) is characterized by multiple small, shallow convolutions on the brain surface. The cortex is thick and may have four layers (rather than six) or be unlayered.[23] In one study[24] PMG was noted in 5% of 500 consecutive autopsies of individuals with mental disability. The area of involvement varies from a small focus to a tumor-like mass (Fig 5) to the entire hemisphere (unilateral megalencephaly).[38] This disorder is thought to occur at 4 to 5 months of gestation.[23] It is often found in association with other NMDs (eg, schizencephaly). PMG is also seen in Zellweger syndrome (an autosomal recessive metabolic disorder), chromosomal disorders, and in association with meningomyelocele and fetal cytomegalovirus infection. PMG has occurred after maternal carbon monoxide exposure at 20 to 24 weeks of gestation, and it may also occur as an isolated problem.[23]

When large areas of the brain are involved with PMG, the individual is retarded and invariably has a seizure disorder. However, focal PMG has been noted incidentally in the autopsy of normal adults, and a focus of PMG was identified in the left temporal region of an adult with dyslexia.[3] Small foci of PMG may be much more common than previously thought, particularly in people with epilepsy. In a recent study, positron emission tomography (PET) detected small foci of PMG missed by MRI.[39] All of the individuals in this study were being evaluated for surgical treatment of intractable epilepsy.

Heterotopias are collections of neurons in abnormal locations; they are thought to result from arrested migration. The causes of heterotopias are varied, as is the case with other NMDs. In fact, heterotopias are seen frequently in association with other NMDs. Nodular subependymal heterotopias cause bulging of the ventricular wall[40] (Fig 6), or heterotopias may project from the cortical surface as brain warts.[23] Their prognostic significance, separate from other neuronal migration disorders, is not known. Barkovich et al[41] recently reported on five patients who may exhibit a new NMD referred to as band heterotopias. MRI of these five children showed symmetric thick bands of apparent gray matter deep to the cerebral cortex. All were severely developmentally delayed and had intractable seizures. The youngest child, age 2 years, was the least delayed.

Agenesis of the corpus callosum (ACC), which is included in this discussion of neuronal migration disorders due to its frequent association with these disorders, is also commonly associated with other CNS malformations.[42,43] The corpus callosum is the major pathway of fibers crossing between the cerebral hemispheres. The first callosal fibers appear at 12 weeks of gestation or thereabouts, and the entire corpus callosum is formed by 17 weeks of gestation.[3,17,44] Barkovich and Norman[43] speculate that failure of development of the group of cells (massa commissuralis) through which the first fibers cross results in redirection of those fibers as longitudinal bundles. ACC can be complete or partial. It is an infrequent congenital anomaly that usually is nongenetic[45]; however, it has been reported in association with chromosomal abnormalities (trisomy 13), genetic (autosomal dominant, autosomal recessive, and X-linked recessive) and nongenetic multiple congenital anomaly syndromes, and as an isolated anomaly with autosomal domi-

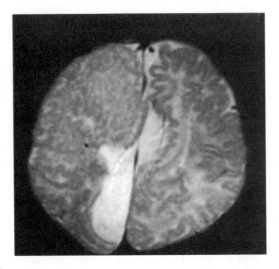

A

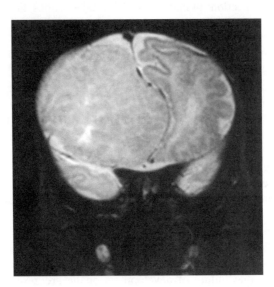

B

Fig 5. (a) Horizontal view of an MRI scan of a 10-month-old girl with acrocallosal syndrome. Note the marked asymmetry between the gyri of the two hemispheres. Polymicrogyria is present in most of the right hemisphere (arrow). (b) Coronal view of the same MRI scan showing a tumor-like mass of PMG extending across the midline.

nant and autosomal recessive inheritance.[45] Fig 6 presents the MRI scan of a female infant with Aicardi syndrome, a probable X-linked dominant disorder that includes ACC, ocular abnormalities, vertebral anomalies, and seizures.[2]

The prognosis for children with ACC associated with an identifiable syndrome is determined by that syndrome. However, the majority of children with apparent isolated ACC are also developmentally delayed and have seizures.[46,47] In fact, children with ACC who present with seizures in infancy are usually severely developmentally delayed. The mental retardation in these children is primarily related to the presence of other CNS malformations, particularly NMDs. In one study,[46] children diagnosed after 4 years of age had a good prognosis for normal intellectual development. ACC has also been noted in normal adults as an incidental finding.

Individuals with isolated ACC and normal intelligence have been reported to have a variety of minor cognitive deficits, including deficits in bilateral coordination,[48] impaired transfer of tactile[49] and visual information,[50] and difficulty with certain aspects of sentence comprehension.[51] Studies using MRI are thus necessary to determine the degree of callosal agenesis, to eliminate subjects with other

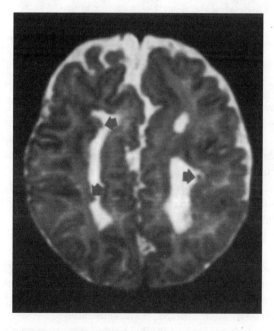

Fig 6a. Horizontal view of an MRI scan of a female infant with Aicardi syndrome. Note the nodular heterotopias extending into the lateral ventricles (arrows). This child also has agenesis of the corpus callosum.

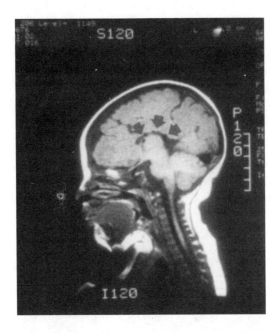

Fig 6b. Sagittal view of an MRI scan of the same child. Note the complete agenesis of the corpus callosum. Arrows indicate normal location of the corpus callosum.

NMDs, and to clarify the actual deficit(s) related to isolated ACC. Isolated ACC, minor degrees of schizencephaly, and small foci of PMG offer the best opportunities for future research studying the correlation of specific functional problems with clearly defined anatomic defects of the brain and the efficacy of specific EI strategies for those problems.

Sarnat[52] also describes disorders of late neuronal migration that are caused by lesions acquired in the perinatal period by premature infants; for example, subependymal hemorrhage or cavitation in subcortical white matter (periventricular leukomalacia). These lesions disrupt the radial glial fibers that then retract from the cortical surface. Neurons can only migrate as far as the radial glial fibers allow, and then they are stranded as collections of heterotopic gray matter or as small foci of cortical dysgenesis. Disorders of late neuronal migration may contribute to the impaired coordination, visual perceptual problems, and seizures experienced by some children born prematurely.

EI professionals should monitor all patients for the presence and frequency of seizures and the potential behavioral side effects of anticonvulsants. Monitoring is particularly important for children with NMDs. The resultant information will help facilitate medical management of the seizures and maximize the child's ability to participate in the EI program.

Organization

The events that characterize brain organization include the selective grouping of neurons (eg, into the six layers of the cerebral cortex), the growth of nerve cell processes (axons and dendrites), the forming of synapses or connections between nerves, the programmed death of excess neurons, and the selective elimination of excess synapses.[3,17,18] These processes begin at 6 months of gestation and last to several years postnatally. Unfortunately, little research information is available concerning possible disorders of brain organization.

Myelination

Myelination is the last major event in the structural development of the brain. It begins at 6 months of gestation with the proliferation of glial or support cells and continues into adult life. The most rapid phase of myelination is from birth to 1 year of age. Myelination within the cerebral hemispheres occurs well after birth and lasts into adulthood.[3,17,18] Little information is available concerning primary disorders of myelination. Two studies[53,54] have documented through MRI a pattern of delayed myelination in some children with unexplained developmental delay. In the first study, this pattern was evident in 9 of 76 children, while in the second study 9 of 30 children showed this pattern. The significance of these findings is not known. A number of inherited, metabolic neurologic disorders that result in a progressive loss of skills cause demyelination and interfere with new myelin formation (eg, metachromatic leukodystrophy). A discussion of these disorders is beyond the scope of this article.

DISCUSSION

It is clear from the preceding text that disorders of brain development have a variety of causes. A single gene mutation or a teratogen may act through a common mechanism that results in disturbance of one or more basic processes of brain development. Except for schizencephaly, all of the disorders reviewed can be part of a genetic syndrome. Therefore an accurate genetic diagnosis is very important for counseling families because it will provide the family with information regarding the recurrence risk, possible associated medical problems, and the natural history of that disorder.

An accurate diagnosis of the primary brain disorder and any associated CNS problems is also important. The MRI scan is superior to the CT scan in diagnosing these disorders.[55,56] It is critical to document the presence or absence of neuronal migration problems, as such problems are associated with the development of mental retardation and seizures.

Most infants and children with disorders of brain development also have associated medical problems. The EI staff should be familiar with the nature and current treatment of these problems including hydrocephalus, seizures, and feeding disorders.

Many children with brain development disorders have a bleak medical and developmental prognosis. They are profoundly impaired and may have a markedly shortened life span. Other children may have normal intelligence and minor developmental dysfunction. Specific prognostic information is necessary for the early intervention professionals who work with these families to establish appropriate goals and expectations for early intervention services. For those children who have a nongenetic brain disorder, information about the timing of the disorder during pregnancy can provide reassurance to parents that a pregnancy problem could not have caused the disorder because it was not temporally related.

Finally, an accurate diagnosis and understanding of the disorders of brain development is important for early intervention research. The benefits as well as limitations of specific intervention strategies for the child or family must be studied with a clear understanding of the social and biologic variables involved.

REFERENCES

1. Jones KL. *Smith's Recognizable Patterns of Human Malformation.* 4th ed. Philadelphia, Pa: WB Saunders; 1988.

2. Gorlin RJ, Cohen MM Jr, Levin LS. *Syndromes of the Head and Neck.* 3rd ed. New York, NY: Oxford University Press; 1990.

3. Volpe JJ. *Neurology of the Newborn.* Philadelphia Pa: WB Saunders; 1987.

4. Lemire RJ, Loeser JD, Leech RW, Alvard EC Jr. *Normal and Abnormal Development of the Human Nervous System.* Hagerstown, Md: Harper & Row; 1975.

5. Anderson SM. Secondary neurologic disability in myelomeningocele. *Inf Young Children.* 1989;1:9–21.

6. Lozes MH. Bladder and bowel management for children with myelomeningocele. *Inf Young Children.* 1988;1:52–62.

7. van der Knapp MS, Valk J. Classification of congenital abnormalities of the CNS. *AJNR.* 1988;9:315–326.

8. Fitz CR. Holoprosencephaly and related entities. *Neuroradiology.* 1983;25:225–238.

9. Warkany J, Lemire RJ, Cohen MM Jr. *Mental Retardation and Congenital Malformation of the Central Nervous System.* Chicago, Ill: Year Book; 1981.

10. Cohen MM Jr. Selected clinical research involving the central nervous system. *J Craniofac Genet Dev Biol.* 1990;10:215–238.

11. Manelfe C, Sevely A. Neuroradiological study of holoprosencephalies. *J Neuroradiol.* 1982;9:15–45.

12. Murray JC, Johnson JA, Bird TD. Dandy-Walker malformation: Etiologic heterogeneity and empiric recurrence risks. *Clin Genet.* 1985;28:272–283.

13. Bordarier C, Aicardi J. Dandy-Walker syndrome and agenesis of the cerebellar vermis: Diagnostic problems and genetic counseling. *Dev Med Child Neurol.* 1990;32:285–294.

14. Maria BL, Zinreich SJ, Carson BC, Rosenbaus AE, Freeman JM. Dandy-Walker syndrome revisited. *Pediatr Neurosci.* 1987; 13:45–51.

15. Blackman JA, ed. *Medical Aspects of Developmental Disabilities in Children Birth to Three.* Iowa City, Iowa: University of Iowa; 1983.

16. Tolmie JL, McNay M, Stephenson JBP, Doyle D, Connor JM. Microcephaly: Genetic counseling and antenatal diagnosis after the birth of an affected child. *Am J Med Genet.* 1987;27:583–594.

17. Sarnat HB. Cerebral dysplasias as expressions of altered maturational processes. *Can J Neurol Sci.* 1991;18:196–204.

18. Herschkowitz N. Brain development in the fetus, neonate and infant. *Biol Neonate.* 1988;54:1–19.

19. Opitz JM, Holt MC. Microcephaly: General consideration and aids to nosology. *J Craniofac Genet Dev Biol.* 1990; 10:175–204.

20. Cowie VA. Microcephaly: A review of genetic implications in its causation. *J Ment Defic Res.* 1987;31:229–233.

21. Sarnat HB. Neural induction and the role of the fetal ependyma. Presented to the Child Neurology Society; October 1991; Portland, Ore.

22. Rakic P. Cell migration and neuronal ectopias in the brain. *Birth Defects.* 1975;11(7):95–129.

23. Barth PG. Disorders of neuronal migration. *Can J Neurol Sci.* 1987;14:1–16.

24. Barkovich AJ, Chuang SH, Norman D. MR of neuronal migration anomalies. *AJNR* 1987;8:1009–1017.

25. Dobyns WB, Stratton RF, Greenberg F. Syndromes with lissencephaly. 1: Miller-Dieker and Norman Roberts syndromes and isolated lissencephaly. *Am J Med Genet.* 1984;18:509–526.

26. Dobyns WB, McCluggage CW. Computed tomographic appearance of lissencephaly syndromes. *AJNR.* 1985;6:545–550.

27. de Rijk-van Andel JF, Arts WFM, Barth PG, Loonen MCB. Diagnostic features and clinical signs of 21 patients with lissencephaly type 1. *Dev Med Child Neurol.* 1990;32:707–717.

28. Gastaut H, Pinsard N, Raybaud C, Aicardi J, Ziflcin B. Lissencephaly (agyria-pachygyria): Clinical findings and serial EEG studies. *Dev Med Child Neurol.* 1987;29:167–180.

29. Barkovich AJ, Koch TK, Carrol CL. The spectrum of lissencephaly: Report of ten patients analyzed by magnetic resonance imaging. *Ann Neurol.* 1991;30:139–146.

30. Hayward JC, Titelbaum DS, Clancy RR, Zimmerman RA. Lissencephaly-pachygyria associated with congenital cytomegalovirus infection. *J Child Neurol.* 1991;6:109–114.

31. Dobyns WB, Pagon RA, Armstrong D, et al. Diagnostic criteria for Walker-Warburg syndrome. *Am J Med Genet.* 1989;32:195–210.

32. Dekaban A. Large defects in cerebral hemispheres associated with cortical dysgenesis. *J Neuropathol Exp Neurol.* 1965;24:512–530.

33. Page LK, Brown SB, Gargano FP, Shortz RW. Schizencephaly: A clinical study and review. *Child's Brain.* 1975;1:348–358.

34. Bird CR, Gilles FH. Type I schizencephaly: CT and neuropathologic findings. *AJNR.* 1987;8:451–454.

35. Barkovich AJ, Norman D. MR imaging of schizencephaly. *AJNR.* 1988;9:297–302.

36. Miller GM, Stears JC, Guggenheim MA, Wilkening GN. Schizencephaly: A clinical and CT study. *Neurology.* 1984;34:997–1001.

37. Zimmerman RA, Bilaniuk LT, Grossman RI. Computed tomography in migratory disorders of human brain development. *Neuroradiology.* 1983;25:257–263.

38. Mikhael MA, Mattar AG. Malformation of the cerebral cortex with heterotopia of the gray matter. *J Comput Assist Tomogr.* 1978;2:291–296.

39. Chugani HT, Shewmon DA, Shields WD, et al. Positron emission tomographic scanning in pediatric epilepsy operation: UCLA experience in 84 patients. Presented to the Child Neurology Society; October 1991; Portland, Ore.

40. Yasumori K, Hasuo K, Nagata S, Masuda K, Fukui M. Neuronal migration anomalies causing extensive ventricular indentation. *Neurosurgery.* 1990;26:504–507.

41. Barkovich AJ, Jackson DE Jr, Boyer RS. Band heterotopias: A newly recognized neuronal migration anomaly. *Radiology.* 1989;171:455–458.

42. Parrish ML, Roessmann U, Levinsohn MW. Agenesis of the corpus callosum: A study of the frequency of associated malformations. *Ann Neurol.* 1979;6:349–354.

43. Barkovich AJ, Norman D. Anomalies of the corpus callosum: Correlation with further anomalies of the brain. *AJR.* 1988;151:171–179.

44. Kendall BE. Dysgenesis of the corpus callosum. *Neuroradiology.* 1983;25:239–256.

45. Young ID, Trounce JQ, Levene MI, Fitzsimmons JS, Moore JR. Agenesis of the corpus callosum and macrocephaly in siblings. *Clin Genet.* 1985;28:225–230.

46. Lacey DJ. Agenesis of the corpus callosum. *AJDC.* 1985;139:953–955.

47. Field M, Ashton R, White K. Agenesis of the corpus callosum: Report of two pre-school children and review of the literature. *Dev Med Child Neurol.* 1978;20:47–61.

48. Jeeves MA, Silver PH, Jacobson 1. Bimanual coordination in callosal agenesis and partial commissurotomy. *Neuropsychologia.* 1988;26:833–850.

49. Jeeves MA, Silver PH. Interhemispheric transfer of spatial tactile information in callosal agenesis and partial commissurotomy. *Cortex.* 1988;24:601–604.

50. Martin A. A qualitative limitation on visual transfer via the anterior commissure. *Brain.* 1985;108:43–63.

51. Sanders RJ. Sentence completion following agenesis of the corpus callosum. *Brain Lang.* 1989;37:59–72.

52. Sarnat HB. Disturbances of late neuronal migrations in the perinatal period. *AJDC.* 1987;141:969–980.

53. Kjos BO, Umansky R, Barkovich AJ. Brain MR imaging in children with developmental retardation of unknown cause: Results in 76 cases. *AJNR.* 1990;11:1035–1040.

54. Harbord MG, Pinn JP, Hall-Craggs MA, Robb SA, Kendall BE, Boyd SG. Myelination patterns on magnetic resonance of children with developmental delay. *Dev Med Child Neurol.* 1990;32:295–303.

55. Byrd SE, Osborn RE, Bohan TP, Naidich TP. The CT and MR evaluation of migrational disorders of the brain. *Pediatr Radiol.* 1989;19:219–222.

56. Byrd SE. Magnetic resonance imaging of supratentorial congenital brain malformations. *J Natl Med Assoc.* 1989;81:873–881.

Developmental implications of intrauterine growth retardation

Marilee C. Allen, MD
Associate Professor, Pediatrics
Eudowood Division of Neonatology
Johns Hopkins School of Medicine
Baltimore, Maryland

OBSTETRICIANS who diagnose poor intrauterine growth of a fetus and pediatricians who make a diagnosis of small for gestational age (SGA) in a newborn infant raise a number of concerns about that infant: Why is he or she so small? When did it occur? Will he or she survive? Will he or she develop complications as a newborn? Most importantly, how will he or she develop neurologically, cognitively, and behaviorally? Each of these concerns must be addressed for each infant who carries a diagnosis of intrauterine growth retardation (IUGR) or SGA.[1] The difficulties that we have in determining an infant's prognosis are related to the uniqueness of each individual's response to an insult or anomaly and to the complexity of the interrelationship between growth and development.

Fetal/infant growth and development are two separate but related processes. Factors that affect one frequently affect the other, but not necessarily in the same way. In addition, each is in some way necessary for the other: Growth of the various organs [especially the central nervous system (CNS)] is necessary for infant development, and frequently development enhances growth (eg, movement is necessary for the continued growth and differentiation of the joints and limbs).

DEFINITIONS

The terms *IUGR* and *SGA* are not entirely synonymous, but they both include an assessment of size and maturity. Size is easier to measure in the newborn infant than in the fetus. Gestational age is best determined early in pregnancy. In some pregnancies, gestational age can be determined with precision (eg, in the case of in vitro fertilization or artificial insemination). In many pregnancies, however, there is some uncertainty. Although postnatal measures of gestational age are available,[2,3] recent research has questioned their accuracy.[4,5] In addition, neurologic maturation may be accelerated in fetuses who are stressed during gestation, leading to further concerns about the accuracy of postnatal gestational age assessments in IUGR infants.[6]

An SGA infant is an infant who is born weighing significantly less than expected for his or her degree of maturity at birth (ie, gestational age). The exact weight cutoff for each week of gestation and the percentile (eg, <3%, <5%, or <10%) used to diagnose SGA varies with the published population norms that the clinician uses.[7–11] Ideally, other parameters (eg, birth length, head circumference, and ponderal index) should be considered, and the population norms used should

Inf Young Children 1992;5(2):13–28
© 1992 Aspen Publishers, Inc.

reflect as nearly as possible the infant's characteristics (eg, race, sex, altitude, and genetic growth potential). Most frequently, however, the diagnosis of SGA is based on the infant's weight at birth compared to general population norms for that gestational age.

IUGR reflects poor fetal growth in utero. In the past, it has been difficult to accurately assess fetal growth or pregnancy duration. Fetal size has traditionally been used to date pregnancies. Establishing a due date is more reliable if a woman registers her pregnancy early (in the first trimester).[12] Accurate dating of a pregnancy is essential for the assessment of the adequacy of fetal/infant growth and/or development.[11,13]

Advances in technology, especially in ultrasound, have brought more accurate methods of assessing fetal growth and thereby of dating a pregnancy.[14,15] Dates for determining fetal maturity can be most reliably determined early in a pregnancy (before 18 weeks). Ultrasound measurements of fetal length (crown-rump length, only useful in the first half of pregnancy), head size (biparietal diameter), femur length, and abdominal circumference have been standardized to population norms and can be used to measure and follow fetal growth.

An IUGR fetus is one who is noted to plateau or decelerate in his or her growth or who is noted to be smaller than expected in comparison to population norms. The obstetrician may decide to evaluate fetal size either because the mother has not demonstrated adequate weight gain and/or abdominal (ie, fundal height) growth or because she may demonstrate one or more risk factors. It is difficult to diagnose IUGR in a mother who presents late in pregnancy because her dates are generally less certain and because the trend of fetal growth is unknown.

All infants who are born SGA must have demonstrated some degree of IUGR, although it may not have been appreciated before birth. IUGR would have to be specifically looked for to be appreciated in many infants who are mildly SGA. An infant who is IUGR may not be SGA at the time of birth. Some infants demonstrate impaired fetal growth (ie, plateauing or deceleration of their growth) but either started out fairly large for their gestational age or were delivered soon enough that they had not fallen below the established population norms[7–10] at the time of birth. These infants are assumed to be at risk for the same morbidities as SGA infants, although perhaps to a lesser degree.

Some make the distinction between symmetric and asymmetric growth retardation. Symmetric growth retardation is when all growth parameters are affected (ie, when length, weight, and head circumference are all less than 5% to 10%). Factors that interfere with fetal nutrient supply tend first to interfere with fat deposit (thereby affecting weight) and only later affect length and then head growth. Asymmetric growth retardation (ie, weight less than 5% to 10%, normal length and head circumference) thus generally signifies a milder and/or later insult, whereas symmetric growth retardation generally signifies an earlier, more severe insult or maldevelopment of the fetus.

FACTORS RELATED TO SURVIVAL AND OUTCOME OF IUGR INFANTS

The term *growth retardation* is generally used to denote an abnormality of the fetus itself or an insult that the fetus has suffered that has impaired growth. This abnormality or insult may be severe enough to cause death of the fetus or infant, may cause damage to the various organ systems, or may make the fetus/infant more vulnerable to subsequent damage (generally at the time of and after birth). Of greatest concern is damage to the CNS leading to long-term impairment (ie, developmental disabilities including cerebral palsy, mental retardation, hearing impairment, visual impairment, minor neuromotor dysfunction, speech and language problems, visual-perceptual deficit, learning disability, attention deficit, hyperactivity, and behavior disorder).

Although the population of IUGR or SGA infants is at higher risk for developmental disability, such disability is by no means a certainty. Small size at birth is merely a marker of risk.[1] Some neonates are small because their parents are small (especially the mother) or because their mother was SGA, and they do not have any higher risk of perinatal complications or developmental disability (although they may remain small for their age).[16] There are various conditions that interfere with fetal growth, and some of these also interfere with fetal development and/or make the fetus more vulnerable to complications at the time of or shortly after birth. The severity of CNS damage is generally related to the etiology of the growth retardation, the duration and severity of the insult (if any), and the nature of any perinatal/neonatal complications.[1]

Etiology

The box, "Etiologies of IUGR," lists some of the conditions that can interfere with fetal growth. The single most predictive factor of survival or developmental outcome of an IUGR/SGA infant is the etiology of the growth retardation.[1] Some conditions carry a known outcome (eg, trisomy 13 and 18 are associated with severe neurologic and cognitive handicap and early death), whereas other etiologies are less certain [eg, asymptomatic congenital cytomegalovirus (CMV) infection] or even appear to be benign (eg, small maternal size and possibly maternal cigarette smoking) with respect to developmental outcome. In addition, some conditions carry recurrence risks that would have important implications for any future children the parents (and perhaps other family members) may have.

Chromosomal abnormalities occur more frequently in SGA infants than in appropriate for gestational age (AGA) infants (2% compared to 0.4%), and up to 11% of SGA infants demonstrate a recognizable chromosomal or dysmorphic syndrome.[17,18] Although not all infants with chromosomal or dysmorphic syndromes are SGA, many of the syndromes (eg, Down and Turner's syndromes and

Etiologies of IUGR

Genetic

Chromosomal [eg, trisomy 13 and 18, Turner's syndrome (XO), various structural rearrangements and ring chromosomes]

Dysmorphic syndromes (eg, Cornelia de Lange, Seckel, Smith-Lemli-Opitz, Prader-Willi, Williams-Campbell, Riley-Day, Bloom, osteogenesis imperfecta, osteochondrodysplasia, Potter, thanatophoric dysplasia)

Metabolic abnormalities: Some inborn errors of metabolism (including some aminoacidurias), hypophosphatasia, leprechaunism, Menkes' syndrome, transient neonatal diabetes

Parental (especially maternal) size, maternal birthweight

Congenital infections

Toxoplasmosis, rubella, CMV, varicella, syphilis, malaria (plasmodia), Chagas' disease

Maternal ingestions

Alcohol (fetal alcohol syndrome or effects), narcotics (heroin, methadone), phenytoin (fetal hydantoin syndrome), antimetabolites (aminopterin, methotrexate), steroids (difficult to separate from effects of maternal illness), coumarin (fetal warfarin syndrome), amphetamines, bromides, trimethadione, phencyclidine, propranolol, polychlorinated biphenyls, cigarette smoke, cocaine)

Maternal conditions

Pregnancy-induced hypertension (preeclampsia), chronic hypertension or renal disease, cyanotic congenital heart disease, sickle cell disease, severe diabetes mellitus, collagen vascular disease, maternal phenylketonuria

Uteroplacental abnormalities

Uterine structural anomalies, abnormalities of insertion of the umbilical cord, hemangiomas of the placenta, twin-to-twin transfusion syndrome, "stuck twin" syndrome, circumvallate placenta, placenta extrachorialis, placenta previa, multiple infarcts of the placenta, syncytial knots, chronic abruption (separation) of the placenta, avascular villi, ischemic villous necrosis, chronic cord compression, fetal vessel thrombosis, chronic antepartum hemorrhage, single umbilical artery

Unknown

some of the sex chromosome disorders) demonstrate a lower mean birthweight and a higher proportion of SGA infants than expected.[19,20] In addition, many SGA infants with chromosomal abnormalities demonstrate early IUGR and symmetric growth retardation.[21] Even if a chromosomal or dysmorphic syndrome is not diagnosed, SGA infants with congenital anomalies (which are more frequent in SGA infants) have a higher risk of neurologic and/or cognitive abnormalities.[22]

Infants with congenital infections (especially toxoplasmosis, rubella, and CMV) are frequently, but not always, SGA.[23-25] The seriousness of these congenital infections is related to their sometimes profound effects on the developing fetus rather than to their prevalence. CMV infection is most common, occurring in up to 15% of pregnant mothers (often as a subclinical or barely noticed infection).[23-25] Frequently, however, the infection does not affect the placenta or the fetus (only about 0.3% to 3.4% of newborns and SGA infants). Even if infected, the fetus may not have any residual of the infection.

The congenital infections may lead to a whole spectrum of effects on the fetus, including death and resorption, spontaneous abortion, stillbirth, premature birth, IUGR, developmental anomalies, acute neonatal illness affecting multiple organ systems, persistent postnatal infection and damage, cerebral palsy, mental retardation, chorioretinitis with subsequent visual impairment, hearing impairment, communication disorder, learning disability, minor neuromotor dysfunction, attention deficit, behavior problems, or no apparent problems at all.[23-27] Severe cases frequently present with IUGR, microcephaly (sometimes with intracranial calcifications), or an acute neonatal illness, and in 40% to 90% of cases the child develops severe multiple handicaps. With congenital CMV infection, the hearing loss can (rarely) be progressive during the infant's first few years.[27] Infants with congenital infections or who have a mild neonatal illness are much less likely to develop major handicaps, but they appear to be at increased risk for subtle, later-appearing CNS defects, especially hearing loss and learning disability.[26,27]

There is a wide range of drugs that, when taken by the mother during pregnancy, can affect the growth of the fetus (see the box, "Etiologies of IUGR"). Some (eg, the antimetabolites) are generally fatal to the fetus. Others (eg, alcohol, hydantoin, trimethadione, and coumarin) can cause specific congenital anomalies and/or dysmorphic features in addition to IUGR, and they generally affect the fetal CNS as well.[20] Fetal alcohol and fetal hydantoin (ie, phenytoin) syndromes can cause a spectrum of effects on the infant, and the number of fetal anomalies or dysmorphic features tends to correlate with the severity of intellectual impairment.[20]

Maternal use of heroin and/or methadone during pregnancy can cause IUGR (15% to 35% of cases), a withdrawal syndrome in neonates (70% to 90% of cases, more common with methadone), and may lead to subtle neurologic abnormalities and/or subtle disturbances of behavior and attention.[28-31] Maternal cocaine use during pregnancy has been associated with lower birthweight, higher incidence of IUGR, microcephaly, abruptio placentae, fetal distress, behavioral and electroencephalographic abnormalities in the newborn, and possibly an increased incidence of cerebral infarction in the fetus or neonate.[32-38] It is extremely difficult, however, to separate the effect of cocaine from that of other factors (eg, other drugs, nutritional status, or lack of prenatal care).[32,33,36,38] Long-term effects of exposure to cocaine in utero are as yet unknown.[38] Maternal cigarette smoking clearly lowers birthweight and length. However, it does not appear to be associated with the child's later intellectual abilities or performance.[39]

Maternal or placental conditions that compromise uteroplacental function, decrease trophoblastic surface, reduce maternal oxygen saturation, or cause maternal metabolic abnormalities can cause IUGR. Approximately half of all SGA infants are born to mothers with obstetric complications or chronic disease, whereas only 1% to 2% are related to placental abnormalities.[40,41] Mothers with severe pregnancy-induced hypertension (ie, preeclampsia), chronic hypertensive vascular disease, and chronic renal failure have the highest risks of producing children with IUGR.[41] Infants born to mothers with pregnancy-induced hypertension tend to have a higher neonatal mortality and morbidity than infants born to mothers with hypertension alone.[42] Untreated maternal phenylketonuria can produce a microcephalic IUGR fetus with cardiac, craniofacial, and CNS defects, and the severity of defects appears to be related to maternal levels of phenylalanine.[20]

Abnormalities that affect the uterus or placenta can cause IUGR (see the Box), but 30% to 50% of the placental mass must be lost before significant growth retardation occurs.[43,44] Severe maternal malnutrition can cause a decrease in birthweight and rarely leads to IUGR, but later cognitive or neurologic effects do not seem to be a significant problem.[45] Newborns with nutritionally induced IUGR (due to maternal malnutrition or uteroplacental insufficiency) tend to demonstrate late (after gestation week 27 or 28) asymmetric growth retardation (ie, with relative sparing of brain and head growth). As Warshaw has suggested,[46(p998)]

> Rather than representing serious pathology, therefore, intrauterine growth retardation can be viewed as an adaptation in which the size of the fetus may be appropriate to the availability of nutrients. Low birthweight may improve the chances for survival with good outcome. The fetus exhibiting intrauterine growth retardation may represent a successful adaption to a substrate-deficient intrauterine environment.

Timing of insult/pattern of intrauterine growth

The pattern of abnormal intrauterine growth is determined by etiology, timing, and severity of the insult. There is little individual variability in fetal growth early in pregnancy, but variability increases by the end of the second trimester.[15] Early, symmetric growth retardation may result from a chromosomal abnormality, an early developmental defect marked by multiple congenital anomalies, or a serious insult (eg, congenital infection or toxin) early in pregnancy. Microcephaly has been associated with a poor prognosis, although poor postnatal head growth is probably a better predictor of outcome.[47–49]

For congenital rubella infection, the risk of fetal damage and the number of organ systems that are likely to be affected are greatest early in pregnancy.[24] For congenital toxoplasmosis, however, the likelihood of transmitting the infection from mother to fetus increases with length of gestation, although severe disease in the fetus occurs only if the infection is acquired during the first two trimesters.[50]

Conditions that are associated with uteroplacental insufficiency tend to cause later (ie, after gestation week 30) asymmetric growth retardation. These children, who have relatively normal head growth, tend to do better than those with symmetric growth retardation. Nevertheless, they are more susceptible to perinatal complications (eg, asphyxia and hypoglycemia) than AGA infants, probably because they have fewer reserves.[41,42,51,52]

Even if infants do not have a known etiology of their IUGR, timing of the IUGR (and presumably of the insult) does appear to be related to later developmental outcome. In longitudinal studies of IUGR infants (infants with chromosomal disorders, congenital infections, and dysmorphic syndromes were excluded), infants who manifested their IUGR before gestation week 26 had significantly poorer intellectual and academic performance, more behavior problems, and more difficulties with concentration than infants who demonstrated IUGR later in pregnancy or AGA controls.[53–56]

Perinatal complications

The SGA neonate is far more vulnerable to a number of perinatal complications (occurring in 65% of SGA neonates compared to 33% of AGA neonates).[42] SGA infants with low ponderal indices and asymmetric growth retardation are especially vulnerable.[42,51,52,57] The following perinatal complications of IUGR can further affect the infant's later development:

- fetal distress during labor,
- perinatal asphyxia,
- meconium aspiration,
- persistent pulmonary hypertension,
- hypothermia,
- hypoglycemia,
- polycythemia/hyperviscosity,
- hypocalcemia, and
- pulmonary hemorrhage.

Many of the perinatal problems that SGA infants encounter can be attributed to or are exacerbated by chronic and/or acute hypoxia (eg, fetal distress during labor, polycythemia, meconium aspiration, persistent pulmonary hypertension, hypothermia, hypocalcemia, hypoglycemia, and massive pulmonary hemorrhage).[58–62] SGA infants have decreased or borderline reserves of oxygen, subcutaneous fat, and liver glycogen but increased surface area and metabolic demands, making them more susceptible to asphyxia, hypothermia, and hypoglycemia.[41,57–59,61,63,64]

Cognitive and neurologic abnormalities in preterm and full-term SGA neonates appear to be strongly associated with CNS depression and asphyxia in the perinatal period.[65–68] Symptomatic hypoglycemia and symptomatic polycythemia (eg, with seizures, lethargy, tremors, apnea, and jitteriness) also carry a higher risk of neurologic and cognitive abnormalities.[69–71]

DEVELOPMENTAL OUTCOME

The most important questions that surround the birth of a growth-retarded infant relate to survival and long-term outcome. Because of their risk for developing severe perinatal complications, SGA infants do have a slightly higher mortality rate than AGA infants.[72,73] Nevertheless, the majority survive.

A number of studies have reported on the developmental outcome of SGA infants. Most studies distinguish between preterm and full-term SGA infants, and most exclude SGA infants with multiple congenital anomalies, chromosomal disorders, recognized dysmorphic syndromes, and congenital infections. How hard each study looks for disability (eg, by including hearing and visual screens in their assessment batteries), the age at which children were assessed, and the criteria used to diagnose disability vary widely among the studies. In addition, the manner in which the growth retardation was diagnosed, the population base from which the study sample was drawn, and the degree to which etiologies were looked for and used for exclusion from the study sample also vary widely. With these limitations in mind, a review of the various existing outcome studies of full-term and preterm SGA infants provides an overview of their short- and long-term outcome.

The full-term SGA infant

As neonates, SGA infants reportedly have lower muscle tone, less activity, poorer head control, less excitability, greater tremulousness, poorer visual fixation, and poorer orientation to visual and auditory stimuli than AGA neonates.[63,74–77] Some primitive reflexes have been reported to be less complete (eg, Moro, standing, and stepping), and others more sustained (eg, asymmetric tonic neck reflex and grasp), in SGA neonates.[74–78] The neonatal neurologic examination, however, is less predictive of infant developmental outcome in SGA than in AGA infants.[79]

During infancy, SGA infants have been reported to score lower than AGA controls on the Bayley mental and physical developmental indices, to be less active, and to have lower energy levels.[80] Three-year-old term SGA children had significantly more hyperactivity, concentration difficulties, fears, behavior problems, and subtle neurologic dysfunction than AGA controls.[81] Other investigators have found no differences on neurologic or cognitive examinations in infants and preschool children.[77,80]

Most prospective studies of full-term SGA infants followed from birth have found no increased incidence of major neurologic handicap,[63,68,80–82] although a few have found a slightly greater incidence of cerebral palsy[84] or seizures.[85] Large retrospective studies of children with cerebral palsy have found no or only a slightly increased incidence of cerebral palsy in SGA children; nowhere near the incidence seen in preterm children.[86,87]

The majority of SGA children have normal intelligence.[22,55,68,80,82–85,88–92] Although a few studies have found significantly lower mean intelligence quotient (IQ) scores, the lower IQ is primarily associated with socioeconomic status[22,68] or gender (lower in boys).[84] One very large prospective study found that SGA children did have a statistically significantly lower mean IQ (despite controlling for various biologic and family factors), but this difference was not clinically significant.[83] Retrospective studies of people with developmental disability have found that an unexpectedly high number of them were IUGR infants.[93,94]

SGA infants do not appear to have a higher incidence of hearing or visual impairment than AGA infants.[79,84] Fitzhardinge and Steven[84] found a strikingly high incidence of speech and language problems in SGA children, especially in boys (31%). They also found a high incidence (25%, compared with 4% in control siblings) of minimal cerebral dysfunction (ie, hyperactivity, short attention span, learning difficulties, hyperreflexia, and poor fine motor coordination). Two studies that compared 5- to 7-year-old full-term SGA and AGA children found higher incidences of mild neurologic abnormalities and more behavior and attention problems in the former.[83,89]

An increased incidence of academic difficulties is a variable finding in studies of full-term SGA children.[68,79,82,84,89] Rubin et al[89] found that more SGA children failed grades (32.5% compared to 11.5%) and required special classes (10.0% compared to 2.5%) than full-term AGA children. Fitzhardinge and Steven[84] found that half the SGA boys and one third of the SGA girls with average intelligence were doing poorly in school (one third of SGA children with IQs higher than 100 were consistently failing at school).

In summary, the vast majority of full-term SGA children have no major handicap. A few large and/or retrospective studies have suggested that the incidence of cerebral palsy and mental retardation may be slightly higher in SGA children. The evidence does clearly suggest, however, that SGA children (even those with normal intelligence and no major neurologic problems) demonstrate a high rate of the more subtle signs of CNS dysfunction (eg, speech and language problems, minor neuromotor dysfunction, learning disability, attention deficits, hyperactivity, and behavior problems).

The preterm SGA infant

The preterm SGA infant certainly appears to be at least at the same risk for developmental disability as full-term SGA infants and preterm AGA infants

(Table 1).[67,87,90–92,95–99] Because they are already expressing their IUGR at the time of their preterm birth, they should probably be viewed as IUGR infants who manifest their growth retardation fairly early in pregnancy (as opposed to those infants who become growth retarded just before term). In addition, preterm SGA infants could be expected to develop the same perinatal complications and risks for developmental disability as preterm AGA infants. Major handicap (ie, cerebral palsy and mental retardation) occurs in approximately 7% to 16% of preterm infants with birthweights less than 1500 g.[100] However, probably because they are often stressed in utero, which leads to accelerated maturation, SGA infants do not have as high an incidence of respiratory distress syndrome or intraventricular hemorrhage as preterm AGA infants of the same gestational age.[101]

In a retrospective study from Sweden of children with cerebral palsy, preterm SGA infants had by far the highest risk of cerebral palsy of all the birthweight/gestational age categories.[87] A number of studies have found a higher incidence of subnormal intelligence and a lower mean IQ than the general population.[22,67,92,95,102] Yet only two of nine studies have found a significantly higher incidence of major handicap in SGA compared to AGA preterm infants.[67,90,95–99]

The retrospective studies suggest that there is at least an additive effect of an infant being both preterm and SGA. Two excellent prospective studies of preterm SGA infants have compared their developmental outcome to that of preterm AGA controls matched by birthweight, and one also compared them to controls matched by gestational age.[90–92] Vohr et al[90] and Vohr and Oh[91] sequentially followed 21 preterm SGA and 20 birthweight-matched preterm AGA infants to age 5. The two groups had a similar rate of major neurologic abnormalities (15% and 12%), but significantly more SGA children had minor neurologic abnormalities (25% compared to 12%). Early on (ie, at 9 months through 3 years), the SGA infants did worse on developmental testing. By ages 4 and 5, however, these differences no longer were observed, which points out the importance of long-term follow-up.

Pena et al[92] compared a group of 35 preterm SGA infants to preterm AGA controls matched for birthweight and to controls matched for gestational age. The SGA infants had a lower mean developmental quotient than both groups of preterm AGA controls. The SGA infants had a similar rate of major neurologic handicap as AGA infants matched for birthweight, but they were smaller, had more neonatal complications, and had more neurologic problems than AGA infants matched for gestational age.

The preterm SGA infant clearly has a higher incidence of major developmental disability than the full-term AGA or SGA infant. It is unclear as to whether the preterm SGA infant has more developmental abnormalities compared to AGA preterm infants matched for small size. When matched to preterm AGA infants of similar maturity at birth, however, the preterm SGA child appears to have more problems. This additive effect of IUGR and prematurity may well be due to the

Table 1. Incidence of major handicap in premature SGA and AGA children

Study	Age	Premature SGA		Premature AGA		
		Number	Handicap	Number	Handicap	Significance
Saint-Anne Dargassies (1977)[96]	2–18 years	24	25%	262	21%	NS*
Koops (1978)[98]	8–23 months	21	24%	67	30	NS
Commey (1979)[67]	2 years	71	49%	—	—	—
Fitzhardinge (1979)[95]	2 years	28	43%	28	11%	$P < 0.01$
Hack (1979)[97]	2 years	43	21%	117	15	NS
Lipper (1981)[47]	7 months	41	17%	86	13	NS
Vohr (1979)[90]	2 years	21	10%	21	5	NS
Vohr (1983)[91]	5 years	19	15%	16	12%	NS
Tudehope (1983)[99]	1 year	33	6%	131	6%	NS
Pena (1988)[92]	1 year	35	23%	35†	26%	NS†
Pena (1988)[92]	1 year	20	30%	20‡	5%	$P < 0.05$‡

* NS, not significant.

† Premature AGA infants matched by birthweight.

‡ Premature AGA infants matched by gestational age.

causes of the growth retardation and the prematurity and to the perinatal complications that occur.

SUMMARY

The vast majority of full-term SGA children have no major handicap, but they do have a greatly increased risk of minimal cerebral dysfunction (language delays or disorders, learning disability, minor neuromotor dysfunction, attention deficit, hyperactivity, and behavioral problems). The risks of developmental disability appear to be additive for IUGR and prematurity, especially when the preterm SGA infant is compared to AGA controls of the same gestational age.

SGA infants with chromosomal disorders, congenital infection, or known dysmorphic syndromes and who are noted to be IUGR early (before gestation week 20) have a higher risk of developmental disability. SGA infants who are growth retarded because of placental insufficiency by and large have a good prognosis (especially if they do not develop perinatal complications). Therefore, infants who were growth retarded on the basis of uteroplacental insufficiency, small maternal size, maternal cigarette smoking, or no definite etiology warrant careful but optimistic developmental follow-up. Even if they do not develop major handicap, all IUGR or SGA children should be followed through school age because of an increased risk for the more subtle CNS abnormalities manifested as school and behavior problems.

In conclusion, there appears to be a spectrum of CNS abnormalities seen in children with growth retardation. These appear to be related to type of CNS insult/ developmental anomaly, severity, timing of the insult, and the development of perinatal complications. The SGA population is an extraordinarily heterogeneous one, with multiple etiologies, patterns of growth retardation, and outcomes. IUGR should be viewed not as a specific diagnosis but primarily as a marker of abnormalities of the fetus and/or the uteroplacental environment and thus of possible CNS abnormality.

RECOMMENDATIONS REGARDING CARE AND FOLLOW-UP OF SGA INFANTS

What, then, are the implications of these findings? How can we use these findings to better evaluate, care for, and follow IUGR and SGA infants? The following recommendations are based on the findings and implications of the studies described above:

1. Complete a diagnostic work-up of each IUGR fetus and each SGA neonate. Elucidate the etiology of the cause of the growth retardation whenever possible, and assess perinatal complications that may contribute to risk. Use

this information to counsel parents about the infant's prognosis and (also important) any risk of recurrence and/or genetic implications for other family members.

2. Anticipate and minimize perinatal complications. Because of their borderline ability to compensate and their limited reserves, growth-retarded fetuses and infants are more vulnerable than AGA infants to a number of perinatal complications, which in turn can further limit their potential. Monitor IUGR fetuses carefully during pregnancy for signs of fetal distress and intervene as indicated to prevent sudden death and to maximize their potential. Delivering an IUGR fetus as soon as the growth retardation is diagnosed only exposes the infant to all the risks of prematurity, and so this option should be reserved only for the fetus who is in danger. Whenever an IUGR infant is delivered or SGA is diagnosed in a neonate, care should be taken to monitor for and to anticipate possible complications (eg, asphyxia and hypoglycemia).

3. Counsel the parents before discharge from the nursery. Parents need to know why their infant was growth retarded, what the significance of the growth retardation is, and what their child's prognosis is. Any recurrence risks or other genetic implications should be discussed at this time (if not earlier). Plans for discharge and follow-up should be formulated. The child's parents, pediatrician, and personnel involved in provision of community services should be included in this planning process whenever possible.

4. Arrange pediatric follow-up of all SGA infants. This should include some assessment of development to ensure early diagnosis and appropriate referrals for evaluation and treatment of infants with developmental disability. Most professionals would agree that early diagnosis of developmental disability is important for helping the child's parents cope with the child's disability and for planning more effectively for the child's habilitation.

5. Arrange for comprehensive developmental follow-up of SGA infants with a significantly increased risk for developmental disability (as determined by etiology, timing of the insult/anomaly, and perinatal complications). Provide these infants and their families with support during the first year, which is a period of great uncertainty. View parents as partners in assessing and planning for their high-risk infant. Honesty during developmental follow-up is the best policy: Parents are already concerned about their child's prognosis, and so avoiding a discussion or minimizing their concerns only serves to make them more scared and angry. On the other hand, most SGA infants do well despite mild neuromotor abnormalities early on that do not lead to functional impairments. A definitive diagnosis of developmental disability should not be made until the evaluator is certain of its presence.

6. Consider early intervention services for infants with a diagnosed condition that carries a high probability of developmental delay. The goal of early intervention would be to help the parents cope with their child and his or her disability, to help maximize the child's potential, and to avoid or minimize any secondary problems (eg, contractures or behavior problems).

7. Consider a multidisciplinary evaluation of each significantly SGA child during the preschool or early school years, because learning disabilities and attention deficits are so common in SGA children. The multidisciplinary team should include a pediatrician, developmental pediatrician, child psychiatrist, or pediatric neurologist; a clinical psychologist; a special educator; and a social worker. The child should undergo evaluation by a speech and language pathologist, audiologist, occupational therapist, physical therapist, or other professional as indicated. Focus on each child's abilities early in the school career to anticipate problems and to begin remediation before he or she experiences multiple failures and subsequent loss of self-esteem .

8. Continue to follow all SGA children through school, paying careful attention to early signs of school and/or behavior problems. Many children with subtle CNS deficits are able to compensate for their difficulties early in their school career. However, as the work becomes more complex, difficult, and time limited, they are no longer able to compensate as effectively, and learning disabilities or attention deficits may become more apparent. Be willing to refer for a multidisciplinary evaluation if these signs develop, even if a previous evaluation was normal or inconclusive.

9. Conduct ongoing research to understand the multiple etiologies of growth retardation, how they work, and what treatment strategies are effective at preventing and minimizing the risks of IUGR.

REFERENCES

1. Allen MA. Developmental outcome and followup of the small for gestational age infant. *Semin Perinatol.* 1984;8:123–155.

2. Dubowitz LMS, Dubowitz V, Goldberg C. Clinical assessment of gestational age in the newborn infant. *J Pediatr.* 1970;77:1–10.

3. Ballard JL, Novak KK, Driver M. A simplified score for assessment of fetal maturation of newly born infants. *J Pediatr.* 1979;5:769–774.

4. Alexander GR, Hulsey TC, Smeriglio VL, Comfort M. Factors influencing the relationship between a newborn assessment of gestational maturity and the gestational age interval. *Pediatr Perinat Epidemiol.* 1990;4:135–148.

5. Saunders M, Allen M, Alexander GR et al. Gestational age assessment in preterm neonates weighing less than 1500 grams. *Pediatrics.* 1991; 88: 542–546.

6. Amiel-Tison C. Possible acceleration of neurological maturation following high-risk pregnancy. *Am J Obstet Gynecol.* 1980;138:303–306.

7. Lubchenco LO, Hansman C, Boyd E. Intrauterine growth in length and head circumference as estimated from live births at gestational ages from 26 to 42 weeks. *Pediatrics.* 1966;37:403–408.

8. Gruenwald P. Growth of the human fetus. *Am J Obstet Gynecol.* 1966;94:1112–1119 .

9. Usher R, McLean F. Intrauterine growth of liveborn caucasian infants at sea level: standards obtained from measurements in 7 dimensions of infants born between 25 and 44 weeks of gestation. *J Pediatr.* 1969;74:901–910.

10. Tanner JM, Thomson AM. Standards for birthweight at gestation periods from 32 to 42 weeks, allowing for maternal height and weight. *Arch Dis Child.* 1970;45:566–569.

11. Van Assche F, Robertson WB. *Fetal Growth Retardation.* New York: Churchill Livingstone; 1981.

12. Andersen HF, Johnson TRB, Barclay ML, Flora JD. Gestational age assessment. *Am J Obstet Gynecol.* 1981;139:173–177.

13. DiPietro JA, Allen MC. Estimation of gestational age: implications for developmental research. *Child Dev.* 1991;62:1184–1199.

14. Robinson HP, Fleming JEE. A critical evaluation of sonar "crown-rump length" measurements. *Br J Obstet Gynaecol.* 1975;82:702–710.

15. Campbell S, Warsof SL, Little D, Cooper DJ. Routine ultrasound screening for the prediction of gestational age. *Obstet Gynecol.* 1985;65:613–620.

16. Hackman E, Emanuel I, van Belle G, Daling J. Maternal birth weight and subsequent pregnancy outcome. *JAMA.* 1983;250:2016–2019.

17. Chen ATL, Falek A, Lester W . Chromosome aberrations in full-term low birth weight neonates. *Humangenetik.* 1974;21:13–16.

18. Anderson NG. A five year survey of small for dates infants for chromosomal abnormalities. *Aust Paediat J.* 1976;12:19–23.

19. Reisman LE. Chromosome abnormalities and intrauterine growth retardation. *Pediatr Clin North Am.* 1970;17:101–110.

20. Jones KL. *Smith's Recognizable Patterns of Human Malformation.* 4th ed. Philadelphia: Saunders; 1988.

21. Kurjak A, Kirkinen P. Ultrasonic growth pattern of fetuses with chromosomal aberrations. *Acta Obstet Gynecol Scand.* 1982;61:223–225.

22. Drillien CM. The small-for-date infant: etiology and prognosis. *Pediatr Clin North Am.* 1970;17:9–24.

23. Panjvani ZFK, Hanshaw JB. Cytomegalovirus in the perinatal period. *Am J Dis Child.* 1981;135:56–60.

24. Alford CA, Pass RF. Epidemiology of chronic congenital and perinatal infection of man. *Clin Perinatol.* 1981;8:397–414.

25. Remington JS, Klein JO. *Infectious Disease of the Fetus and Newborn Infant.* 2nd ed. Philadelphia: Saunders; 1983.

26. Hanshaw JB, Scheiner AP, Moxley AW, Gaev L, Abel V, Scheiner B. School failure and deafness after "silent" congenital cytomegalovirus infection. *N Engl J Med.* 1976;295:468–470.

27. Stagno S, Reynolds DW, Amos CS, et al. Auditory and visual defects resulting from symptomatic and subclinical congenital cytomegaloviral and *Toxoplasma* infections. *Pediatrics.* 1977;59:669–678.

28. Zelson C, Lee SJ, Casalino M. Neonatal narcotic addiction. *N Engl J Med.* 1973;289:1216–1220.
29. Stone ML, Salerno LJ, Green M, Zelson C. Narcotic addiction in pregnancy. *Am J Obstet Gynecol.* 1971;109:716–723.
30. Wilson GS, McCreary R, Kean J, Baxter JC. The development of preschool children of heroin-addicted mothers: a controlled study. *Pediatrics.* 1979;63:135–141.
31. Lifschitz MH, Wilson GS, Smith EO, Desmond MM. Factors affecting head growth and intellectual function in children of drug addicts. *Pediatrics.* 1985;75:269–274.
32. Bingol N, Fuchs M, Diaz V, Stone RK, Gromisch DS. Teratogenicity of cocaine in humans. *J Pediatr.* 1987;110:93–96.
33. Oro AS, Dixon SD. Perinatal cocaine and methamphetamine exposure: maternal and neonatal correlates. *J Pediatr.* 1987;111:571–578.
34. Doberczak TM, Shanzer S, Senie RT, Kandall SR. Neonatal neurologic and electroencephalographic effects of intrauterine cocaine exposure. *J Pediatr.* 1988;113:354–358.
35. Chasnoff IJ, Griffith DR, MacGregor S, Dirkes K, Burns KA. Temporal patterns of cocaine use in pregnancy. *JAMA.* 1989;261:1741–1744.
36. Fulroth R, Phillips B, Durand DJ. Perinatal outcome of infants exposed to cocaine and /or heroin in utero. *Am J Dis Child.* 1989;143:905–910.
37. Hadeed AJ, Siegel SR. Maternal cocaine use during pregnancy: effect on the newborn infant. *Pediatrics.* 1989;84:205–210.
38. Roland EH, Volpe JJ. Effect of maternal cocaine use on the fetus and newborn: review of the literature. *Pediatr Neurol.* 1989;15:88–94.
39. Hardy JB, Mellits ED. Does maternal smoking during pregnancy have a long-term effect on the child? *Lancet.* 1972;2:1332–1336.
40. Bjerre B, Bjerre I. Significance of obstetric factors in prognosis of low birthweight children. *Acta Paediatr Scand.* 1976;65:577–583.
41. Low JA, Galbraith RS. Pregnancy characteristics of intrauterine growth retardation. *Obstet Gynecol.* 1974;44:122–126.
42. Ounsted M, Moar V, Scott WA. Perinatal morbidity and mortality in small-for-dates babies: the relative importance of some maternal factors. *Early Hum Dev.* 1981;5:367–375.
43. Elliott K, Knight J, eds. *Size at Birth* (Ciba Foundation Symposium 27). New York: Excerpta Medica; 1974.
44. Poma PA. Intrauterine growth retardation associated with uterine malformations. *JAMA.* 1982;8:745–748.
45. Stein Z, Susser M, Saenger G, Marolla F. Nutrition and mental performance. *Science* 1972;178:708–713.
46. Warshaw JB. Intrauterine growth retardation: adaptation or pathology? *Pediatrics.* 1985;76:998–999.
47. Lipper E, Lee K, Gartner LM, Grellong B. Determinants of neurobehavioral outcome in low-birthweight infants. *Pediatrics.* 1981;67:502–505.
48. Gross SJ, Oehler JM, Eckerman CO. Head growth and developmental outcome in very low-birthweight infants. *Pediatrics.* 1983;71:70–75.
49. Hack M, Breslau N, Fanaroff AA. Differential effects of intrauterine and postnatal brain growth failure in infants of very low birth weight. *Am J Dis Child.* 1989;143:63–68.
50. Desmonts G, Curvreur J. Congenital toxoplasmosis. *N Engl J Med.* 1974;290:1110–1116.

51. Kurjak A, Latin V, Polak J. Ultrasonic recognition of two types of growth retardation by measurement of four fetal dimensions. *J Perinat Med.* 1978;6:102–108.

52. Villar J, Belizan JM. The timing factor in the pathophysiology of the intrauterine growth retardation syndrome. *Obstet Gynecol Surv.* 1982;37:499–506.

53. Fancourt R, Campbell S, Harvey D, Norman AP. Follow-up study of small-for-dates babies. *Br Med J.* 1976;1:1435–1437.

54. Parkinson CE, Wallis S, Harvey D. School achievement and behavior of children who were small-for-dates at birth. *Dev Med Child Neurol.* 1981;23:41–50.

55. Harvey D, Prince J, Bunton J, Parkinson C, Campbell S. Abilities of children who were small-for-gestational-age babies. *Pediatrics.* 1982;69:296–300.

56. Parkinson CE, Scrivener R, Graves L, Bunton J, Harvey D. Behavioural differences of school-age children who were small-for-dates babies. *Dev Med Child Neurol.* 1986;28:498–505 .

57. Walther FJ, Ramaekers LHJ. Neonatal morbidity of SGA infants in relation to their nutritional status at birth. *Acta Paediatr Scand.* 1982;71:437–440.

58. Jones MD Jr, Battaglia FC. Intrauterine growth retardation. *Am J Obstet Gynecol.* 1977;127:540–549.

59. Scott KE, Usher R. Fetal malnutrition: its incidence, causes, and effects. *Am J Obstet Gynecol.* 1966;94:951–963.

60. Warshaw JB. The growth retarded fetus. *Clin Perinatol.* 1979;6:353–363.

61. Low JA, Boston RW, Pancham SR. Fetal asphyxia during the intrapartum period in intrauterine growth-retarded infants. *Am J Obstet Gynecol.* 1972;113:351–357.

62. Tsang RC, Gigger M, Oh W, Brown DR. Studies in calcium metabolism in infants with intrauterine growth retardation. *J Pediatr.* 1975;86:936–941.

63. Low JA, Galbraith RS, Muir D, Killen H, Karchmar J, Campbell D. Intrauterine growth retardation: a preliminary report of long-term morbidity. *Am J Obstet Gynecol.* 1978;130:534–545.

64. Cefalo RC. The hazards of labor and delivery for the intrauterine growth-retarded fetus. *J Reprod Med.* 1978;21:300–304.

65. Hagberg G, Hagberg B, Olow I. The changing panorama of cerebral palsy in Sweden 1954–1970. III. The importance of fetal deprivation of supply. *Acta Paediatr Scand.* 1976;65:403–408.

66. Kyllerman M. Dyskinetic cerebral palsy. II. Pathogenetic risk factors and intra-uterine growth. *Acta Paediatr Scand.* 1982;71:551–558.

67. Commey JOO, Fitzhardinge PM. Handicap in the preterm small-for-gestational age infant. *J Pediatr.* 1979;94:779–786.

68. Westwood M, Kramer MS, Munz D, Lovett JM, Watters GV. Growth and development of full-term nonasphyxiated small-for-gestational-age newborns: follow-up through adolescence. *Pediatrics.* 1983;71:376–382.

69. Koivisto M, Blanco-Sequeiros M, Krause U. Neonatal symptomatic and asymptomatic hypoglycaemia: a follow-up study of 151 children. *Dev Med Child Neurol.* 1972;14:603–614.

70. Lucas A, Morley E, Cole TJ. Adverse neurodevelopmental outcome of moderate neonatal hypoglycaemia. *Br Med J.* 1988;297: 1304–1308.

71. Black VD, Lubchenco LO, Luckey DW, et al. Developmental and neurologic sequelae of neonatal hyperviscosity syndrome. *Pediatrics.* 1982;69:426–431.

72. Koops BL, Morgan LJ, Battaglia FC. Neonatal mortality risk in relation to birth weight and gestational age: update. *J Pediatr.* 1982;101:969–977.

73. Starfield B, Shapiro S, McCormick M, Bross D. Mortality and morbidity in infants with intrauterine growth retardation. *J Pediatr.* 1982;101:978–983.

74. Michaelis R, Schulte FJ, Nolte R. Motor behavior of small for gestational age newborn infants. *J Pediatr.* 1970;76:208–213.

75. Schulte FJ, Schrempf G, Hinze G. Maternal toxemia, fetal malnutrition, and motor behavior of the newborn. *Pediatrics.* 1971;48:871–882.

76. Als H, Tronick E, Adamson L, Brazelton TB. The behavior of the full-term but underweight newborn infant. *Dev Med Child Neurol.* 1976;18:590–602.

77. Leijon I, Finnstrom O, Nilsson B, Ryden G. Neurology and behaviour of growth-retarded neonates. Relation to biochemical placental function tests in late pregnancy. *Early Hum Dev.* 1980; 4/3:257–270.

78. Fredrickson WT, Brown JV. Gripping and Moro responses: differences between small-for-gestational-age and normal weight term newborns. *Early Hum Dev.* 1980;4/1:69–77.

79. Leijon I, Billstrom G, Lind I. An 18-month follow-up study of growth-retarded neonates. Relation to biochemical tests of placental function in late pregnancy and neurobehavioural condition in the newborn period. *Early Hum Dev.* 1980;4/3:271–285.

80. Low JA, Galbraith RS, Muir D, Killen H, Pater B, Karchmar J. Intrauterine growth retardation: a study of long-term morbidity. *Am J Obstet Gynecol.* 1982;142:670–677.

81. Walther FJ, Ramaekers LHJ. Developmental aspects of subacute fetal distress: behavior problems and neurological dysfunction. *Early Hum Dev.* 1982;6:1–10.

82. Babson SG, Henderson NB. Fetal undergrowth: relation of head growth to later intellectual performance. *Pediatrics.* 1974;53:890–894 .

83. Neligan GA, Kolvin I, Scott DM, et al. *Born Too Soon or Born Too Small. A Follow-up Study of Seven Years of Age.* Philadelphia: Lippincott; 1976.

84. Fitzhardinge PM, Steven EM. The small-for-date infant. II. Neurological and intellectual sequelae. *Pediatrics.* 1972;50:50–57.

85. Winer EK, Tejani NA, Atluru NL, DiGiuseppe R, Borofsky LG. Four- to seven-year evaluation in two groups of small-for-gestational age infants. *Am J Obstet Gynecol.* 1982;143:425–429.

86. Ellenberg JH, Nelson KB . Birthweight and gestational age in children with cerebral palsy or seizure disorders. *Am J Dis Child.* 1979;133:1044–1048.

87. Hagberg B. Epidemiological and preventive aspects of cerebral palsy and severe mental retardation in Sweden. *Eur J Pediatr.* 1979;130:71–78.

88. Wiener G. The relationship of birth weight and length for gestation to intellectual development at ages 8 to 10 years. *J Pediatr.* 1970;76:694–699.

89. Rubin RA, Rosenblatt C, Balow B. Psychological and educational sequelae of prematurity. *Pediatrics.* 1973;52:352–363.

90. Vohr BR, Oh W, Rosenfield AG, Cowett RM. The preterm small-for-gestational-age infant: a two-year follow-up study. *Am J Obstet Gynecol.* 1979; 133:425–431.

91. Vohr BR, Oh W. Growth and development in preterm infants small for gestational age. *J Pediatr.* 1983;103:941–945.

92. Pena IC, Teberg AJ, Finello KM. The premature small-for-gestational-age infant during the first year of life: comparison by birth weight and gestational age. *J Pediatr.* 1988;113:1066–1073.

93. Collins E, Turner G. The importance of the "small for dates" baby to the problem of mental retardation. *Med J Aust.* 1971;2:313–315.

94. Sabel KG, Olegard R, Victorin L. Remaining sequelae with modern perinatal care. *Pediatrics.* 1976;57:652–658.

95. Fitzhardinge PM, Kalman E, Ashby S, Pape KE. Present status of the infant of very low birth weight treated in a referral neonatal intensive care unit in 1974 (Ciba Foundation Symposium 59). New York: Excerpta Medica; 1979.

96. Saint-Anne Dargassies S. Long-term neurological follow-up study of 286 truly premature infants. I: Neurological sequelae. *Dev Med Child Neurol.* 1977;19:462–478.

97. Hack M, Fanaroff AA, Merkatz IR. The low-birthweight infant—evolution of a changing outlook. *N Engl J Med.* 1979;301:1162–1165.

98. Koops BL. Neurologic sequelae in infants with intrauterine growth retardation. *J Reprod Med.* 1978;21:343–351.

99. Tudehope DI, Burns Y, O'Callaghan M, Mohay H, Silcock A. The relationship between intrauterine and postnatal growth on the subsequent psychomotor development of very low birthweight (VLBW) infants. *Aust Pediatr J.* 1983;19:3–8.

100. Allen MC, Jones MD Jr. Medical complications of prematurity. *Obstet Gynecol.* 1986;67:427–437.

101. Procianoy RS, Garcia-Prats JA, Adams JM, Silvers A, Rudolph AJ. Hyaline membrane disease and intraventricular haemorrhage in small for gestational age infants. *Arch Dis Child.* 1980;55:502–505.

102. Francis-Williams J, Davies PA. Very low birthweight and later intelligence. *Dev Med Child Neurol.* 1974;16:709–728.

Glossary

Abdominal circumference—measurement of fetal size; circumference of the abdominal cavity.

Abruptio placenta—separation of the placenta from the uterine wall, causing blood loss generally from the maternal side and occasionally from the fetal side of the placenta.

Antimetabolites—a class of drugs that interfere with cell metabolism, often used as chemotherapy for cancer.

Apnea—time period when an infant does not ("forgets to") breathe.

Appropriate for gestational age (AGA)—an infant who is born with a weight that is expected for his or her degree of maturity (ie, gestational age) compared to population norms.

Asphyxia—inadequate oxygenation and/or circulation to the tissues of the body, especially to the lungs, kidneys, gastrointestinal tract, and CNS.

Asymmetric growth retardation—in a fetus or newborn, weight is significantly below that expected for gestational age compared to population norms. Head circumference is usually spared (normal for gestational age); length is variable.

Biparietal diameter—measurement of fetal head size; diameter of the head (roughly, from ear to ear).

Chorioretinitis—inflammation of the choroid and retina of the eye, often due to a congenital infection (eg, toxoplasmosis, rubella, CMV).

Congenital anomaly—an unusual or irregular physical trait that is established during intrauterine life.

Congenital infection—an infection that is present in the mother during pregnancy and is passed along to the fetus (eg, syphilis, toxoplasmosis, rubella, CMV, HIV).

Coumarin—a medication used to discourage the blood from clotting or to "thin the blood."

Crown–rump length—measurement of the fetus from the top of the head to the buttocks.

Cytomegalovirus—cytomegalic inclusion disease virus, a human virus in the herpes family, that causes mild symptomatology in children and adults but, if passed from mother to fetus in utero, can cause malformations and illness in the fetus.

Dysmorphic—features that are abnormally shaped. They may occur singly or in combination. A few dysmorphic features frequently have no clinical significance, but certain combinations may signify a chromosomal disorder or a dysmorphic syndrome with a known etiology and/or prognosis.

Femur length—measurement of fetal size; length of the thigh bone.

Fetal distress—sign that the fetus is in trouble and that injury and/or death is imminent.

Gestational age—age of a fetus as calculated from the mother's last menstrual period (or best obstetric estimate of it).

Hydantoin (Dilantin, phenytoin)—medication used to treat a number of problems, especially seizures.

Hypocalcemia—low blood calcium.

Hypoglycemia—low blood glucose (sugar).

Hypothermia—abnormally low body temperature; can cause severe problems (eg, hypoxia, acidosis, poor circulation) in the newborn.

Hypoxia—decreased tissue oxygen; may be acute (sudden) or chronic (lasting over a period of time).

Intracranial calcifications—precipitation of calcium salts in brain tissue; generally a result of inflammation or other injury.

Intrauterine growth retardation (IUGR)—plateauing or deceleration in fetal growth, or a fetus that is smaller than expected compared to population norms.

Intraventricular hemorrhage—bleeding into the ventricles and/or the tissue of the brain; a complication of prematurity.

Lethargy—inactivity, sluggishness.

Meconium aspiration—a fetus or newborn infant who inhales his or her first stool (meconium) with inspiration. Generally the first stool is passed in relation to fetal distress (thus meconium aspiration is viewed as a sign of fetal distress). The meconium can be irritating to lung tissue and can cause a pneumonia.

Microcephaly—smaller head circumference than expected for age compared to population norms.

Persistent pulmonary hypertension—condition in a newborn infant in which the circulation does not switch over from fetal circulation (in which the lungs are virtually bypassed and all blood goes through the placenta) to circulation required for life outside the uterus (in which virtually all blood goes through the lungs). The vessels bringing blood to the lungs remain constricted, and the infant is cyanotic (blue).

Phenylalanine—a common amino acid in protein.

Phenylketonuria—a congenital deficiency of an enzyme necessary to metabolize phenylalanine. Accumulation of phenylalanine during the developmental period produces damage to the brain (eg, seizures, severe mental retardation). Autosomal recessive inheritance.

Polycythemia—an increase in the concentration of red blood cells, often associated with a thickening of the blood (ie, hyperviscosity) and sludging of the blood in small vessels.

Ponderal index—birthweight divided by the cube of the length at birth (BW/L3); a measure of nutritional status at birth.

Pregnancy-induced hypertension (preeclampsia)—a disorder of pregnancy that includes elevated blood pressure, edema, increased weight gain, and protein in the urine and may also include headache, visual disturbances, liver and kidney abnormalities, and, when very severe, seizures (then called eclampsia). The mortality rate is high with this disorder, and treatment includes delivery of the infant.

Pulmonary hemorrhage—bleeding into the lungs.

Respiratory distress syndrome—difficulty with breathing due to immaturity of the lungs in preterm infants.

Ring chromosomes—circular chromosomes, generally due to abnormalities in the division process, often with loss of chromosomal tissue.

Rubella—an acute viral illness with rash and enlargement of the lymph nodes; it is caused by an RNA virus. If passed from mother to fetus in utero, can cause malformations and illness in the fetus.

Small for gestational age (SGA)—an infant who is born weighing significantly less than expected for his or her maturity compared to population norms.

Symmetric growth retardation—a fetus or newborn in whom all growth parameters (length, weight, head circumference) are significantly below those expected for gestational age compared to population norms .

Toxoplasmosis—disease caused by *Toxoplasma gondii*, a parasite. The only known person-to-person transmission is from infected mother to fetus; it can result in infection and severe anomalies in the fetus.

Trimethadione—a medication used to treat seizures.

Trisomy—condition in which there is an extra (third) chromosome of a pair; for example, in trisomy 13 the cells of the body all have three, not two, of chromosome 13.

Turner's syndrome—a chromosomal anomaly in which the individual's cells all have only 45 chromosomes, with only one sex (X) chromosome. Anomalies include short stature, webbed neck, shield-shaped chest, and infertility with abnormal ovaries.

Uteroplacental insufficiency—condition in which something within the placenta has interfered with adequate delivery of nutrition, circulation, and/or oxygen to the fetus.

Etiology of developmental disabilities

I. Leslie Rubin, MD
Director of Pediatrics
Developmental Evaluation Center
The Children's Hospital
Assistant Professor of Pediatrics
Harvard Medical School
Boston, Massachusetts

THE TERM "developmental disabilities" describes a group of conditions that are permanent, have a neurodevelopmental basis, and have some effect on functioning ability.[1] Included in this term are a diverse group of diagnostic entities, such as:

- cerebral palsy,
- mental retardation,
- syndromes of multiple congenital anomalies,
- autism and pervasive developmental disorder of childhood,
- epilepsy,
- sensory impairment (deafness and blindness),
- serious learning disabilities, and
- hyperactivity syndrome with attention deficit disorder.

Although these conditions may seem quite specific and even clinically discrete, one characteristic they share is the fact that society has mobilized a variety of resources toward enhancing and optimizing the physical, emotional, and social well-being of children with such disabilities.

The establishment of an etiological diagnosis is an integral part of the clinical assessment of a child with developmental disabilities.[2] For the scientific community, the pursuit of an accurate etiological diagnosis aids the understanding of pathological mechanisms and hence the prevention of specific conditions (eg, congenital infections, perinatal asphyxia, lead toxicity). Knowledge and understanding of etiology also allows for a greater appreciation of the manifestations of each condition when anticipating medical, therapeutic, and educational needs.

The pursuit of an etiological diagnosis is also of importance to a child's parents; it gives them a greater understanding of causality and helps to ease their sense of guilt and blame. Greater understanding of etiology helps parents to adapt to their child's needs and to feel better, stronger, and more confident in an optimal future for their child. A specific etiological diagnosis is also absolutely and indisputably relevant to genetic counseling for the parents, siblings, and other family members who consider childbearing. The pursuit of a firm diagnosis can be an ongoing process. Advances in the clinical and technical aspects of the genetics of developmental disabilities may reveal new diagnostic entities, as has been seen in this last decade with the discovery of the Fragile X syndrome.[3]

Although a clear and unequivocal etiological diagnosis is always desirable, it may be an elusive challenge. With or without a clear diagnosis, it is important to convey to parents an understanding of how the pathology manifests in the func-

Inf Young Children 1990;3(1):25–32
© 1990 Aspen Publishers, Inc.

tional deficits they see or will see in their children. In order to do this, it helps to have a simplified, unifying concept of the diverse group of clinical entities that the term "developmental disabilities" represents.

ETIOLOGICAL SUBSTRATE

At its most basic level, the underlying etiological substrate is the brain or the CNS. Apart from the important basic physiologic functions essential to life, the CNS controls and determines other functions vital to personal and social function. These functions are numerous and extremely complex but, if conceptually simplified, can be more clearly understood.

The functions of the CNS can be viewed as layers of increasing complexity. The most fundamental layer consists of those functions that relate to intact sensory systems (notably, vision and hearing), cognition (the ability to interpret information, store it, and generate an appropriate response), motor (the ability to move in space in response to an external or internal need or stimulus), and socialization (the ability to interact in a meaningful and culturally predictable manner with other individuals in society). The layer at the next level of complexity contains more sophisticated functions, such as those of speech (which involves cognitive, motor, and social components) and learning in a classroom setting (which involves all the above-mentioned components plus a set of age-specific, culturally specific, and group-related expectations).

The concept of etiological substrate holds that if there is something wrong with how the brain works, then the consequence will be manifested in a dysfunction, with a resultant disability. In addition, the dysfunction may result in a specific disability, whether motor, cognitive, or social. There are prototypical clinical conditions for dysfunction in each of these specific areas—the motor disorder that is a consequence of CNS dysfunction is cerebral palsy; the cognitive dysfunction, mental retardation; and the socialization disorder, autism[4] (Fig 1). Not all conditions are clinically pure; it is not unusual for more than one manifestation of CNS dysfunction to be present in any individual, particularly if the CNS dysfunction is severe. Consequently, a child may have CNS dysfunction that manifests in both cerebral palsy and mental retardation, or in both autism and mental retardation. A child may have a list of problems in addition, including epilepsy, visual impairment and hearing impairment.

There is a quantitative as well as a qualitative element in this consideration. The degree of functional impairment is a reflection of the extent of CNS involvement or damage. Children with more severe involvement have the diagnostic labels mentioned above, while children with less severe or even minimal dysfunction have milder manifestations, including perceptual disorders, disorders of motor coordination and planning, or behavioral disorders of activity or attention.

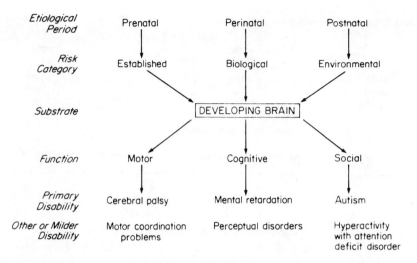

Fig 1. Simplified concept of etiology of developmental disabilities and the derivation of some of the clinical terminology. This construct overlooks the more basic physiologic and sensory functions and the more complex ones of speech and learning.

CAUSES OF CNS DYSFUNCTION

There are three major periods during which one or more CNS functions can be adversely affected by a pathologic alteration in either anatomy or physiology: (1) prenatal (before birth), (2) perinatal (during or around the time of birth), and (3) postnatal (after birth)[4] (Table 1).

Prenatal

The prenatal period can be further subdivided into the preconceptual, periconceptual, embryogenesis, and fetal growth and maturation periods.

Preconceptual

The potential cause of preconceptual disabilities existed before conception took place. Heredity plays a major role, and a genetic mechanism is likely to have been elucidated.[3] Although preconceptual conditions have been studied extensively and are best understood pathophysiologically, they only represent approximately 5% of all causes of developmental disabilities. Preconceptual disabilities can be examined from genetic and pathophysiologic points of view.

Table 1. Causes of developmental disabilities

Onset of dysfunction	Percentage
Preconceptual	5
Prenatal	30
Perinatal	10–15
Postnatal	20–25
Unknown (Presumably prenatal, or at least combined.)	30

Adapted with permission from Crocker AC. The causes of mental retardation. *Pediatr Ann.* 1989;18:623.

Autosomal recessive conditions imply that the gene is carried by both parents, neither of whom has any clinical manifestations. Inborn errors of metabolism in general and phenylketonuria (PKU) in particular are classic examples of this mode of transmission. A double dose of the gene is necessary for the condition to become manifest. A parent who has a single dose of the gene, but does not have the clinical features, is called a "carrier."

Autosomal dominant conditions imply that the gene is carried by one of the parents; the parent does not necessarily manifest any of the neurodevelopmental features. Indications of carrier status in the parent can be detected by subtle clinical signs, as in the case of neurofibromatosis or tuberous sclerosis. These conditions, called "neurocutaneous syndromes," indicate the presence of both neurological and skin manifestations. While the affected parent may have some skin lesions that can be detected only by close scrutiny, the child may have major neurodevelopmental consequences.

Sex-linked conditions imply that the gene is carried on the X chromosome. As in autosomal recessive conditions, the presence of the gene on only one of two X chromosomes (ie, in females) constitutes carrier status and causes no or minor manifestations. Males who have the gene have the potential for full manifestation of the condition, as the gene on the single X chromosome is unsuppressed by the small Y chromosome. The most common example is the Fragile X syndrome, a condition characterized by a constellation of physical features (notably, large testes in the adult) and a fragile site on the X chromosome detectable under specific laboratory conditions.

Translocation of chromosomal material can be present in asymptomatic parents when the total chromosomal complement is balanced. In the offspring, however, the chromosomal complement will be unbalanced, with a little extra or a little missing. Translocation in the 21st chromosome results in Down syndrome in approximately 5% of all populations.

Periconceptual

Conditions that arise at the time of conception relate mostly to chromosome number, usually as a result of abnormalities in cell division. The most common example in this category is the extra chromosome 21 in Down syndrome, which confers on the child characteristic physical features, clinical features, and developmental patterns.

Embryogenesis

During embryogenesis, a variety of factors can influence organ development and result in syndromes of multiple congenital anomalies, including abnormalities in brain development.[5,6] The nature and extent of the abnormalities relate to some polygenic elements as well as some external factors and the timing of the insult. For example, myelodysplasia (spina bifida) is an abnormality in CNS development that occurs at the time of closure of the spinal cord. Familial associations suggest a polygenic element operating as well as possible environmental factors that increase the likelihood of occurrence. In contrast, agenesis of the corpus callosum is a condition that arises earlier in embryonic life when the brain is in the process of dividing into two hemispheres. Myelodysplasia can be readily clinically identified, and agenesis of the corpus callosum can be diagnosed by computed tomography.

Probably the most common abnormality in CNS development arises after brain and spinal cord development is complete, when the neurons migrate from their original periventricular position to their eventual destination in precise layers of the cerebral cortex. Abnormalities in neuronal migration have been described in experimental animals as well as in autopsy material in a variety of clinical situations. There may be adverse influences (eg, alcohol) during early pregnancy or other nonspecific but diagnostic clinical syndromes, especially mental retardation.[6,7] Specific abnormalities in cell size, number, and position have been described in association with infantile autism.[8]

Fetal growth and maturation

During fetal growth and maturation, various factors can adversely affect CNS structure and function. Intrauterine infections, most notably congenital rubella, but also toxoplasmosis, cytomegalovirus, and herpes, can have serious damaging effects each with characteristic diagnostic features.[6]

Physical or chemical agents such as alcohol and certain medications (eg, Dilantin or phenytoin) can result in specific diagnostic syndromes (ie, fetal alcohol syndrome and fetal dilantin syndrome).[5] Intrauterine exposure to narcotics and other nonmedicinal drugs, usually in combination, with or without cigarette smoking, can seriously affect fetal growth and development with permanent CNS consequences. Cigarette smoking by itself is also associated with significant morbidity and even mortality.

Maternal illness can affect the fetus metabolically, most dramatically in the case of diabetes. Preeclampsia, a common disorder, can indirectly affect fetal well-being by impairing placental function. A diseased or damaged placenta (eg, from infarctions) will not adequately support the growing fetus; although this condition may not necessarily cause CNS damage directly, it may well render the fetus more vulnerable to stresses such as hypoxia or hypoglycemia during or immediately after birth. This pathologic situation may also increase the likelihood of premature birth.[9]

Clinical syndromes with diagnosable prenatal etiology affect approximately 30% of all children with developmental disabilities, while in an additional 30%, unknown factors with at the least some prenatal elements are felt to be etiologically responsible. Thus, the causal origins of two thirds of developmental disabilities occurred before the children were born.[2]

Perinatal

Hypoxic-ischemic encephalopathy

Over the last 50 years there has been a dramatic shift in the world of newborn medicine, changing the perspective on etiology of developmental disabilities.[10] Fifty years ago perinatal trauma and asphyxia neonatorum in full-term infants were the more common causes of clinical conditions such as cerebral palsy. Advances in prenatal care and obstetric management of fetal well-being and of the delivery itself have successfully reduced the risk of hypoxic-ischemic injury to full-term healthy infants, thus preventing permanent CNS consequences.[11] Although CNS damage as a result of hypoxic-ischemic injury does still occur, it represents only a small number of all causes.[9]

Prematurity

The advances in neonatal intensive care for smaller and smaller infants over the same period has resulted in survival of ever-smaller premature infants who are born alive.[4,11] Most children whose developmental disabilities have their origins in the perinatal period were born prematurely. The vulnerability of the premature (especially the extremely premature) infant lies in the immaturity of its organ systems, most significantly pulmonary. Respiratory distress syndrome (RDS), also known as hyaline membrane disease, adversely affects metabolic and hemodynamic factors that ultimately determine the nature and degree of CNS damage.

Although hypoxic-ischemic CNS injury is probably responsible for most of the long-term consequences in this group, the presence and extent of intraventricular

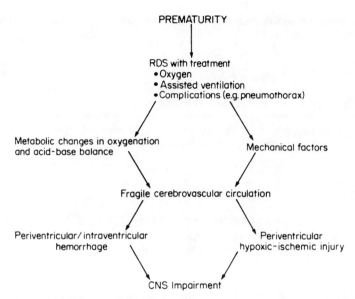

Fig 2. Schema of pathway to CNS injury in premature infants who have respiratory distress syndrome.

hemorrhage is now used as the index of risk (Fig 2).[12] Advances in radiologic studies of intracranial phenomenology in the newborn infant, at first with computed tomography and subsequently with ultrasound, have allowed professionals to examine the significance of the size and extent of intraventricular hemorrhages as well as associated factors such as ventricular dilatation, with or without hydrocephalus. While exact predictions cannot be made, prematurity is associated with an increased risk for developmental disabilities. The more complications there are, and the greater the extent of the intraventricular hemorrhage, the greater the likelihood of developmental disabilities (Table 2).

The vulnerability of premature infants in their growth and development is exacerbated by adverse socioeconomic circumstances. Conversely, an infant who has been rendered vulnerable by premature birth will benefit from a positive home environment and parental support through early intervention programs.

Other perinatal problems can cause CNS damage and associated consequences, including metabolic disorders, such as hypoglycemia, hyperbilirubinemia, or hypothermia, and infections, most importantly meningitis. This group is small and diverse. In all, perinatal etiologies are behind only about 10% to 15% of developmental disabilities.

Table 2. Grading of periventricular/intraventricular hemorrhage and risk of CNS injury with developmental consequences.

Grade of hemorrhage	Risk of CNS injury
Grade I (small): Isolated germinal matrix hemorrhage	
Grade II (small): Intraventricular hemorrhage with normal ventricular size	Low
Grade III (moderate): Intraventricular hemorrhage with ventricular dilation	Moderate
Grade IV (severe): Intraventricular with parenchymal hemorrhage	High

Postnatal

Postnatal etiologies account for approximately 20% to 25% of developmental disabilities. There are four major categories (1) CNS infections, (2) accidents, (3) lead toxicity, and (4) psychosocial vulnerability.

CNS Infections

Meningitis, encephalitis, and bacterial, viral, or other organisms constitute a decreasing number of etiologies since the use of antibiotics has improved. Tuberculosis, meningitis, and measles encephalitis are still problems in third-world countries.

Accidents

Head injury from motor vehicle accidents has been reduced since parents have been required to firmly secure infants traveling in cars in appropriate seats with seat belts. Head injury also results from child abuse (eg, shaken baby syndrome). Accidental ingestion of poisons or other toxins; cardiorespiratory arrests, either spontaneous or associated with serious illnesses; and near-drowning can produce permanent CNS damage. Accidents cause the most severe developmental consequences for children.

Lead toxicity

Lead toxicity is associated with significant encephalopathy. Even after effective treatment and complete elimination of circulating lead in the blood, permanent CNS damage may remain. Chronic exposure to lead even at subclinical levels produces temporary and very likely some permanent impairment of CNS function.[13] Lead toxicity is a significant public health concern; legislation has been necessary to reduce the risk of exposure from leaded gasoline and leaded paint. Unfortunately, inner-city children living under low socioeconomic circumstances, who are already at risk for developmental disabilities, are also at greatest risk for lead exposure.

Psychosocial vulnerability

Children who are physically and emotionally deprived suffer neurodevelopmentally and have major problems in adapting to society. Children living in poverty constitute the largest group at risk for developmental disabilities with postnatal etiologies.[4,9,14,15] Children in low socioeconomic circumstances suffer the damaging effects of poverty at different developmental stages in different ways, and the effects are very likely cumulative.

Teenage pregnancy, inadequate prenatal care, and substance abuse increase the risk of intrauterine stresses and premature birth. The increased vulnerability of the premature infant to medical complications and CNS sequelae prevents bonding between mother and infant; the infant's responses are reduced, and the infant may require a long stay in the neonatal intensive care unit before being released from the hospital. Once at home, mother and infant continue to require support. Society has not met the obligation to ensure that each infant has community resources to supplement what the family cannot provide. The risk for cognitive, educational, and social dysfunction is therefore compounded for infants born into low socioeconomic conditions, and the chances are great that once these infants reach childbearing age, they will repeat the cycle (Fig 3).

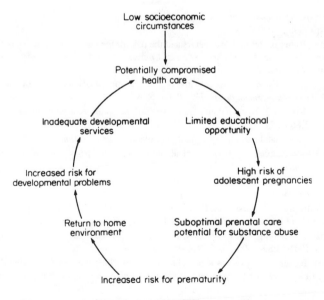

Fig 3. Vicious circle of poverty and the morbidity of prematurity.

Publicly funded resources are inadequate for infants and their families who are psychosocially vulnerable. The single greatest impact on prevention of developmental disabilities could be achieved by developing services that provide optimal educational and social programs to this population, ultimately benefitting the society as a whole.

•   •   •

The conceptual understanding of developmental disabilities is important in determining etiology. Once etiology is understood, infant care professionals can identify the causes of developmental disabilities and implement an approach that optimizes outcomes for this generation and prevents developmental disabilities in future generations.

REFERENCES

1. Crocker AC. The spectrum of medical care for developmental disabilities. In: Rubin IL, Crocker AC, eds. *Developmental Disabilities: Delivery of Medical Care for Children and Adults.* Philadelphia, Pa: Lea & Febiger; 1989.
2. Crocker AC. The causes of mental retardation. *Pediatr Ann.* 1989;18:623–629.
3. Meryash DL. The genetic approach. In: Rubin IL, Crocker AC, eds. *Developmental Disabilities: Delivery of Medical Care for Children and Adults.* Philadelphia, Pa: Lea & Febiger; 1989.
4. Rubin IL. Infant follow up, tracking, and screening. In: Rubin IL, Crocker AC, eds. *Developmental Disabilities: Delivery of Medical Care for Children and Adults.* Philadelphia, Pa: Lea & Febiger; 1989.
5. Jones KL. *Smith's Recognizable Patterns of Human Malformation.* 4th ed. Philadelphia, Pa: W.B. Saunders; 1988.
6. Golden NL, Rubin IL. Intrauterine factors and the risk for the development of cerebral palsy. In: Thompson GH, Rubin IL, Bilenker RM, eds. *Comprehensive Management of Cerebral Palsy.* New York, NY: Grune & Stratton; 1983.
7. Banker BQ, Bruce-Gregorios J. Neuropathology. In: Thompson GH, Rubin IL, Bilenker RM, eds. *Comprehensive Management of Cerebral Palsy.* New York, NY: Grune & Stratton; 1983.
8. Bauman M, Kemper T. Histoanatomic observation of the brain in early infantile autism. *Neurology.* 1985;35:866–874.
9. Rubin IL. The perinatal period: Antecedents and sequelae. *Pediatr Ann.* 1989;18:653–661.
10. O'Reilly DE, Walentynowicz JE. Etiological factors in cerebral palsy: An historical review. *Dev Med Child Neurol.* 1981;23:633–642.
11. Rubin IL. Perinatal factors. In: Thompson GH, Rubin IL, Bilenker RM, eds. *Comprehensive Management of Cerebral Palsy.* New York, NY: Grune & Stratton; 1983.
12. Papile LA, Burnstein J, Burstein R, Coffler H. Incidence and evolution of subependymal hemorrhage: A study of infants with birth weight of less than 1,500 gms. *J Pediatr.* 1978;92:529–534.
13. Needleman HL, Bellinger D, Leviaton A. Does lead at low dose affect intelligence in children? *Pediatrics.* 1981;68:894–896.
14. Moser HW. Prevention of psychosocial mental retardation. In: Thompson GH, Rubin IL, Bilenker RM, eds. *Comprehensive Management of Cerebral Palsy.* New York, NY: Grune & Stratton; 1983.
15. Wise PH, Kotelchuck M, Wilson ML, Mills M. Racial and socioeconomic disparities in childhood mortality in Boston. *N Eng J Med.* 1985; 313:360–366.

Medical problems in infants and young children with Down syndrome: Implications for early services

Don C. Van Dyke, MD
University Hospital School
Division of Developmental
  Disabilities
Department of Pediatrics
The University of Iowa Hospitals and
  Clinics
Iowa City, Iowa

DOWN SYNDROME (DS) occurs in approximately one in 1,000 births in the United States.[1] It is one of the major presenting diagnoses in both genetics and developmental clinics.[1-5] The medical problems of DS are multiple and have a significant effect on the provision of clinical care, on the family's management of stress, and on the level of participation and benefit from both educational and developmental programs.[4] Early identification and integration of the multiple medical problems of the DS infant and child will lead to more sophisticated care and a greater understanding of the problems that are associated with DS.

This article will discuss areas of common medical concern in the DS infant and child, including heart disease, gastrointestinal (GI) tract problems, endocrine dysfunction, genitourinary (GU) abnormalities, leukemia and cancer, infection, skin problems, eye problems, ear, nose, and throat (ENT) problems, dental problems, neurologic/developmental concerns, feeding problems, and musculoskeletal problems. Subsequent sections deal with the medical problems of DS and its impact on care and delivery of services. In addition, some of the alternative and controversial therapies that have been proposed for the treatment of DS will be discussed.

MEDICAL PROBLEMS IN DS

Heart disease

The prevalence of congenital heart disease in the DS population is approximately 35% to 40%.[3,4] Some of these individuals have single defects, while others have multiple cardiac defects.[3,4] The most common are septal defects, such as ventricular septal defects (hole between the bottom two chambers of the heart), atrial septal defects (hole between the top two chambers of the heart), and endocardial cushion defects (connections between the top and the bottom chambers of the heart).[6,7] Many other congenital heart malformations are also seen in infants and young children with DS.[4,7-9] Congenital cardiac abnormalities may and often do present in the newborn period. The most common presentation is the presence of a heart murmur on initial newborn examination; however, the presence of increased

The author acknowledges MJ Soucek, BGS, SS Eberly, MA, and ML Wolraich, MD.

Inf Young Children 1989;1(3):39–50

pulmonary resistance or another protective lesion may not make the initial presentation obvious. The absence of a murmur does not rule out the presence of congenital heart disease in the DS infant. As a result most institutions recommend baseline studies in the newborn nursery prior to discharge of infants with DS. Normally a high percentage of septal defects such as ventricular septal defects (VSDs) close spontaneously, and the patients can be discharged from routine follow-up. However, the VSD in DS is often different from that seen in non-DS children, and a large percentage of these children will need serial echocardiograms, Doppler studies, and cardiac catheterization to fully document their specific cardiac lesions to provide optimal clinical management.[6,9,10] Prevention of subacute bacterial endocarditis (infection of the heart) is an issue that must always be addressed with the DS child who has congenital heart disease. Parents and caregivers must understand recommendations for prophylaxis prior to any dental or surgical procedures. In short, infants and young children with DS and heart disease need to be on antibiotics prior to any dental, surgical, or invasive procedure that would allow bacteria to be released into the blood and possibly to travel to the heart.

It is important to understand the medical recommendations for an infant with congenital heart disease who is participating in a developmental or educational program. Some of these children tire easily, are difficult feeders, and do not tolerate temperature changes. Any child who has a sudden change in feeding, an increased lethargy, a change in skin coloration, and a poor growth needs to be seen by his or her primary care medical provider.

Congenital abnormalities of the GI tract

Congenital abnormalities of the GI tract have been noted with increased incidence in children with DS. The most common of these are aganglionic megacolon (lack of appropriate neural innervation), small-bowel obstruction due to either an annular pancreas or small-bowel malformation, and esophageal malformation.[3,11-13] Thus any child who presents in the newborn period with recurrent episodes of vomiting or other signs of GI tract obstruction needs immediate evaluation. The presence of pneumonia in the newborn period must raise suspicions of esophageal abnormalities or tracheoesophageal fistula (a connection between the trachea and esophagus). Obviously the physical examination of the DS newborn should be detailed enough to rule out the possibility of any rectal abnormalities. Ongoing clinical management of chronic constipation is likely to be required. Because of variations in autonomic patterns, constipation can be a severe problem, and because of the increased incidence of abnormal neural innervation associated with DS, a few of the more severe constipation problems require more detailed diagnostic studies to rule out this possibility.[11,12]

GU abnormalities

The most common GU abnormalities reported in the literature are small penis and undescended testes.[3,13] More recently, however, investigators report that the frequency of an undescended testis in males with DS is actually not different than that of the general population.[14] In the male with DS, penile length and testicular volume have been shown to be below the norm, and males with DS are sterile.[3,13,14] It is felt that this is secondary to primary gonadal deficiency and is progressive from birth to adolescence.[14] The specific etiology of sterility, however, is unknown.

Recent studies have reported DS individuals with an abnormal position of the urethral orifice. In a study by Lang et al,[15] 12% of males (or a 40-fold increase) were noted to have a double urethral orifice. One urethral opening led to a blind pouch. Diagnostic studies in these patients did not demonstrate any anatomic abnormalities of the bladder, urethra, ureter, or kidneys.[15]

Endocrine dysfunction

In DS individuals the incidence of thyroid dysfunction increases with age.[16,17] Most of the studies report the incidence of low thyroid function as being from 15% to 20%.[16] However, congenital low-thyroid function may be present at birth.[16] Since many of the physical characteristics of low thyroid function are also associated with DS, thyroid function studies must be done as part of the initial evaluation of all DS infants. Follow-up assessments of thyroid functions are also needed because physical and clinical symptoms are rarely helpful in identifying those individuals developing low thyroid function.

Leukemia

The coincidence of DS and leukemia was first reported by Brewster and Cannon[18] in 1930. In 1956 Krivit and Good[19] proposed that DS children might be at increased risk for acute leukemia. Epidemiologic studies now place the frequency of acute leukemia in DS at 10 to 20 times that expected on the basis of chance alone.[20] Compounding the difficulty of detecting congenital leukemia among newborns with DS is the occurrence of a transient white cell reaction or leukemia-like picture in infants with DS.[21,22] In addition, it has been shown that infants with DS are approximately 19 times as likely to develop elevated red cell counts as are infants without DS.[22]

In a ten-year study by the Child Cancer Study Group, 2.1% of the subjects were children with DS.[23] Of these children with DS, 95% had acute lymphocytic leukemia (ALL), confirming that ALL is the most common form of leukemia in children with DS.[23] Children with DS who have lymphocytic leukemia seem to differ dramatically from children without DS in their remission/induction rates. DS children with leukemia are far more likely to die, usually from infection during the initial phase of chemotherapy.[24] If the DS child survives this initial phase of treatment, however, there appears to be a lower rate of relapse among DS children with ALL than among non-DS children with ALL. Bone marrow transplantation has recently been used in children with DS. In a case report by Rubin et al[25] of four cases of children with DS and acute leukemia treated with bone marrow transplantation, three died posttransplantation from infections and their complications. The investigators concluded that DS individuals were at higher risk for toxicity, pneumonia, and mortality associated with this type of therapy.[25] However, the study was small, and further evaluation is needed. In addition, children with DS who have ALL have poor tolerance to anticancer drugs.[26] The metabolism of anticancer drugs such as methotrexate differs in children with DS and in non-DS children. Children with DS show a lower average of drug clearance and a greater incidence of toxicity.[26] Thus the treatment of ALL in the patient with DS poses a challenge, not only because of lower rates of remission and increased incidence of infection but also because of poor tolerance to conventional doses of anticancer drugs.

Other cancers have also been reported to occur with higher-than-normal frequency in patients with DS.[27] Some investigators have reported a possible association between DS and testicular cancer, while others have suggested an association with malignant tumors of the eye.[28,29]

Infection

Investigations of individuals with DS have shown a number of immune problems.[30,31] Abnormalities of cellular and humoral function have been described, including poor lymphocyte proliferation, undefined T-cell defects, and alterations of interferon-receptor function.[30-33] The clinical findings and presentation in children with DS have been inconsistent.[30,34] These inconsistencies have been variously attributed to such factors as age, variability between subjects and controls, and exposure to frequent infections in group living circumstances found in institutions.

Frequent, repeated, and chronic respiratory infection has commonly been reported in children with DS.[34,35] In one study 40% of DS patients had chronic nasal drainage on examination.[36] Otitis media is also highly prevalent among children with DS. A study by Schwartz and Schwartz[37] of institutionalized children with DS found that 50% had at least a unilateral middle-ear effusion. In a study by Samuelson and Nugyen[38] of 138 DS patients, 39 had ear disease, with 63% having middle ear effusion. There is a high frequency of hepatitis B carriers in the DS population.[39,40] Other infections, such as skin infections and fungal infections, also occur at a high frequency. Thus persons with DS should probably be considered immunocompromised, with a higher susceptibility to infections and a higher mortality rate from infectious disease than non-DS persons. Their compromised immune systems may also place them at a higher risk for malignancies (as discussed earlier) and autoimmune types of problems, such as those associated with thyroid antibodies.

The management of the DS child in a day-care situation may present additional problems because of the increased risk of infections. An infection in the DS infant and child should not be treated as "just another respiratory infection." The DS child with infections such as those affecting the upper respiratory tract should, at the very least, have been discussed by the parent with the child's primary care medical provider. The increased incidence of hepatitis B carriers among older children with DS may present an increased concern for staff members caring for these individuals.[39,40] Good hand-washing technique, proper facilities, and good technique for changing diapers are always a necessity.

Skin problems

Children with DS may commonly present with severely dry skin. Some skin problems may be due to an increased sensitivity to environmental factors, while others are secondary to a greater susceptibility to skin infection. In a few instances dry skin may be secondary to thyroid dysfunction, so the presence of severely dry skin should always raise questions regarding thyroid status. If there is no specific etiology (ie, infection or thyroid dysfunction), this dermatologic problem usually responds to moisturizing products such as Eucerin. However, a few DS patients require further evaluation by a dermatologist for more aggressive dermatologic intervention.

Eye problems

A number of visual, ocular, and orbital problems appear in DS individuals.[41,42] The most noticeable are the variations in orbital size, abnormal position of palpebral fissures, and the presence of epicanthal folds and conjunctival inflammation.[41,42] Lens opacities are common, but should not be confused with the two to three percent occurrence of cataracts in children with DS.[43] The frequent occurrence of abnormal eye movements and jerking of the eyes (nystagmus) have been well documented in DS individuals.[43-45] These may be of neuromuscular origin, or they may be due to significant visual error.[45] Jerky eye movements are common in the DS population, especially in children under 3 years of age. Ophthalmologic examination in this patient population has demonstrated optic nerve underdevelopment and significant refractive error.[44] Refractive error may be due to astigmatism, nearsightedness, or farsightedness. Abnormal eye movements are a fairly common clinical finding, usually manifested as in-turning of the eye and occasionally as out-turning of the eye.[45] Because of the many eye findings and the importance of vision in all educational and developmental programs, DS children should have a baseline eye examination early in life to verify the normality of their vision and to determine if appropriate ophthalmologic intervention is required.

ENT

Children with DS present with significant ENT problems, particularly recurrent ear infections, chronic sinusitis, chronic discharge from the nose, and ear wax impaction. Hearing problems are common, and congenital anomalies of the palate, midface, and external auditory canal are frequently reported.

Palates in DS adults appear to be appreciably smaller in all dimensions than those of adults without DS, but they are usually not high arched.[46] Clefts of the palate occur with a greater frequency in DS, with a reported frequency of cleft palate of 4.6% (0.4% in the general population) and of submucous cleft of 0.78%.[47]

Sinusitis with chronic nasal drainage was a frequent finding in one study by Strome[36]; 40% of DS individuals in this study had chronic nasal discharge. Treatment with antibiotics was usually satisfactory. Sleep apnea has been documented in the DS population; consequently DS children with abnormal sleep patterns, significant facial features of DS, and obesity should be considered for a sleep study.[48]

The external auditory canals of DS individuals are small, with an increased incidence of canal narrowing.[36] In addition, middle ear abnormalities have been noted and are an important cause of sensorineural hearing loss.[49,50] The smallness of the ear canal is what has led to greater difficulty in dealing with the increased incidence of excessive accumulation of ear wax. A study by Dahle and McCollister[51] found impaction of ear wax to a significant degree to be a frequent medical problem, with the hearing losses due to ear wax impaction averaging 24 dB.

Otitis media is highly prevalent. In one study of institutionalized DS individuals the frequency ranged between 40% and 80%.[37,38] In a survey of 106 DS children, bilateral hearing loss was noted in 68%, with 78% having a hearing loss in one or both ears.[36,50] In some DS individuals, myringotomies and tubes provide relief of serous otitis media. Despite this surgical procedure, however, some DS individuals have been noted to have recurrences.[52]

The hearing problems and related speech problems of DS children must be treated aggressively. Initial medical management is indicated, and in some cases long-term medical management and prophylactic antibiotics are required. Some children need surgical intervention with myringotomies and tubes.[52] Some investigators feel that any language delay in DS children should be promptly treated as part of a generalized developmental/educational program with a home language-stimulation program; in more severe cases amplification through use of a hearing aid should be considered.[52] Estimates of hearing loss have ranged between 40% and 77%, with most hearing losses being conductive.[53,54]

Dental problems

Dental problems, particularly inflammation of the gums, are widespread in the DS population.[55] Gum inflammation may be so prevalent that it progresses to bone loss, tooth mobility, and eventual tooth loss.[55] The most common teeth affected in this manner are the lower incisors, upper incisors, and upper and lower first permanent molars, in that order. Clinical studies have shown that the bacteria of the dental plaque are the primary agent of gum disease and that gum disease begins at an early age in the DS child.[55,56] The specific reason for this is unknown, and there may be a variety of factors, such as differences in salivary composition and in salivary pH and in the structure of the teeth in the DS child.

The teeth of the DS child are also different from those of the non-DS child. The child with DS is best characterized by over-retained primary teeth, unerupted primary teeth, missing teeth, and anomalies in tooth size, shape, and enamel.[13] In most cases the primitive teeth display true, generalized, small size. DS individuals demonstrate large deviations in contact relationships and a number of different malocclusions, the most characteristic being mesioclusion, open bite, and posterior crossbite.[56–58]

Oral hygiene in the DS individual must be aggressive. The child with DS should undergo dental evaluation early and probably at more frequent intervals than are usually recommended for the non-DS child, particularly if gum inflammation is developing. The presence of malocclusion may necessitate early pediatric dentistry or orthodontic intervention.

Neurologic/developmental concerns

Although seizures have been documented in the DS population, their frequency is no higher than it is for seizures found in the general population.[13] The most common type of seizures experienced are infantile spasms, a generalized motor-type seizure.

Children with DS demonstrate a wide variation in mental and motor development, with a range of attainment of developmental milestones. Research has indicated that motor skill development follows a normal but slower sequential pattern of progression.[59–61] Infants with DS follow the normal content and sequence of progression in gross motor activities, the difference being that they are slower in reaching milestones. Many factors affect their rates of motor development, the most frequent being hypotonia or other neurologic deficits. Other problems that have significant impact are the increased extensibility of the joints and the complications of congenital heart disease.[60]

Cognitive development in children with DS is characterized by some level of mental retardation, usually in the mild-to-moderate range.[60] The rate of development is definitely slower and possibly different from that in children who do not have DS, but the linearity of the rate of mental development with DS is still not clear. Some authors have found a linear relationship, while others have found a deceleration between 10 months and 2 years of age.[59,60] Most investigators agree that the mental developmental profile in children with DS is different from that of normal children and may even be different from that of other children with similar degrees of cognitive deficits.[60-64]

Feeding problems

Studies of feeding patterns have supported the idea that normal development follows a systematic timetable. In children with DS this sequence of development may be delayed. Multiple craniofacial skeletal differences in the DS individual may have significant impact on feeding skills. These physical anomalies are primarily the short palate, underdevelopment of the maxilla, and abnormal tongue size. Generalized facial and oral hypotonia may also contribute to poor lip closure, poor sucking ability, poor tongue control, and difficulties with jaw stability. In a study by Pipes and Holm,[65] 80% of children with DS had difficulties related to food or feeding. A study by Calvert et al[66] identified feeding problems that included difficulties using eating utensils, eating meat or chewing foods, drinking from a cup, sucking, and regurgitating. Children with moderate or severe heart defects were more often delayed in chewing or feeding than those children with mild heart defects.[67]

Although eating problems are common in DS children, they are usually minor, and by adulthood most DS individuals are independent in feeding. The most common oral problems have been slight oral hypotonia, tongue thrust, difficulties in chewing, poor lip closure, and choking or gagging on foods. The success of feeding programs are an important part of development programs for DS individuals. These programs are in part responsible for a large number of DS individuals becoming independent in feeding and having only minor, although frequent, feeding problems.

Musculoskeletal problems

Most orthopedic problems in the DS population are acquired, resulting from increased joint extensibility due to soft-tissue laxity and muscle hypotonia. Some investigators[68] estimate that approximately 26% of the DS population has one or more orthopedic deformities.

The orthopedic problem that is receiving the most attention recently is atlantoaxial subluxation, which is instability of the space between the first two cervical vertebrae, sometimes resulting in high spinal-cord compression.[69] Other reported orthopedic anomalies are scoliosis (curvature of the spine), spondylolisthesis (instability of the lower lumbar vertebrae), spina bifida occulta (nonfusion of the back of one of the lumbar vertebrae), slipped capital femoral epiphysis (movement of the growth center at the head of the femur), recurrent patella (knee cap) dislocation with chondromalacia (degenerative changes of the cartilage), flat feet, and a number of forefoot deformities (primarily absent longitudinal arch), and calcaneovalgus (abnormal position of the foot) deformities.[68-71]

Several investigators have documented evidence of foot deformities in DS individuals.[68,71,72] Surgical intervention has been described, but only recently has there been interest in orthotic management of these types of deformities. The flat foot is felt to be universal in individuals with DS.[71] Calcaneovalgus deformities are another common finding that may affect ambulation and motor development.

Scoliosis may occur in up to 50% of individuals with DS.[70] Curves are usually 20% or less and are equally distributed between a left and right thoracic curve. Spinal curves appear to be related to soft-tissue insufficiency; they are rarely progressive, and bracing is seldom required.[70]

Arthropathies (inflammation of the joints) have been reported in children with DS. In a study by Yancey et al,[73] the prevalence figure of arthritis in the DS population was approximately 1.2%, or 1,200 per 100,000 children. This prevalence is much higher than that of juvenile rheumatoid arthritis (JRA) in the general population, which has been suggested to be approximately 0.2 to 1 per 1,000 children.[74] Of significant clinical importance in children with the arthropathy of DS is the relationship of the arthropathy to the involvement of the cervical spine. Since a C1-2 subluxation is well documented in both DS and JRA, this complication should be carefully evaluated in children who have a combination of DS and arthritis.[69,75-78]

Atlantoaxial instability has been a relatively frequent finding in DS, with a reported incidence of between 10% and 20%.[69,79] Although the number of individuals having C1-2 instability is significant, the number who are symptomatic and require surgery is small (1% to 2%).[79] A recent bulletin of the Special Olympics requiring cervical spine radiographs of all participating children with DS has raised several questions.[80] However, more than 85% of individuals with DS show no evidence of C1-2 instability and can participate in all physical education and sports activities. For the 10% to 15% with asymptomatic C1-2 instability, special precautions need to be taken and follow-up provided.[79] There appear to be some differences of opinion between the American Academy of Pediatrics Committee on Sports Medicine and the Special Olympics, the latter having a restrictive recommendation that prohibits individuals with DS and C1-2 instability from training or participation in gymnastics, butterfly (strokes in swimming), diving, high jump, decathlon, soccer, and warming-up exercises that put pressure on the head and neck muscles.[80]

ALTERNATIVE AND CONTROVERSIAL THERAPIES

Some alternative therapies that are offered to the parents of children with DS are considered controversial. These therapies are often based on the use of dietary supplements, physical therapy, or injections of various materials. The therapies have included thyroid hormone therapy, dimethyl sulfoxide therapy (DMSO), cell therapy (sicca cell therapy), orthomolecular therapy (a form of vitamin therapy), and the administration of a large number of vitamins and other substances, including glutamic acid, DMSO, vitamin B_6, and serotonin (Table 1). Two areas that have generated significant interest and controversy are cell therapy, initiated by Dr. Paul Nehan in the 1930s, and megavitamin therapy.

Cell therapy involves injection of freeze-dried cells from the organs of fetal sheep, cows, and rabbits. The unproven theory is that these cells become the nucleus for tissue regeneration. The success claimed for cell therapy is based on the assumption that there is an affinity between the cells of a particular organ for the embryonic donor and the corresponding organ of the child. This has never been proven. Programs, as postulated by Schmid,[81,82] have consisted not only of

Table 1. Alternative therapies in Down syndrome

Therapy	Researcher	Year of study
Cell therapy	Schmid	1983
B_6, 5-hydroxytryptophan	Pueschel, Reed, Cronk, et al.	1980
Serotonin	Coleman	1973
Megavitamin	Harrell, Capp, Davis, et al	1981
	Turkel	1975
Thyroid	Benda	1960
DMSO	Aspillage, Morizon, Vendano	1975
Patterning		
Dehydroepiandrosterone	De Moragas	1958
Craniofacial surgery	Holher	1978
	Rozner	
	Feurstein	1983

cell therapy injections but of speech therapy, sound framing, physical therapy, vitamin preparations, minerals, tryptophan, and other teaching measures. Investigators, both in this country and in Germany, have not found any significant difference between the experimental group (ie, those receiving cell therapy) and a control group.[83,84]

Orthomolecular therapy is the use of various combinations of vitamins, minerals, enzymes, and hormones. Turkel[85] has postulated that these combinations are important for the treatment of the mental disorder because they provide an optimal molecular environment for the mind, especially optimum concentrations of substances normally found in the human body. Since 1940 Turkel[86] has been confirmed the proponent of the U-series as a means of ameliorating the condition of DS. Harrell et al[87] stimulated recent interest in vitamin therapy when preliminary reports showed children with DS improving in growth and cognitive development from megavitamin and mineral therapy. Later replication of Harrell's work did not support these preliminary results.[88] Thus while families of DS individuals may be more vulnerable and more amenable to embracing unorthodox or unproven approaches to treatment and management of DS, there continues to be no scientific support for megavitamin therapy in DS.

There is no scientific evidence or support for such therapies as orthomolecular therapy, cell therapy, thyroid supplement, and a long list of vitamins and other supplemental therapies. However, other areas, such as plastic surgery, continue to be an area of active investigation and discussion.[89–91]

Recent results from plastic surgery include more attractive appearance, improved speech, and less drooling.[90] Preliminary studies reported in 1987 demonstrate that craniofacial surgical procedures appear to have no effect on the auditory quality of speech, with minimal improvement in chewing and biting. Some DS children had less mouth breathing, others had decreased upper respiratory infections, and there were no significant changes in IQ.[92] Long-term studies are now in progress.

• • •

If there are to be early services for infants and young children with DS, all professionals must understand and recognize the common medical problems of the DS infant and child and the problems for their families. There will be increasing pressure from medical and parent groups and increasing resistance from third party payers to cover the provision of early preventive health care for children with DS and other developmental and disabling disorders. With improved education and communication, perhaps medical problems and needs can be identified early, and efforts can be directed toward mobilizing resources to maximize the potential for individuals with DS.

REFERENCES

1. Adams MM, Erickson JD, Layde PM, et al: Down's syndrome: Recent trends in the United States. *JAMA* 1981;246(7):758–760.

2. Penrose LS, Smith GF: *Down's Anomaly.* London, J and A Churchill Ltd, 1966.

3. De La Cruz FF, Gerald PS (eds): *Trisomy 21 (Down Syndrome) Research Perspective.* Baltimore, University Park Press, 1981.

4. Smith DW: *Recognizable Patterns of Human Malformations.* Philadelphia, Saunders, 1982.

5. Pueschel SM: The child with Down syndrome, in Levine MD, Carey WB, Crocker AC, et al (eds): *Developmental-Behavioral Pediatrics.* Philadelphia, Saunders, 1983, pp 353–362.

6. Buckley LP: Cardiac assessments, in Pueschel SM (ed): *The Young Child with Down Syndrome.* New York, Human Sciences Press, 1984, pp 351–361.

7. Rowe RD: Cardiac malformation in mongolism. *Am Heart J* 1962;64:567–569.

8. Rowe RD, Uchida IA: Cardiac malformation in mongolism: A prospective study of 104 mongoloid children. *Am J Med* 1961;31:726–735.

9. Park SC, Matthews RA, Zuberbuhler B Jr, et al: Down syndrome with congenital heart disease. *Am J Dis Child* 1977;131:29–33.

10. Greenwood RD, Nadas AS: The clinical course of cardiac disease in Down syndrome. *Pediatrics* 1976;58(6):893–897.

11. Knox GE, Bensel RW: Gastrointestinal malformations in Down's syndrome. *Minn Med* 1972;55(6):542–549.

12. Kilcoyne RF, Taybi H: Conditions associated with congenital megacolon. *Am J Roentgenol* 1970;108:615–620.

13. Smith FR, Berg JM: *Downs Anomaly.* New York, Churchill Livingston, 1976.

14. Hsiang YH, Berkovitz GD, Bland GL, et al: Gonadal function in patients with Down syndrome. *Am J Med Gen* 1987;27:449–458.

15. Lang DJ, Van Dyke DC, Heide F, et al: Hypospadias, and urethral abnormalities in Down syndrome. *Clin Pediatr* 1987;26(1):40–42.

16. Pueschel SM, Pezulo JC: Thyroid dysfunction in Down syndrome. *Am J Dis Child* 1985;139(6):636–639.

17. Fort P, Lifschitz F, Bellisario R, et al: Abnormalities of thyroid function in infants with Down syndrome. *J Pediatr* 1984;104(4):545–549.

18. Brewster HF, Cannon HE: Acute lymphocytic leukemia: Report of a case of an eleven-month old monogolian idiot. *New Orleans Med Soc J* 1930;82:872–875.

19. Krivit W, Good RA: Simultaneous occurrence of leukemia and mongolism: Report of four cases. *Am J Dis Child* 1956;91:218–222.

20. Miller RW: Childhood cancer and congenital defects: A study of US birth certificates during the period 1966-1969. *Pediatr Res* 1969;3:389–397.

21. Miller RW: Neoplasia in Down syndrome. *Ann NY Acad Sci* 1970;171:637–644.

22. Miller RW, Fraumeni JF: Down's syndrome and neonatal leukemia. *Lancet* 1988;2:204.

23. Robinson LL, Wesbit ME, Sather HW, et al: Down syndrome and acute leukemia in children: A ten-year retrospective study from Children's Center Study Group. *J Pediatr* 1984;105(2):235–242.

24. Stowens D: Down syndrome in acute leukemia. *Lancet* 1973;1:53.

25. Rubin CM, O'Leary M, Koch PA, et al: Bone marrow transplantation for children with acute leukemia and Down syndrome. *Pediatrics* 1986;78(4):688–691.

26. Garre ML, Relling NV, Kalwinsky D, et al: Pharmokinetics in toxicity of methotrexate in children with Down syndrome and acute lymphocytic leukemia. *J Pediatr* 1987;111(4):606–612.

27. Holland WW, Doll R, Carter CO: The mortality from leukemia and other cancers among patients with Down's syndrome (mongols) and among their parents. *Br J Cancer* 1962;16:177–186.

28. Braun DL, Green MD, Rausen AR, et al: Down's syndrome in testicular cancer: A possible association. *Am J Pediatr Hemotol Oncol* 1985;7(2):208–210.

29. Jackson EW, Turner JH, Klauber MR, et al: Down syndrome: Variation of leukemia occurrence in institutionalized populations. *J Chronic Dis* 1968;21:247–253.

30. Burgio GR, Ugazio A, Nespoli L, et al: Down syndrome: A model of immunodeficiency. *Birth Defects* 1983;19(3):325–327.

31. Levin S, Nir E, Mogilner BM: T system immune deficiency in Down syndrome. *Pediatrics* 1975;56:123–126.

32. Lockitch G, Singh VK, Puterman ML, et al: Age-related changes in humeral and cell-mediated immunity in DS children living at home. *Pediatr Res* 1987;22(5):536–540.

33. Burgio GR, Ugazio AG, Nespoli L, et al: Derangements of immunoglobulin levels, phytohemagglutin responsiveness and T and B cell markers in Down's syndrome at different ages. *Eur J Immunol* 1975;5:600–603.

34. Palmer S: Influence of vitamin A nutriture on the immune response: Findings in children with Down's syndrome. *Int J Vitam Nutr Res* 1978;48(2):188–216.

35. Oster J, Mikkelsen M, Nielsen A: Mortality and life tables in Down's syndrome. *Acta Paediatr Scand* 1975;64(suppl):322–326.

36. Strome M: Down's syndrome: A modern otorhinolaryngological perspective. *Laryngoscope* 1981;91(10):1581–1594.

37. Schwartz DM, Schwartz RH: Acoustic impedance in otoscopic findings in children with Down syndrome. *Arch Otolaryngol* 1978;11(104):652.

38. Samuelson ME, Nugyen VT: Middle ear fusion in Down's syndrome. *Nebr Med J* 1980;65:83–84.

39. Sutnick AI, London WT, Gerstley BJ, et al: Anicteric hepatitis associated with Australia antigen. *JAMA* 1968;205(10):670–674.

40. Ugazio AG, Jayakar S, Marcioni AF, et al: Immunodeficiency in Down syndrome: Relationship between presence of human thyroglobulin antibodies and HBsAg carrier status. *Eur J Pediatr* 1977;126(3):139–146.

41. Falls HF: Ocular change in mongolism. *Ann NY Acad Sci* 1970;171:627–636.

42. Eissler R, Longnecker LP: The common eye findings in mongolism. *Am J Ophthalmol* 1962;54:398–402.

43. Pueschel SM, Tingey C, Rynders JE, et al: *New Perspectives On Down Syndrome.* Baltimore, Paul H. Brookes, 1987.

44. Woillez M, Dansaut C: Les manifestations occularies dans le mongolisme. *Arch Ophthalmol* 1960;30:810–828.

45. Hiles DA, Hoyme SH, McFarlane F: Down syndrome and strabismus. *Am Orthop J* 1974;24:63–68.

46. Redman RS, Shapiro BL, Borlin RJ: Measurement of normal and reportedly malformed palatal vaults III Down syndrome (trisomy 21 mongolism). *J Pediatr* 1965;67:162–165.

47. Shendelsa SA, Gorlin RJ: Frequency of cleft uvula and submucous cleft in patients with Down's syndrome. *Dent Res* 1974;53(4):840–843.

48. Kavanagh KT, Kahane JC, Rordon B: Risk and benefits of adenotonsillectomy for children with Down syndrome. *Am J Ment Defic* 1986;91(1):22–29.

49. Walby AP, Schuknecht HF: Concomitant occurrence of cocheosaccular dysplasia in Down's syndrome. *Arch Otolaryngol* 1984;110(7):477–479.

50. Balkany TJ, Mischke RE, Downs MP, et al: Ossicular abnormalities in Down's syndrome. *Otolaryngol Head Neck Surg* 1979;87(3):372–384.

51. Dahle AJ, McCollister FP: Hearing and otologic disorders in children with Down syndrome. *Am J Ment Defic* 1986;90(6):636–642.

52. Downs MP, Jafek B, Wood RP II: Comprehensive treatment of children with recurrent serous otitis media. *Otolaryngol Head Neck Surg* 1981;89(6):658–665.

53. Keiser H, Montague J, Wold D, et al: Hearing loss of Down syndrome adults. *Am J Ment Defic* 1981;85(5):467–472.

54. Maurizi M, Ottaviani F, Paludetti G, et al: Audiologic findings in Down syndrome. *Int J Otorhinolaryngol* 1985;9(3):227–232.

55. Keyes PH, Bellack S, Jordan HV: Studies on the pathogenesis of destructive lesions of gums and teeth in mentally retarded children. Dentobacterial plaque infection in children with Down syndrome. *Clin Pediatr* 1971;10(12):711.

56. Cohen MM, Winer RA: Dental and facial characteristics in Down's Syndrome (mongolism). *Bull Acad Dent Handicap* 1065;3(1):18–27.

57. Jenson GM, Clear JF, McCloskey TC: Craniofacial complex in trisomy 21 (Down syndrome). *Am J Orthodon* 1973;64:609–618.

58. Jenson GM, Cleall JF, Yip AF: Dentoalveolar morphology and developmental changes in Down's syndrome (Trisomy 21). *Am J Orthodon* 1973;64(6):607–618.

59. Carr J: Mental and motor development in young mongoloid children. *J Ment Defic Res* 1970;14:205–220.

60. Schell R: Psychomotor development, in Pueschel S (ed): *The Young Child With Down Syndrome.* New York, Human Sciences Press, 1984, pp 207–276.

61. Zausma E, Schea A: Motor development, in Pueschel S (ed): *The Young Child With Down Syndrome.* New York, Human Sciences Press, 1984, pp 143–206.

62. Carr J: *Young Children With Down Syndrome.* London, Butterworths, 1975.

63. Morss J: Cognitive development in the Down's syndrome infant: Slow or different? *Br J Ed Psych* 1983;53:40–47.

64. Silverstein AB, Legutki B, Friedman SL, et al: Performance of Down syndrome individuals on the Stanford-Binet Intelligence Scale. *Am J Ment Defic* 1982;8615:548–551 .

65. Pipes PL, Holm VA: Feeding children with Down's syndrome. *J Am Diet Assoc* 1980;77(5):277–281.

66. Calvert SD, Vivian VM, Calvert GP: Dietary adequacy, feeding practices and eating behavior of children with Down's syndrome. *J Am Diet Assoc* 1976;69(2):152–156.

67. Cullens M, Cronk CE, Pueschel SM, et al: Social development and feeding milestones of young Down syndrome children. *Am J Ment Defic* 1981;85(4):410–415.

68. Golberg MJ, Ampola MG: Birth defect syndromes in which orthopedic problems may be overlooked. *Orthop Clin North Am* 1976;7(2):283.

69. Hreidarsson S, Magram G, Singer H: Symptomatic atlantoaxial dislocation in Down syndrome. *Pediatrics* 1982;69(5):568–571.

70. Diamond LS, Lynne D, Sigman B: Orthopedic disorders in patients with Down syndrome. *Orthop Clin North Am* 1981;12(1):57–71.

71. Scheffler NM: Down's syndrome and clinical findings related to the foot. *J Am Pediatr Med Assoc* 1973;63(1):18–21.

72. Mahan KT, Diamond E, Brown D: Podiatric profile of Down's syndrome individual. *J Am Pediatr Med Assoc* 1983;73(4):173–179.

73. Yancey CL, Zimjewski C, Athreya BH, et al: Arthropathy of Down syndrome. *Arthritis Rheum* 1984;27(8):929–934.

74. Gewanter HL, Roghmann KJ, Baum J: The prevalence of juvenile arthritis. *Arthritis Rheum* 1983;26(5):599–603.

75. Martel W, Uyham R, Stimson CW: Subluxation of the atlas causing spinal cord comprehension in a case of Down syndrome with a "manifestation of occipital vertebrae." *Radiology* 1969;93:839–840.

76. Curtis BH, Blank S, Fisher RL: Atlantoaxial dislocation in Down syndrome. *JAMA* 1968;205(25):461–465.

77. Schaller JG: Arthritis in immunodeficiency. *Arthritis Rheum* 1977;20(suppl):443–445.

78. Athreya BH, Yancey CL: Rheumotologic emergencies, in Fleisher G, Ludwig S (eds): *Textbook of Pediatric Emergency Medicine.* Baltimore, Williams & Wilkins, 1983, pp 66–70.

79. Pueschel SM, Scola FH: Atlantoaxial instability in individuals with Down syndrome: Epidemiologic, radiographic, and clinical studies. *Pediatrics* 1987;80(4):555–559.

80. Special Olympics Incorporated: *Participation by individuals with Down syndrome who suffer from atlantoaxial dislocation conditions* (bulletin). Washington, DC, Special Olympics Incorporated, March 31, 1983.

81. Schmid F: *Cell Therapy. A New Dimension in Medicine.* Thoune, Switzerland, Ott Publishers, 1983.

82. Schmid F: *Mongolism syndrome.* Dettehhebamman Z 1976a;28:169–173.

83. Bardon LE: Sicca cell treatment in mongolism. *Lancet* 1964;2:234–235.

84. Bremer JH: Discussion of cell therapy in children with relationship to pediatric metabolic issues. *Mschrkinderheik* 1976;123:674–675.

85. Turkel H: Medical treatment of mongolism. *Proceedings. Second International Congress on Mental Retardation*, 1963;1:409.

86. Turkel H: Medical amelioration of Down's syndrome incorporating the orthomolecular approach. *J Orthomol Psychiatry* 1975;4:1–14.

87. Harrell RF, Capp RH, Davis DR, et al: Can nutritional supplements help mentally retarded children? An exploratory study. *Proc Natl Acad Sci USA* 1981;78(1):574–578.

88. Golden GS: Controversies in therapies for children with Down syndrome. *Pediatr Rev* 1985;6(4):116–120.

89. Lemperle G, Radu D: Facial plastic surgery in children with Down's syndrome. *Plast Reconstr Surg* 1980;66(3):337–345.

90. Rozner L: Facial plastic surgery for Down's syndrome. *Lancet* 1983;1(8387):1320–1323.

91. Olbrisch RR: Plastic surgical management of children with Down's syndrome: Indications and results. *Br J Plast Surg* 1982;35:195–200.

92. Lefebvine A: Should retarded people have surgery? The psychological aspects of craniofacial problems. Surgery Is Not Enough. Dallas, Conference at the International Craniofacial Institute, 1987.

Management of developmentally disabled children with chronic infections

Richard D. Andersen, MD
Associate Professor
Division of Infectious Disease
Department of Pediatrics
University of Iowa Hospitals and
  Clinics
Iowa City, Iowa

CARING FOR children with developmental disabilities can expose caregivers to a multitude of infectious diseases, the majority of which are the same acute respiratory and gastrointestinal disorders experienced by the general population. Although most of these illnesses require only minimal and temporary adjustments by the caregivers, a small number of infectious agents have the capacity to produce extended, or chronic, infection. Brought into sharper focus by the emergence of acquired immunodeficiency syndrome (AIDS) and related diseases, these special circumstances pose more difficult and long-term questions of management. It is the purpose of this article to review the nature of chronic infections in developmentally disabled children and the implications for care providers and other children.

THE NATURE OF CHRONIC INFECTION

Numerous microorganisms exist in all parts of the earth that are capable of causing human infection. While thousands of different infectious agents have been noted to cause disease, most can be classified into four general categories: viruses, bacteria, fungi, and parasites. In developed countries, viral and bacterial diseases are predominant.[1]

Viruses can be viewed as fragments of living forms that are dependent on human (or other host) cells for survival. In contrast, bacteria are much more complex, are independent, and can grow in the absence of host cells. The human body is covered with bacteria, most notably on the surface of the skin and in the gastrointestinal and upper respiratory tracts. These constitute the so-called normal flora of the body and only under highly unusual circumstances cause disease. Most viruses, on the other hand, are encountered transiently; most of the routine respiratory and gastrointestinal diseases of young children (and adults) are caused by viruses. Finally, from the standpoint of therapy, a crucial difference between viruses and bacteria is that few viruses are susceptible to drug (antiviral) therapy, whereas virtually all bacteria are susceptible to various antibiotics.

This final difference implies that bacterial disease in general can be arrested by the appropriate antibiotics. Moreover, in a person with a normal immune system, the causative agent in general can be fully eradicated. In contrast, viral disease is treatable with drugs in only a small number of situations. Thus, the virus runs its course and if the host's immune defense system is to prevail, it must be without drug assistance.

Inf Young Children 1988;1(1):1–9

In several viral infections, however, the host's defense system inhibits but does not eradicate the virus after its initial introduction into the body. In these special situations, viral invasion can be limited by the virus's inability to thrive in most host cells and also by the immune attack. But chronic infection regularly ensues with certain agents because they are not completely eradicated. With some viruses, such as herpes simplex virus (HSV), permanent integration into host tissue is the rule; with others, such as hepatitis B virus, only a minority of patients go on to be chronically infected. In addition, certain viruses, such as HSV, are entirely latent (ie, dormant or inactive between episodes of reactivation), while others are continuously active and produce a more chronic, smoldering infection, as with chronic hepatitis.

VIRAL AGENTS

Because of the special characteristics of viral infection, it is not surprising that the key issues regarding chronic infection in developmentally disabled children all involve viruses. At present, there are four viral agents that provoke the most concern: HSV, cytomegalovirus (CMV), hepatitis B virus, and human immunodeficiency virus (HIV), the cause of AIDS and AIDS-related disorders.

Herpes simplex virus

HSV is a member of the herpesvirus family and is the cause of cold sores in the lip area and similar sores in the genital area. The virus is divided into two distinct types: type 1, which causes most but not all oral herpes infections, and type 2, which causes most but not all genital herpes infections. The vast majority of humans encounter type 1 HSV during their lifetime, while a much smaller proportion, perhaps 10% to 20%, encounter type 2.

A key feature of HSV infection is that after the initial encounter the virus becomes integrated, apparently for life, into the host's neural tissue beneath the skin. The first (primary) encounter can produce no symptoms or can result in primary herpetic gingivostomatitis or primary genital herpes, both of which are often accompanied by fever and enlarged lymph nodes.[2] Primary gingivostomatitis is a relatively common manifestation of initial infection and involves painful ulceration of the mouth and sores around the mouth. As with primary genital herpes, it may persist for one to two weeks. Recurrences of either cold sores or genital sores during subsequent reactivations of the virus tend to be a mild annoyance of several days' duration.

While infants and toddlers can experience primary oral herpes and cold sores similar to those in adults, newborns have a much greater vulnerability to widespread or fatal infection. Newborns acquiring HSV at the time of delivery are often born to mothers with no known history of genital herpes since the infection commonly occurs without symptoms. Roughly 1% of all pregnant women shed the virus from the uterine cervix at the time of delivery. Fortunately, most newborns avoid overt infection even when the virus is present in the birth canal and, thus, neonatal HSV infection is very uncommon. When it does occur, however, the infection can be serious or fatal. While early diagnosis and antiviral therapy can be lifesaving, infection of the brain typically produces neurologic sequelae in survivors even when treatment is prompt. Skin lesions in infected newborns are randomly distributed over the body (not merely in oral or genital regions) and tend to recur very frequently on various skin surfaces during childhood.

Recent legal controversies have arisen because of the perceived risk of these children to other children and caregivers in group situations. In general, an understanding of the biology of the virus has facilitated the incorporation of children into usual activities. The central issues regarding HSV for caregivers, then are the management of primary gingivostomatitis and cold sores and the management of a child's recurring skin lesions following infection as a newborn. It is theoretically possible for any herpetic sore to communicate the virus through direct contact to another child or caregiver. Policies designed to minimize the risk to other children and care providers should take into account the ubiquitous nature of HSV. Because most children will encounter HSV during childhood, its occasional presence in a particular child need not greatly disrupt the usual activities of the group.[3]

Given the limited risk of transmission, it is still reasonable and consistent with other hygienic practices to exclude a child with active lesions of the skin or oral cavity from center-based programs for the period that the lesions are present. In a home-based setting, caregivers should wear gloves when in contact with active skin (oral or genital) lesions. When the lesions are crusted or absent, the risk to other children and care providers is immeasurably low and the child should be allowed to participate fully in activities.[3]

Cytomegalovirus

CMV is another member of the herpesvirus family capable of causing serious disease early in life. Whereas HSV tends to infect newborns during birth, CMV produces its most severe consequences *before* birth. Infections of the pregnant woman that are transmitted to the fetus are termed congenital infections. While the majority of agents causing the usual maternal respiratory and gastrointestinal illnesses do not affect the fetus, a few viruses, bacteria, and other microbes occasionally do. CMV is clearly the most important of these causes of congenital infection in this country.

As in the case of HSV, most people become infected with CMV during their lifetime. CMV infection occurs in all age groups and all countries of the world.

Infection is more likely to occur in crowded settings such as developing countries, urban areas, and group childcare facilities than in situations where people are more isolated. As with HSV, the primary infection may be followed by a reactivation later in life, though the site and nature of the latent CMV is more obscure. Importantly, most CMV infections produce no symptoms (ie, are clinically silent). In a host with normal immunity, a primary or reactivated CMV infection is thus of no apparent consequence, though occasionally infectious mononucleosis-like symptoms (fatigue, swollen lymph nodes, etc.) result during primary infection.

Because an increasing awareness of CMV has emerged in the last 10 to 15 years, diagnostic techniques have become more widely used. At the same time, an estimation of the risk to pregnant women and their fetuses in various settings has become more clearly quantified.[4] The risk to the fetus appears to be linked to primary but not reactivated maternal infection. Approximately one in a hundred women experience primary CMV infection during pregnancy. Of those pregnant women with CMV, roughly one half will transmit the virus to the fetus, as determined by newborn urine cultures taken shortly after delivery. Fortunately, the majority of these CMV-infected newborns show no overt evidence of brain damage or other organ injury from congenital infection, although there appears to be an increased risk of hearing loss in those without symptoms at birth. But of all infected newborns, 5% to 10% will demonstrate clear evidence of disease at birth. They will most often have substantial involvement of multiple organ systems, including the liver, spleen, brain, and other organs, the most critical of which is the brain. The newborn exhibiting the many signs of this so-called cytomegalic inclusion disease will generally have substantial neurologic injury and subsequent developmental disabilities.

Since most of the overtly affected newborns will require special developmental interventions, caregivers must be aware of several features of the infection. First, the children will generally excrete the virus for years after birth, and should be assumed to be shedding the virus in their urine and, to a lesser extent, their saliva throughout the early years of life. Second, it is important to recall that for every child known to be excreting CMV, many more children are excreting the virus without symptoms: CMV infections are simply very common early in life.[5]

A major area of current interest is the occurrence of CMV infection in group childcare settings, where a large percentage of children experience CMV infection. Most studies of group child care suggest that at any given time, many of the children—from 10% to 40%—will have positive CMV urine cultures,[5] and the majority will encounter and excrete the virus with no symptoms or obvious ill effects to themselves. Of equal interest, then, is the estimation of risk to those persons most intimately involved with the children—the parents and care providers. One study of parent contacts of culture-positive children in group child care showed a 40% rate of infection in parents who had no prior CMV infection.[6] Some cautionary commentary has emerged regarding the potential for maternal CMV infection in this setting. Some authors suggest that parents should be made aware of this risk in their decision making regarding pregnancy and group care of their children.

More reassuring are studies of hospital personnel caring for young children and of care providers in group and special care environments.[7] In one study of personnel serving disabled children, fewer than 5% of staff members with child contact experienced a primary CMV infection over a one-year period, which was not significantly greater than those without contact. In light of their findings, the authors of that study suggest that a small, cumulative risk of CMV infection cannot be excluded, but that the overall risk to such personnel is low. Another study found no evidence of CMV infection over a one-year period in 55 caregivers who were working with developmentally disabled children.[8]

Given the high frequency of unrecognized CMV infection in childhood and the low frequency of clear-cut congenital CMV infection with sequelae, two strategies appear to be appropriate. First, because CMV and other herpesviruses are destroyed by soap, washing one's hands provides the most crucial and reliable barrier for persons dealing with young children. Second, it is prudent that pregnant women avoid direct contact with children with known congenital CMV infection; they should also be particularly scrupulous in washing their hands while caring for other children.[5] In future years, screening for CMV immune status and even immunization, may become feasible components of strategies aimed at reducing the risk of congenital CMV infection.

Hepatitis B virus

Hepatitis A and hepatitis B are both infections of the liver, but they are caused by two different viruses, each with very different implications. The fecal-oral spread and epidemic patterns, especially related to food handlers, long ago gave hepatitis A the name "infectious hepatitis." While hepatitis A is a common problem in group day-care settings, it seldom causes symptoms in young children, and chronic virus carriage does not occur. In contrast, hepatitis B (formerly termed "serum hepatitis") has a much lower level of communicability because its transmission usually requires exposure to blood or through sexual intercourse. Of more concern is that after hepatitis B infection, chronic and possible lifelong virus carriage can occur. Most of the risk to child-care providers comes from children whose serum demonstrates chronic hepatitis B virus carriage.[9]

The identification of hepatitis B virus carriage in young children is difficult because there are no symptoms. Immigrants arriving from certain parts of the world—notably southeast Asia, China, Korea, and Taiwan, which have high endemic rates of hepatitis B carriage—are generally screened to determine their hepatitis B status. Regardless of the child's ethnic origin, if the mother was a chronic carrier prior to becoming pregnant, the newborn is likely to become a chronic carrier unless special interventions are undertaken at the time of delivery. But ethnic origin and maternal history do not identify all children carrying the hepatitis B virus, and there is no universal screening of children in this country.

When a child is identified as a chronic carrier of the hepatitis B virus, he or she is not likely to pose a significant risk to others in the environment. The rate of transmission is low because the virus is not highly communicable through saliva, urine, or feces. Few data are available to determine the risk in group child care, although children in residential care institutions do appear to have a higher risk of illness than other children.[10]

Within the past decade, the advent of safe, effective immunization for hepatitis B has provided an excellent alternative for prevention. Its cost precludes mass immunization at present, but people who work in hospitals and residential institutions should be immunized because of their increased likelihood of exposure. Family contacts who have not experienced hepatitis B infection are also potential candidates for the vaccine if a carrier lives within the household. As more becomes known about the risk of transmission in group child-care settings and as the cost of the vaccine decreases, immunization recommendations may become more inclusive.

When blood spills occur, whether or not the person is a carrier of hepatitis B, cleaning with routine disinfectants (eg, a bleach solution) is prudent. As in the case of other agents discussed earlier, a person's status with respect to hepatitis B is generally not known. If care is taken to disinfect all blood spills, this route of contagion for hepatitis B will be eliminated.[11]

Human immunodeficiency virus

Since it was first reported in 1981, AIDS has taken on enormous significance worldwide. The explosive increase in the number of persons infected with the virus has prompted massive research and educational activities in an attempt to contain this global epidemic. Because of the growing number of children infected with the virus, consistent policies for dealing with such children in the school or day-care environment are imperative.

AIDS is a disease in which HIV infects and impairs certain immune cells of the body. The resulting vulnerability to opportunistic infectious agents and cancerous growths represents the chief manifestation of "true" AIDS. At least 40,000 cases of AIDS have arisen in the United States in the 1980s. Hundreds of thousands of people, however, have some symptoms related to HIV infection, but not true AIDS, and thus are classified as having AIDS-related complex. Finally, there is an even larger number of people—probably more than 1 million, according to public health officials— who are infected with HIV but exhibit no symptoms of any illness. These people are believed to carry the virus because they are seropositive for antibodies against the virus.

Despite the rapid increase in the number of infected persons, the distribution of HIV infection in subsets of the US population has remained relatively stable. AIDS has afflicted primarily homosexual or bisexual men, intravenous drug users, prostitutes, and hemophiliacs. HIV infection in children is generally acquired through blood products (for those with hemophilia) or from transmission during pregnancy and delivery. Because of the screening improvements in clotting factor preparations, the number of new hemophilic children infected with the virus is likely to decline dramatically in the next decade; in contrast, the number of children born to HIV-infected mothers is likely to increase substantially in coming years.

Most public concern and confusion related to the danger of AIDS are derived from two apparently conflicting areas: (1) the rate of HIV infection is increasing dramatically and (2) HIV cannot be transmitted among humans, except by sexual contact or infusion of infected blood from another person. The dramatic increase in the number of those infected in this country in less than a decade seems to contradict the relatively limited communicability of HIV infection. The facts can be reconciled only by recognizing the high level of male homosexual activity in the late 1970s and early 1980s, as well as the continuing high frequency of needlesharing by intravenous drug users.

Because of the limited means of transmission, children have constituted no more than 1% to 2% of AIDS patients in this country. However, because of the increasing number of HIV-infected women of childbearing age, the problem of AIDS in preschool children will increase in the foreseeable future. There is a striking geographic concentration of HIV infection in pregnant women (eg, in New York City) that reflects the concentration of intravenous drug users. When an HIV-infected woman becomes pregnant, one of three outcomes is likely:

1. A small percentage of fetuses will be infected in utero and will exhibit clinical features of the congenital HIV syndrome. Because of the high frequency of brain involvement with this syndrome, persons caring for the developmentally disabled may encounter a disproportionate number of such children, especially in areas with a large number of HIV-infected pregnant women.

2. In the majority of pregnancies complicated by HIV infection, the newborn is overtly normal at the time of delivery. It appears that roughly one half of such newborns will be infected with the virus and become symptomatic early in life.[12]

3. The third outcome, then, is that of a healthy, normal infant who does not become infected before or during birth.

The chief indicator of infection is the presence of serum antibody against HIV because culturing the virus itself is difficult and somewhat unreliable. Antibody levels in newborns are difficult to interpret because of the passage of maternal antibody across the placenta. Thus, all newborns of HIV-infected mothers must be regarded initially as HIV-infected themselves. Techniques to differentiate the truly infected from those with maternal antibody may well emerge in the near future. Since maternal antibody to most other agents disappears in the first year of life, the persistence of antibody to HIV beyond the first 12 to 15 months of life is believed to reflect true HIV infection of the infant.

In roughly 40% to 50% of newborns of HIV-infected mothers, clinical symptoms and changes in the immune system may become manifest during the first year of life. In contrast to seropositive adults who exhibit no symptoms and greatly outnumber the patients with AIDS, most truly infected infants become symptomatic in the early years of life. Thus, at present the management issues related to HIV-infected children can be divided into three general age categories: (1) newborns and preambulatory infants with a possible HIV infection, (2) infants and toddlers with a definite HIV infection, and (3) school-age children (mostly with hemophilia) who are proven or presumed to have an HIV infection.

In all age groups, it appears that child-to-child transmission does not occur. Studies of siblings of patients with AIDS reveal no evidence for sibling-to-sibling transmission of HIV. This is particularly noteworthy in light of the crowded circumstances and intimate sibling interaction (eg, sharing of toothbrushes) in many such settings.[13] Similarly, data from health care workers exposed to HIV suggest an exceedingly low risk of HIV transmission, even in the instance of needle-stick exposure. The few cases where transmission to health care workers has occurred have involved highly unusual circumstances or substantial quantities of blood.[14] At least 99% of needlesticks from HIV-infected patients in health care workers produce no evidence of HIV infection in the recipient.

In managing school-age children with HIV infection, then, the issues are straightforward. Children with HIV infection should be allowed to attend school or special education classes when their health permits. If classroom epidemics place such children in jeopardy (eg, if a child with AIDS is exposed to chickenpox), parents and other caregivers should be notified. In the rare instance of a child known to bite, however, the possibility of transmission justifies consideration of alternative, individualized education programs. If such a child exhibits urinary or fecal incontinence, disposable diapers or well-fitting rubber pants are appropriate solutions. Blood spills, from this *or any* child, should be handled with gloves. Good hand-washing practices should be observed with exposure to other bodily secretions or fluids. Importantly, these standard hygienic measures do not constitute stringent or special adaptation to the school-age child with AIDS. The prevention of hepatitis B and other conditions is a more realistic rationale for stringent hygienic practices than the highly remote risk of HIV transmission.

In addressing the problem of newborns and infants (or their developmental equivalents) with HIV infection, a similarly permissive approach appears to be reasonable. For several reasons, however, public health officials have suggested more caution in policy making and individualization of education.[15] First, infants and toddlers in group care exhibit an extremely high frequency of contagion with many infectious agents. Second, biting behavior and urinary and fecal incontinence are common, and the theoretical chance of contagion is indeed greater. The reassuring data with respect to sibling transmission and the absence of evidence of HIV transmission in group child care suggest that it is reasonable to allow these children to participate in day-care and center-based programs. The usual hygienic measures cited above for school-age children are adequate to eliminate the hypothetical possibility of HIV transmission. The presence of a caregiver with open cuts or abraded skin, or a child with diarrhea makes prudent the use of disposable gloves during diaper changes. When a special risk (eg, biting behavior) is determined to be present with ambulatory HIV-infected infants and toddlers, a special review and consultation with health officials should be undertaken. Similarly, with the child with symptomatic HIV infection, caregivers must weigh the social advantages against the potentially harmful results of numerous encounters with infectious agents.

•   •   •

The management of developmentally disabled children with chronic infections can be accomplished with only minimal disruption of their daily routine and with very limited risk to caregivers. The importance of frequent handwashing, particularly after exposure to bodily fluids of any child cannot be overemphasized. As a general rule, consistently observing standard hygienic measures in all circumstances is likely to be more effective than instituting special adaptations for a child with a known chronic infection.

REFERENCES

1. Andersen RD, Bale JF, Blackman JA, et al: Introduction: Infectious disease in children, in *Infections in Children: A Sourcebook for Educators and Child Care Providers*. Rockville, Md, Aspen Publishers, 1986.

2. Baker DA, Amstey MS: Herpes simplex virus: Biology, epidemiology and clinical infection. *Semin Perinatol* 1983;7:1–15.

3. Blackman JA, Andersen RD, Healy A, et al: Management of young children with recurrent herpes simplex skin lesions in special education programs. *Pediatr Infect Dis* 1985;4:221–224.

4. Stagno S, Whitley RJ: Characteristics of cytomegalovirus infection in pregnancy. *N Engl J Med* 1985;313:1270–1273.

5. Bale JF, Blackman JA, Murph J, et al: Congenital cytomegalovirus infection. *Am J Dis Child* 1986;140:128–131.

6. Pass RF, Hutto C, Ricks R, et al: Increased rate of cytomegalovirus infection among parents of children attending day-care centers. *N Engl J Med* 1986;314:1414–1418.

7. Blackman JA, Murph JR, Bale JF Jr: Risk of cytomegalovirus infection among educators and health care personnel serving disabled children. *Pediatr Infect Dis* 1987;6:725–729.

8. Jones LA, Duke-Duncan PM, Yeager AS: Cytomegaloviral infections in infant-toddler centers: Centers for the developmentally delayed versus regular day care. *J Infect Dis* 1985;151:953–955.

9. American Academy of Pediatrics: *Report of the Committee on Infectious Diseases,* ed 20. Elk Grove Village, Ill, American Academy of Pediatrics, 1986.

10. Krugman S, Katz SL: Viral hepatitis, in *Infectious Diseases of Children.* St. Louis, Mosby, 1981.

11. Andersen RD, Bale JF, Blackman JA, et al: Gastrointestinal disease and hepatitis, in *Infections in Children: A Sourcebook for Educators and Child Care Providers.* Rockville, Md, Aspen Publishers, 1986.

12. Rubenstein A, Bernstein L: The epidemiology of pediatric acquired immunodeficiency syndrome. *Clin Immunol Immunopathol* 1986;40:115–121.

13. Committee on Infectious Disease: Health guidelines for the attendance in day care and foster care settings of children infected with human immunodeficiency virus. *Pediatrics* 1987;79:466–471.

14. Centers for Disease Control: Update: Human immunodeficiency virus infections in health-care workers exposed to blood of infected patients. *MMWR* 1987;36:285–289.

15. Rogers MF: AIDS in children: A review of the clinical, epidemiologic and public health aspects. *Pediatr Infect Dis* 1985;4:230–236.

Bladder and bowel management for children with myelomeningocele

Marcia Henderson Lozes, RN, MA, CPNP
Pediatric Nurse Practitioner
Division of General Pediatrics
Spina Bifida Program
Childrens Hospital of Los Angeles
Los Angeles, California

BLADDER AND bowel dysfunction is a common problem for children with myelomeningocele and their families. Its effects are significant in terms of the misery and frustration due to incontinence, odor, breakdown of the skin, infections, social immobility, isolation, loss of self-esteem, depression, and refusal of entry into certain mainstream schools. In extreme cases, it can lead to renal failure and death. This type of bladder or bowel dysfunction is termed *neurogenic* or *neuropathic impairment* and is also present in children who have other forms of myelodysplasia (an abnormality of the spinal cord and nerve roots), such as lipomyelomeningocele, sacral agenesis, spinal dysraphism, caudal regression syndrome, or neuroenteric cysts.[1]

Myelomeningocele is a congenital malformation in which a sac containing the meninges (the membrane covering the spinal cord and brain), portions of the spinal cord and nerve roots, and cerebrospinal fluid protrudes through defective vertebrae (Fig 1). Irreparably damaged or congenitally malformed nerve roots indicate a lack of innervation of the motor and sensory lumbosacral nerve roots involving the bladder and bowel. Other conditions resulting in a neurogenic bladder or bowel include traumatic paraplegia, cerebral palsy, and spinal cord disease. The severe neuropathic lesions are present at birth but occasionally will escape detection until the child is referred for evaluation of daytime and nighttime incontinence.[2]

The neurologic lesion in children with myelodysplasia is complex and difficult to categorize. A lower motor neuron lesion or interruption of the spinal reflex arc (Fig 2) causes several complications of the urinary tract: a partial or total inability to empty the bladder, urinary tract infections, upper urinary tract deterioration, renal failure, and incontinence.[3] The effect of the lesion on lower extremity function correlates with the degree of functional ability and the level of the lesion, but its effect on bladder function has not been found to correlate well with the degree of neurologic deficit or lower limb competence.[4,5] In fact, further involvement of the spinal cord in some cases may increase rather than decrease the chance of continence.[1] Secondary factors, such as an overfilled bladder, can modify bladder function before birth. These complications suggest that the neurologic lesion may be a dynamic or progressive disease process rather than a static entity; in fact, there have been recent reports of suspected progressive denervation in older children with myelomeningocele.[6] Progressive urinary tract problems are also noted in the "tethered cord" syndrome, in which traction on the cord from linear growth and scarring at the site of the defect damages the cord and nerve roots. Changes in

Inf Young Children 1988;1(1):52–62

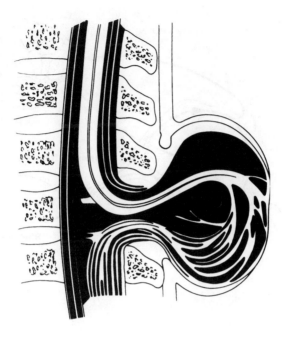

Fig 1. Myelomeningocele.

bladder or bowel dysfunction are sometimes a presenting symptom prior to pain, gait disturbances, foot deformities, and progressive scoliosis.[7]

An upper motor neuron lesion such as that seen in children with cerebral palsy may cause an upper motor neuron type of neuropathic bladder with exaggerated sacral reflexes and uninhibited bladder contractions. Some children with cerebral palsy show both upper and lower motor neuron urinary tract neuropathy, suggesting that they suffered a spinal cord injury at the same time as the cerebral insult.[2]

Lack of nerve root innervation to the bowel is termed *neurogenic bowel* or *bowel paralysis*. Its effects include constipation or diarrhea, more frequent bowel movements, fecal incontinence, prolapse of the bowel, and a predisposition to fissures.[8]

NORMAL BLADDER AND BOWEL FUNCTION

The urinary tract

The upper urinary tract comprises the kidneys, which produce urine, filter blood, control concentration, and excrete metabolic end products, and the ureters, which transport urine to the bladder by peristalsis. Where the ureter enters the

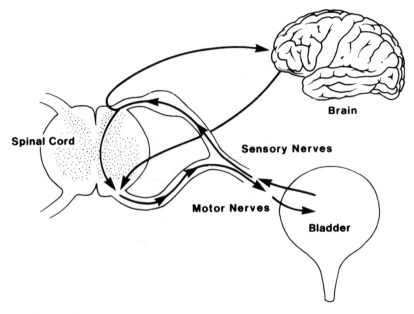

Fig 2. Spinal reflex arc.

bladder, a valvelike mechanism prevents the reflux of urine. The lower urinary tract comprises the bladder, the bladder wall musculature, the bladder neck, and the external sphincter mechanism. The bladder serves to store and expel urine through the urethra. Within the urethra are three sphincter components that maintain urinary control: (1) an internal or involuntary sphincter that remains contracted until the person decides to urinate; (2) intrinsic urethral resistance, which is another involuntary sphincter under sympathetic control that stays contracted until the person urinates; and (3) an external or voluntary sphincter that the person chooses to contract or relax (Fig 3).[8]

The musculature of the lower urinary tract is controlled by several areas in the nervous system: (1) the supraspinal centers in the cerebral cortex, thalamus, hypothalamus, basal ganglia, and cerebellum; (2) the spinal centers in the T-11, T-12, and S-2 through 4 segments; and (3) the hypogastric, pelvic, and pudendal nerves (Fig 4).

In the presence of a neurologic lesion, the components of the lower urinary tract fail to act in unison, causing improper urinary storage, increased or decreased bladder tone, and inadequate or increased resistance of the bladder neck and urethra.[2] Improper urinary storage means that urine remains in the bladder, thus providing a good medium for the growth of bacteria usually found close by (ie, the

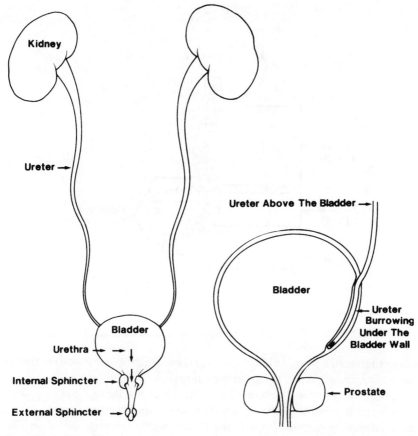

Fig 3. The urinary tract.

rectal and diaper area in children). Because bacteria grow very rapidly in this situation, urinary tract infections often result, accompanied by a high fever, abdominal pain, and nausea and vomiting.

Although urination is under the control of various centers in the nervous system, it is also influenced by maturation. In the normal infant, urination is a simple cord reflex, with the bladder emptying automatically when a certain volume of urine is reached. As the child becomes older and toilet training becomes a consideration, certain maturational milestones must occur: The bladder must increase in size and capacity, and the child must develop voluntary control of the periurethral muscles necessary to stop urination and of the muscles necessary to contract and relax the bladder.[9] The child with bladder neuropathy has little or no sensation of

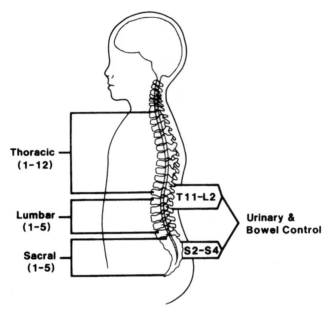

Fig 4. Spinal centers controlling the urinary tract.

bladder fullness, a poor bladder capacity, no awareness of urine passing through the urethra, and no ability to stop urinary flow.

In the male, sexual and reproductive function is controlled by the innervation of the same cord segments as the urinary tract, so that the same urologic studies will aid in counseling parents or young men about specific functions such as erection and ejaculation.[2] In the female, the denervation of cord segments can cause decreased genital sensation, but the menses and fertility are not affected.

The gastrointestinal tract

The motor-sensory innervation of the bowel also arises from the S-2 through 4 spinal cord segments. The upper gastrointestinal tract in children with a neurogenic bowel is usually normal and the gastrocolic reflex, which is stimulated by food, liquids, activity, and anxiety, stimulates peristalsis of the bowel and filling of the rectum. The stretch caused by rectal filling allows the child to become aware of the pressure of the feces as they are pushed into the anal canal. The internal or involuntary sphincter automatically relaxes, allowing the stool to come into contact with the sensory nerves of the anal canal and produce the urge to defecate. The child can then voluntarily relax the external or voluntary anal sphincter and expel stool by the Valsalva maneuver, which requires the ability to increase intraabdominal pressure and contract the diaphragm and abdominal and perineal muscles. Although impaired innervation is the primary cause of the neurogenic bowel, other contributing problems include poor abdominal tone, immobility, dehydration, dietary alterations, and drugs (which may increase or decrease peristalsis).[10]

TECHNIQUES FOR BLADDER CONTINENCE

A few children who have only partial neurogenic bladders will benefit from timed or scheduled voidings to empty their bladder and maintain dryness. Occasionally, the timed voiding is augmented with a medication to increase bladder capacity or urethral resistance so the child can hold urine longer. Since the child lacks sensory awareness of the voiding mechanism and does not know when the bladder is full, the schedule must be adhered to rigidly.

Another technique, clean, intermittent catheterization (CIC), allows for complete emptying of the bladder several times a day to control and prevent urinary tract infections. First described in 1966[11] and well accepted by 1972, the technique was found not only to reduce infections and improve renal function, but also to improve urinary continence. The parent or, eventually, the child inserts a small, clean catheter into the urethra for the two to five minutes it takes to empty the bladder every three to four hours. The technique is not painful to the majority of children and does not require complex equipment or maneuvers. Parents are able to learn the procedure in one demonstration.

CIC is not associated with any major complications, but its minor complications (often caused by incorrect technique) include difficulty in passing the catheter, a sore urethra or swelling of the penis, urethral discharge, urethral tears, and bleeding.[12] Even though CIC significantly reduces the incidence and severity of urinary tract infections, it does not eliminate them completely, and urinalysis and renal function studies must be a regular part of routine visits.

Medications can be used with CIC to increase bladder capacity and urethral resistance. The combination of these techniques is successful in the achievement of continence 26% to 78% of the time.[13] The most commonly used medications are oxybutynin chloride (Ditropan) and propantheline bromide (ProBanthine), anticholinergic agents; pseudoephedrine hydrochloride (Novafed, Sudafed), phenylephrine hydrochloride (Neo-Synephrine), and bethanecol chloride (Duvoid, Myotonachol, Urecholine), cholinergic agents; and imipramine hydrochloride (Imavate, SK-Pramine, Tofranil), tricyclic antidepressants.[14] Combinations of drugs are frequently used. The side effects of these medications are usually minimal, but therapists and teachers may need to know whether a medication has any behavioral side effects that might reduce endurance or the child's functioning. The common side effects include dry mouth, blurred vision, drowsiness, dizziness, weakness, nervousness, rapid heart rate, headache, skin flushing, and constipation.

However, as a relatively simple technique with some success in achieving continence, CIC has been met with varying degrees of acceptance. Twenty-five percent of parents in one center found CIC to be unacceptable.[12] Certain ethnic populations find manipulating external genitalia and passing a catheter to be extremely unacceptable. In addition, 16.5% of schools in one study found CIC to be unacceptable to only slightly acceptable, which means parents are faced with the problem of noncompliance when the child is at school.[12]

External appliances such as rubber pubic pressure or condom-type appliances can be used in boys for whom timed voiding or CIC does not work. Appliances provide children with freedom from wetness, an opportunity to wear more normal underclothing, and a better ability to care for skin and odors. Adapted and extraabsorbent underclothing is also available.

Surgical diversions such as the ileal conduit that were used in the past for continence or preservation of upper urinary tracts were found to have many long-term complications, including progressive deterioration, infection, stoma problems, and renal stones.[15] Since the complications outweighed the benefits, few surgical procedures were performed for continence management for many years, and the use of conservative techniques increased considerably.

However, the development of the artificial urinary sphincter in recent years has been received with a great deal of interest for use in the adolescent population. The use of the artificial sphincter is limited to a small population selected on the basis of type of bladder, failure of other techniques, and predicted compliance with a strict maintenance regimen. Experience with the sphincter has shown that it has many complications and requires many revisions. The preparation for the insertion of the artificial sphincter involves surgical procedures that permanently change the lower urinary tract so that previously used techniques (CIC and augmentation drugs) can no longer be used. Therefore, in the event of sphincter failure, there will be fewer management options available to the young person. For this reason, the artificial sphincter should be considered last for the attainment of continence.

Another surgical procedure with less negative features is the continent ileal reservoir, or Kock pouch. Like the artificial sphincter, this procedure is selected for young persons when conservative techniques have failed to achieve social continence. A small piece of intestine is isolated to create a pouch with two intussusceptive nipples. The pouch is placed beneath the lower right abdominal wall and the ureters are transplanted to the pouch instead of to the urinary bladder. The pressure of urine in the pouch keeps one nipple closed, and the other nipple prevents urine from flowing back to the upper tracts. The stoma is very small and requires no bags or appliances for dryness. The person catheterizes the pouch every two to six hours. The procedure has been successful in achieving continence without urinary tract infections, although some patients have had to undergo subsequent operations to reform the continence valves (ie, the nipples).[16]

An alternative approach is urethral lengthening and reimplantation with a one-way valve allowing a catheter to be passed into the existing bladder.[17] Individual selection of a more reversible procedure will offer the adolescent and young adult another option for achieving urinary continence.

Other treatments, such as operant conditioning, biofeedback, electrical stimulation, and gastroileal reflux training, have limited application in bladder or bowel management in children with myelomeningocele.[18]

TECHNIQUES FOR BOWEL CONTROL

Regulating the consistency of the stools by medication so that it is neither too hard nor too soft is one of many techniques to control bowel function. Another technique suitable for some children is scheduling bowel movements and taking advantage of the gastrocolic reflex (ie, activated peristalsis) after meals. Rectal suppositories (once or twice a day or with meals) can be used in combination with such scheduling. The expansion enema (in which a small amount of a hypertonic solution is given quickly to stimulate the colon), has been used with some children.[8] By far one of the most common methods of regulating the stool to prevent accidents is digital stimulation of the rectum and/or manual evacuation of the stool.

Dietary manipulation is commonly used to treat constipation, and parents are taught early which foods, bulk additives, and fluids will help soften the stool. Dietary manipulation alone, however, is not successful in changing stool consistency as might be expected in a person with normal bowel tone. In addition, it is helpful to remember that children have more constraints and are more particular in their personal eating habits than adults, who might willingly consume a large daily dose of bran or large hourly doses of water or juice. The child with a neurogenic bowel is more sensitive to certain foods, and a large serving of a favorite but problematic food can suddenly change a controllable, firm stool into an uncontrollable, liquid stool overnight. Some medications to increase stool firmness and slow peristalsis are also frequently used in conjunction with certain evacuation methods.

DEVELOPMENTAL INTEGRATION OF MANAGEMENT TECHNIQUES

Infants

The primary goal of urologic management of the infant is to identify congenital structural problems or evidence of upper or lower tract damage by radiographic studies. Intervention is started at the first signs of bladder overfilling or reflux (the backward flow of urine to the kidneys). This can be accomplished by CIC or a temporary cutaneous vesicostomy (in which the bladder wall is brought to a skin stoma to drain freely).[2]

Bowel management includes dietary regulation to prevent constipation since hard or large stools can cause fissures or prolapse of the bowel. Normal straining by an infant with a soft stool can also cause bowel prolapse.

Constant wetness from dribbling or urine and/or constant stool soiling can cause more problems with diaper rashes and breakdown of the skin than in the normal infant. The infant who wears abduction hip braces or who is unable to change his or her position even slightly is at greater risk for skin problems. Many medical recommendations cannot be separated from early infant intervention efforts: Positioning, skin care, bracing, and appliances can be affected by the need for frequent diaper changes, skin airing, or CIC.

Toddlers

By 12 to 18 months of age, the pyramidal tracts are completely myelinated, allowing for the retention of more urine in the bladder, voluntary sphincter release, some sphincter control with urgency, and more regularity of bowel movements. The acquisition of these neurologic functions signals the beginning of the child's ability to impose social control over automatic functions depending on his or her physical limitations (such as trunk control for sitting), cognitive abilities, and emotional maturity. When the child does not give any physical cues of his or her readiness to initiate toilet training, such as an awareness of voiding or defecation or a sensation of being soiled or wet, it is important to know the child's level of developmental and emotional maturity (eg, an ability to focus attention and ignore distracting stimuli, and a willingness to please and imitate others). The parents can then be counseled about how to position the child, what instructions to give to the child, which behaviors to praise (eg, sitting on the potty and attempting to urinate or defecate), and which behaviors to ignore (eg, failing to pass urine or stool).

If the lower urinary tract and the act of urination are predictably impaired, one might wonder what gains can be made from scheduled toilet training. Toilet training is recognized as a social skill and as one of the functional tasks children learn in becoming independent. Toilet training and independence are also important developmental stages between the ages of 1½ to 4 years, and parents may feel they have some control over this area of their child's care. The child's own beginning awareness of the differences in others may make him or her conscious of wearing diapers. Working on the task of being free from diapers is an important developmental milestone to the child and his or her parents.

The acquisition and maintenance of toilet training skills is greatly influenced by a conducive environment, proper positioning, parental education, and appropriate expectations.

School-age children

The school-age developmental stage is marked not by the traditional entry of school but rather by the achievement of developmental skills of a 5-year-old child. At this stage, the child is more ready to accept the manipulation of his or her toilet activities and the imposition of techniques to control continence, and is more motivated to be like other children.

It has been accepted that a child with a high-level lesion and the associated severe physical disability might be slower in achieving certain independent toilet and hygiene skills. However, 50% of children with low-level lesions in one study achieved socially acceptable toilet skills at age 7 to 9 years at the earliest, which is later than the normal child, and their delayed toilet skills were found to be unrelated to abnormal neurologic function or poor eye-hand coordination.[19] Children with higher lesions cannot be expected to learn independent toilet skills until 17 to 18 years of age. Although these expectations do not apply to every child, knowledge about general delays in this population is helpful in planning appropriate intervention.

Adolescents

The young person with a low lesion who may not appear to be physically disabled is likely to perceive bladder and bowel dysfunction as a severe handicap and may then perceive himself or herself as severely handicapped.[20] Accidents and odor are now described as the worst handicaps associated with neurogenic bladder and bowel. The adolescent is more interested in continence issues and more vocal in making choices to disguise the problem, being more like his or her peers, or denying the problem. The point of view of the young person may make him or her less compliant than previously and requires the staff to be sensitive to the fact that older boys and girls with normal urethral sensation may dislike CIC or may have difficulty even inserting catheters because of problems with self-esteem and issues of sexuality. The two most attractive choices for many adolescents are the Kock pouch (continent ileal reservoir) and the artificial sphincter.

The dependent adolescent needs to be monitored continually for his or her degree of continence. Parents and professionals need to understand the usual progress in achieving toilet skills so they are neither too aggressive nor too lenient in their expectations.

INTERDISCIPLINARY MANAGEMENT

Achieving continence and independent toilet skills are difficult goals to meet because of the nature of the neurologic lesion and the child's IQ, physical mobility, manual dexterity, motivation, and compliance. Additional causes of failure and delays in bladder and bowel programs include family disruption, hospitalization, surgery, irritable bowels, emotional problems, and failure of the school to comply.[19] Achieving continence is somewhat elusive in a population in which every child is affected. However, persistence, education, and interdisciplinary management do yield encouraging results in selected children.

Information—both the acquisition and transmission of it—is always the primary interdisciplinary focus. A tremendous amount of complex information about anatomy and physiology needs to reach both parents and professionals. Bladder and bowel dysfunction is not a visible problem to the parents, and is only radiographically visible to the urologist. How to time and transmit this information to parents and therapists is an ongoing task requiring patience and different methods of presentation. Educational meetings help the staff update their knowledge about other systems in order to coordinate their goals for the family.

With regard to psychosocial issues, parental readiness for certain parts of the program depends on the parents' feelings, past experiences, and perceptions of current issues. Parents may not understand why prevention is important, they may fear radiographs, they may not divulge their financial inability to carry out recommendations, or they may be concerned that catheterization will sexually violate their child. This kind of information needs to be discovered and disclosed to caregivers who are planning radiographic studies, prevention, or early intervention. Parents who see each other in the clinic or in parents' groups share a pipeline of information that is shaped by parental perceptions, newsletters, gossip and "wives' tales," and consumer resources. The information may be very positive or very negative and is important to know for planning teaching methods and predicting or improving compliance.

Gradually the intervention team acquires information about the developmental level and the cognitive, linguistic, adaptive, motor, social, and emotional strengths of each child. Therapists translate this information into the child's readiness to learn toilet skills, as well as all activities of daily living. Together with nursing and medical team members, they can develop a plan for toilet performance.

•   •   •

Improved medical care of the urinary system has resulted in fewer urinary tract infections and complications that can lead to renal failure and death. Previously life-threatening problems of bladder and bowel management have become part of the social and educational issues faced by the child or young person. These life-long issues of working toward independent toilet skills and continence will involve not only the child, but also the school system, extended family members, and temporary caretakers. Persons outside the home may be sensitive to these issues and may need additional education and supervision. Therapists or others may find themselves administering medical procedures such as CIC previously reserved for medical personnel. Learning the procedures may be necessary to know how to better educate parents to teach their child and how to better adapt the procedures to public areas, awkward positioning, braces, clothing, and other physical limitations. Working through these problems and adapting the child to the public domain or the least restrictive environment involves dedicated teamwork.

REFERENCES

1. Spindel M, Bauer S, Dyro F, et al: The changing neurologic lesion in myelodysplasia. *JAMA* 1987;258:1630–1633.
2. Bauer S: Urodynamic evaluation and neuromuscular dysfunctions, in *Clinical Pediatric Urology.* Philadelphia, Saunders, 1985.
3. Bauer S: Management of neurogenic bladder dysfunction in children. *J Urol* 1984;132:544–545.
4. Wyndalle JJ, De Sy WA: Correlation between the findings of a clinical neurologic examination and the urodynamic dysfunction in children with myelodysplasia. *J Urol* 1985;133:638–640.
5. Kaplan W: Urological dynamics in the management of the child with spina bifida. Presented at the Annual Conference of the Spina Bifida Association of America, Detroit, MI, June 3–8,1986.
6. Kroovand RL: Myelomeningocele, in *Campbell's Urology.* Philadelphia, Saunders, 1986.
7. Helstrom W, Edwards M, Kogan B: Urological aspects of the tethered cord syndrome. *J Urol* 1986;135:317–320.
8. Sullivan-Bolyai S: Practical aspects of toilet training the child with a physical disability. *Issues Compr Pediatr Nurs* 1986;9(2):79–96.
9. Koff S, Lapides J, Piazza J: The uninhibited bladder in children: A cause for urinary obstruction, infection and reflux, in Hudson J (ed): *Reflux Nephropathy.* New York, Masson, 1979.
10. Coffman S: Description of a nursing diagnosis: Alteration in bowel elimination related to neurogenic bowel in children with myelomeningocele. *Issues Compr Pediatr Nurs* 1986;9(2):179–191.
11. Schoenberg H, Meador M: Analysis of 48 children with myelodysplasia. *J Urol* 1982;127:749–750.
12. Cass AS, Luxenberg M, Gleich P, et al: Clean intermittent catheterization in the management of the neurogenic bladder in children. *J Urol* 1984;132:526–528.
13. McGuire E: Neuromuscular dysfunction of the lower urinary tract, in *Campbell's Urology.* Philadelphia, Saunders, 1986.
14. Borzyskowski M: Management of neuropathic bladder in childhood. *Dev Med Child Neurol* 1984;26:401–404.
15. Cass AS, Luxenberg M, Gleich P, et al: A 22 year followup of ileal conduits in children with a neurogenic bladder. *J Urol* 1984;132:529–531.
16. Lieskovsy G, Skinner D: Use of intestinal segments in the urinary tract, in *Campbell's Urology.* Philadelphia, Saunders, 1986.
17. Kropp K, Angwafo F: Urethral lengthening and reimplantation for neurogenic incontinence in children. *J Urol* 1986;135:533–536.
18. Okamoto G, Sousa J, Telgrow R, et al: Toileting skills in children with myelomeningocele: Rates of learning. *Arch Phys Med Rehabil* 1984;65:182–185.

19. Sullivan-Bolyai S, Swanson M: Toilet training the child with neurogenic impairment of bowel and bladder function. *Issues Compr Pediatr Nurs* 1984;7(1):33–43.

20. Blum R: The adolescent with spina bifida. *Clin Pediatr* 1983;22:331–335.

Index

A

Accidents, head injury, 228
Agenesis of corpus callosum, 191, 193–194
Aicardi syndrome, 193
AIDS
  clinical features of, 84–89
  diagnosis of, 89–90
  epidemiology, 84
  historical background, 82
  neurologic disorders in, 85–89
  prognosis, 91
  treatment approaches, 90–91
  virology in, 83
  See also HIV infection
Alternative therapies, for Down syndrome, 240–241
Anencephaly, 183–184
Antioxidants, as lung therapy, 129
Arthropathies, in Down syndrome, 239
Asphyxia, foods causing problems, 99
Assessment of Preterm Infant Behaviors, 162
Atlantoaxial instability, in Down syndrome, 239
Attachment problems, and fetal alcohol syndrome, 23–24
Attention deficit hyperactivity disorder (ADHD), behavioral signs of, 23

B

Autism
  fetal alcohol syndrome, 24
  fragile X syndrome, 52, 60–61
Autosomal dominant disorders, 146–147, 224
Autosomal recessive disorders, 147, 149, 224
AZT, in AIDS, 90–91

B

Barriers, infection control, 74, 76, 77–78, 79
Bayley Scales of Infant Development, 115, 131–132
Behavioral evaluation, brain injury infants, 162–163
Behavioral problems
  fetal alcohol syndrome, 21–22, 24
  fragile X syndrome, 61–62
Birth defects
  multifactorial, 149–150
  See also Genetic disorders
Bites, human, and bloodborne pathogens, 70–71, 73
Bloodborne pathogens
  HBV infection, 68
  HIV infection, 67
  and human bites, 70–71, 73